On
Healing

On Healing

Finding Wholeness
Beyond the Limits of Medicine

Amitha Kalaichandran, MD

Heliotrope Books
New York

Printed in the United States of America
First Edition

ISBNs: 978-1-956474-53-4 (paperback); 978-1-956474-55-8 (hardcover); 978-1-956474-54-1 (eBook)

Most Heliotrope books are available at special quantity discounts for bulk purchase for sales promotions, premiums, fundraising, and educational needs. Special books or book excerpts also can be created to fit specified needs. For details, contact us at heliotropebooks@gmail.com.

Heliotrope Books, LLC
heliotropebooks.com

Parts of this book appeared in earlier form in *The New York Times* and other publications. Please see "Permissions," page 343.

Cover design by Mykola Shelepa
Illustrations by Kaitlin Walsh

For the doctors, both past and future,
who are committed to healing the world and themselves.

For Rob Sargeant — the best mentor a medical student could ask for.

In memory of Ryan Seguin — I wish we had met.

Time is generally the best doctor — Ovid

Note About the Font:

The font used throughout this book is Baskerville, a classic serif typeface designed in 1757 by English printer and typographer John Baskerville. Known for its elegant, high-contrast strokes and refined letterforms, Baskerville was created to enhance readability and bring a sense of sophistication to printed works. Its clean, crisp lines made it a popular choice in the world of publishing, and it has been admired for its timeless design ever since. Recently, this iconic typeface was adapted by Jony Ive for LoveFrom, demonstrating its continued relevance and ability to merge tradition with modern design.

Table of Contents

Introduction

"And though she be but little, she is fierce."
— Shakespeare

1.

So this is how it ends, I thought. The uncertainty, the confusion, all of it. Here, in an office with fluorescent overhead lights, wood paneling, and commercial carpet on College Street in Toronto, I'd get the answers and re-calibrate. I had arrived at Dr. Bends' office early, at 2 pm, to fill out the required paperwork. His administrative assistant, Cathy, smiled as she handed me five neatly printed pages. I was familiar with these, having filled out so many for my patients: screening tools to self-assess mental health and well-being prior to the doctor's assessment. I couldn't have a diagnosable issue, I thought. I was under stress, definitely, but could it be more than that?

I completed the questions, reading each one slowly:

★ Have you lost interest in activities you used to enjoy?
★ Has your mood been low most days over the last two weeks?
★ Are you having trouble concentrating?
★ Do you feel more irritable than usual?
★ Do you feel anxious or afraid on most days?
★ Do you feel an impending "sense of doom"?

The questions were straightforward, but the answers were not. I replied to most in the affirmative, mindful that the condition my answers were describing was likely linked to my time in an academic medical setting, particularly in one unit. I noticed I felt much better when I was working elsewhere, even in other parts of the same hospital.

Dr. Bends, a psychiatrist specializing in physician workplace health, called me in. He looked younger than I expected, with a slight tan. He reviewed my survey answers and asked me a round of follow-up questions. He thought the symptoms I described of new stress and recent mood changes were restricted to one specific environment. I was just beginning to process what exactly I had experienced in one specific academic medicine environment and the impact it was having on me.

A month later, I reviewed Dr. Bends' report and the results of some blood tests with my family doctor. I was shocked at the clinical affirmation of what I thought of as mild stress and problems with my focus as something else: Dr. Bends had provided the diagnosis of "workplace-induced anxiety and depression." Above all, he recommended I transfer to work in a different hospital environment. My symptoms had abated after a break from that environment. If I went back, I'd risk the symptoms returning, and if they worsened, I might require medication just to survive.

I had cared for depressed and anxious patients before during my psychiatry rotation in medical school. I had spent my evenings finding tools and techniques to help them manage and overcome their distress. But I didn't quite understand depression, and I often wondered why my patients couldn't just be happy, as though it were a choice. And anxiety: was it not just the result of an overactive, albeit pessimistic, imagination?

My anxiety wasn't the only struggle I was facing: I was also on the verge of spiraling into physical disease. My lab results showed that I had a high level of cholesterol in my blood. Thanks to my active lifestyle and healthful diet, my total cholesterol was still one point below the level at which the American Heart Association guidelines advise taking a statin (a cholesterol-lowering medication), but my doctor still offered a prescription to prevent the kind of build-up in my arteries that could result in a heart attack.

The evidence was clear: over the previous two years, both my body and mind had been under significant strain. I found myself shifting from a calm and confident person into someone who was hypervigilant, nervous, irritable, and struggling with focus to the point that even my short-term memory was affected. Even after stepping away from one particularly challenging environment within the hospital—a setting that presented unique pressures—my mental fog persisted. Over time, I would come to understand how stress could impact physical health, even contributing to poor cholesterol metabolism, something I was already predisposed to due to my family history.

Here I was in my early thirties, facing two diagnoses—workplace-induced depression and anxiety, along with hypercholesterolemia—two big signs that something desperately needed to change. How on earth had my body veered so far off course?

2.

One thing was for sure: if I could help it, I was not ready to begin a lifelong regimen of prescription drugs to address my problems. Though I knew that the biomedical model I was taught in medical school emphasized the role of drugs and surgery, it suddenly felt limiting, as there was no medicine or surgical procedure that could heal me.

Coincidentally, two years before I noticed a decline in my well-being, I had begun asking the families of my pediatric patients what sorts of treatments they were using in addition to doctor-prescribed medicines and therapies. I had become intrigued by parent after parent telling me, often only after I'd probed after sensing there was more under the surface, that they were adding to their children's care with things like amber teething necklaces, acupuncture, Chinese medicine, and special foods. Most of these therapies had limited-to-no scientific evidence to support their effectiveness, although some mind-body approaches, like guided imagery or hypnosis, specific forms of exercise, and changes in diet, *did* have a basis in science. My project research team, consisting of a pediatric integrative medicine physician, a pediatric emergency medicine physician, and a variety of statisticians and epidemiologists, set out to quantify how many parents were seeking alternative approaches to common ailments and how effective families perceived these treatments to be. We decided to focus on families we encountered in the children's hospital emergency department, one of the busiest pediatric emergency departments in the country. We talked to over 300 parents over a six-month period, and what we found (which we published) was surprising, to say the least.

Just over 60 percent of parents we surveyed said they used complementary health approaches (CHAs), with vitamins and minerals and massage being the most common. Parents with university-level education were *more* likely to use CHAs compared to those with less education, and most parents perceived these alternatives as effective. We then asked parents if they had used a specific CHA for the acute condition that brought their child into the emergency room in the first place. About one-third said they did, most commonly for stomach issues such as gastroenteritis (stomach flu). For these acute conditions, there was absolutely no association with parental education.

I had spent four years at a relatively progressive medical school in Toronto, which I loved, but our classes never explored why people were seeking other options for healing. We had learned to start with a patient history, examine the body's system in question, order specific diagnostic tests, come up with a diagnosis, and discuss a treatment plan with the medical team (and, ideally, the patient). This protocol was supported by a foundation in anatomy (structures of the body), physiology (how those structures function), and a bit of biochemistry. But we didn't cover much about the role of non-medicinal methods for alleviating our patients' suffering—exercise, nutrition, mind-body approaches—or even how our social and physical environments affect our health. Over the span of four years, I estimate we spent a total of two hours on these issues.

Here I stood: faced with two drastic issues inflicting my mind and body. They were intertwined, I sensed, between what American essayist and novelist Susan Sontag calls the "two kingdoms" of the well and the sick, where neither a pill nor surgical procedure seemed appropriate. Why had I not given much thought to this dilemma while on the other side of the curtain as a doctor? In my early training, I focused on healing patients using the structured toolbox provided during medical school—an approach that, while useful, felt limited in scope. My practice initially followed what amounted to a formulaic application of protocols and guidelines, leaving little room for personalized care or deeper understanding of each patient's unique context. An unexpected lesson on belonging from a South American zoo helped ground me in understanding where to start.

3.

Mara didn't fit in. She was different—and so she was targeted by the other elephants or just left out altogether.* As reported in the *New York Times*, she was an elephant kept in captivity. She was 50 years old—far from elderly for an elephant—and had been born in a work camp in India. She was sold to a zoo in Hamburg, Germany, and then an Argentinian family purchased her and sold her to a South American-based circus, where the other elephants were African. That's when, seemingly out of frustration, she killed an animal trainer. She was chained in a parking lot as her punishment. Over time, she was moved to an enclosure that resembled a Hindu temple. Mara wasn't just challenged with being held captive; she was blamed for reacting to an unusual environment.

And she had no way of escaping; that is, until a movement began years later to free her. This culminated in the decision to move her to an elephant sanctuary in Brazil in March 2020. Once Mara was out of the enclosure, she changed. Mara became as gentle as a pachyderm weighing several tons could be. Indeed, by changing her *environment*, everything about her shifted. Perhaps the same applied to me.

In India, baby elephants are domesticated by chaining one or both of their hind legs to a tree. As the elephant ages, it does not stray from its owners because the chains stay on even though the elephants are no longer tied to the tree. The irony here is that in Hinduism, the elephant god, Ganesha (or Ganesh), is meant to represent the defeater of obstacles. Like Mara, I, too, had obstacles within and around me. My faith, and Ganesh perhaps, helped me realize that healing myself was a crucial yet small part of the journey ahead—and if I could finally free myself from this situation that was harming my physical and emotional health, I could help free others.

---

* Brooke Jarvis' masterful reporting about Mara can be found in the New York Times, https://www.nytimes.com/2020/08/09/science/coronavirus-elephants-wildlife-zoo.html

Healing the system of medical culture would be a gargantuan task, one best left to those who were stronger and more resilient. But what if part of my own healing was *earning* this resilience, and the trade-off was that I used it to facilitate change? Could I do it? Now, it was time to rethink what it really meant *to heal* and, in the process, heal myself.

4.

What does it even mean "to heal"? The answer can differ from culture to culture. In Tamil, the South Indian and Sri Lankan language my parents spoke when they were growing up, to heal is "குணப்படுத்த" (Kunnappatutta), which can mean "to comfort"—though in another context, it can mean "to be suppressed." In English, the word "heal," which is the basis of "health," is often attributed to the Old English word "*haelan*," which can also mean "to cure, save, greet, salute," or the Proto-Germanic "*hailijana*," which means "to make whole, or save."

Our wounds, as the 13th-century poet, scholar, and theologian Rumi wrote, are "where the light enters you." The essay, "The Body and the Earth" by American novelist and poet Wendell Berry, beautifully portrays healing as a return to "wholeness":

> To be healthy is to be whole. ...If the body is healthy, then it is whole. But how can it be whole and yet be dependent, as it obviously is, upon other bodies, and upon the earth, upon all the rest of Creation in fact?

Even though human physiology the world over is roughly the same, different cultures have different ideas about what it means to heal, and those differences affect how our governments approach healthcare. Based on data from 2022, in the U.S., 14.6% of the Gross Domestic Product (GDP)—$3.8 trillion dollars—is spent on healthcare (of which 31% is based on hospital-based care). Even in Canada, which is close to providing universally accessible healthcare, hospital spending remains the most expensive part, comprising 25% of its healthcare budget (which was $308 billion). The U.K., which has a fully funded National Health Service (NHS), spends about $214 billion dollars (10% of its GDP), of which 25% was spent on hospital-based care. Australia also spends 10% of its GDP on healthcare (a figure of $185 billion). Japan has a model in which universal healthcare exists, but it's topped up most often by workplace-supported private healthcare; it spends 10.9% of its GDP on healthcare. Many of the countries that fared better during the COVID-19 pandemic provided access to universal healthcare: access means fewer barriers to obtaining a diagnosis and treatment. Indeed, refining healthcare systems to streamline spending should involve a total re-envisioning of *where* healing occurs—it certainly isn't restricted to hospitals—and *what* healing modalities can be added to our currently very limited toolbox.

Healing is usually thought of as *repair*. The body or mind gets injured, and the medical system primarily uses medications or surgery to restore things to the way they were, to approximate what the patient's body or mind would do naturally. *Healing* is also used interchangeably with *curing*, to the detriment of our healthcare systems globally, as the latter often places the onus on invasive treatments.

In recent years, the term "wellness" has permeated our culture to mean everything from self-help to a more holistic version of healthcare, as an extension of what we understand as "healing. " The word "wellness" is said to have been coined by Sir Archibald Johnston, a Scottish politician in the 1500s, who remarked, "I blessed God…for my daughter wealnesse"—the original spelling was clearly not popularized. Centuries later, wellness was described in 1975 by Johns Hopkins University's John W. Travis, a preventative medicine resident, during the opening of the wellness resource center in Mill Valley, California. When Dan Rather interviewed Travis in 1979, Rather remarked, "Wellness, that's not a word you hear every day." Halbert Dunn, chief of the U. S. National Office of Vital Statistics, wrote that the environment should "encourage you to live to the very full," which provided a crucial lesson I was never taught in medical school.

Now, I sought my own version of this wellness, centered on regaining "wholeness." It would take a ten-year journey, bringing me to more than ten countries in order to come to grips with what that actually meant, healing myself in the process. It became clear to me that there were twelve components that are crucial to healing:

1. understanding our place in history and our story
2. optimal cell and tissue repair
3. our environments
4. our social connections
5. our minds and mindset
6. what and when we eat
7. our faith and spirituality
8. how we exercise
9. the cultures of our workplaces
10. appropriate use of plant medicines
11. whether we prioritize rest and sleep
12. whether we come to terms with letting go when we must

I would become intimately familiar with each of these concepts as I struggled to regain wholeness. The non-emergent nature of my issues allowed me a chance to figure out how to repair the problems without resorting to the quick fixes our medical system too heavily relies upon and, perhaps, to employ healing modalities that are often overlooked by the conventional healthcare system.

I was determined, if possible, to heal myself.

As a scientist first, though, I tend to be skeptical of many things, from the latest research study to the latest wellness trend. My training in both conventional medicine and several integrative approaches to healing has informed my point of view while also forcing a sense of intellectual humility. I've changed my mind countless times over the course of researching the healing modalities presented here.

This book is an invitation to come along on my journey as I seek scientific evidence of what it means to heal in the 21st century, in a post-pandemic world, while being confronted by the unique tension between the conventional medical establishment and various new and emerging stakeholders. I've made it clear where the research still hasn't reached a consensus about the value of these approaches and what questions remain. But as medicine evolves, recommendations change. The "Notes" section at the end is an offering for further examination of the sources I've found to be most helpful, and the Appendix includes an article I wrote for *The New York Times* about assessing medical research, especially that found in the popular press.

Along the way, we'll meet an endangered Mexican salamander that's helping scientists improve how we can regenerate parts of our brain or limbs. We'll encounter a revolutionary architect in Sweden who uses design to help patients heal faster, and we'll stop over in Milan to visit a scientist who uses a fasting diet protocol as a method to improve cancer outcomes post-chemotherapy. We'll look at how major sports organizations like the National Basketball Association (NBA) are rethinking the role of rest for their players' recovery and how this translates to other professions. We'll meet a former gymnast from Nashville who used movement to help her recover from paralysis. We'll learn why a palliative care doctor in Toronto dedicated his career to caring for the homeless at the end of their lives. And we'll take a journey into why we must sometimes let go: why true healing may, paradoxically, involve complete surrender to that which ails us.

But this is, perhaps most crucially, a book about the people who dared to see healing differently after their own brush with the medical system and who then had the courage to rethink dogma and change how we understand the ways we heal.

I hope this book empowers you to take responsibility for your own healing by thinking of tools beyond conventional medicine while contributing to the healing of others. A healer is not only someone who treats a patient within the walls of a hospital, but it can be anyone who might want to contribute to restoring wholeness. So, let's begin in the basement of the school where I studied medicine before we pan back to understanding how medicine lost its way over a century ago.

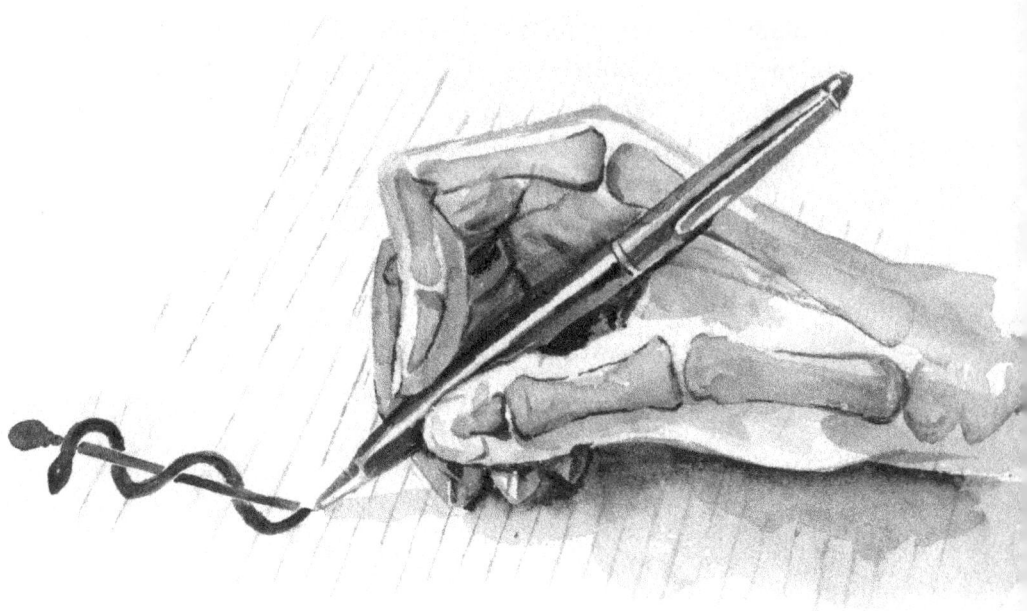

CHAPTER ONE

Healing Stories

*"Illness is the night-side of life, a more onerous citizenship. Everyone who is
born holds dual citizenship, in the kingdom of the well and in the kingdom of
the sick."*

— Susan Sontag in *Illness as a Metaphor*

1.

J oe was a burly man. I wasn't certain of his name, of course. My fellow
lab-mates—there were six of us sharing Joe—might have had their own
private names for him, or maybe to them he was just "a cadaver." But to
me, in that dank room in the basement of the medical sciences building at the
University of Toronto, I decided I'd call him by a name, and to me, he looked
like a Joe.

Joe had decided at some point in his life that when he died, he would donate
his body to science, in this case, to medical education. We met as he lay on
his back. A stark white sheet respectfully draped his generous abdomen, hips,
and private area. His yellowish-grey skin would have sloughed off by now if
not for the formaldehyde that preserved it. Joe was almost bald, save for a few
curly wisps of white hair framing a matte and freckled scalp. My labmates and
I weren't given any information about him except his age: 68. We surmised
that his cause of death might have been a heart attack. It wasn't clear whether
his history was kept from us to prevent us from becoming distracted by the life
behind the body or for the sake of Joe's privacy in case one of us were to find

1

out that he had been the uncle or father of a friend. At the time, we wondered if it was a mix of both.

On that warm August afternoon, our gaggle of first-year medical students had shuffled from an upstairs classroom, where anatomy had meant a stack of notes and hand-drawn pictures, to the basement anatomy lab. It was a ritual of sorts, entering the bowels of the medical sciences building, an area very few people would ever see—voluntarily, at least. Soon, wearing crisp white lab coats, we'd become familiar with the smell and fluorescent glare of the lab and what would eventually become second nature: slicing human flesh.

In my group, Cary was the first to go. We were dissecting the arm. The blood had been drained, so it was effectively just skin, muscles, and a layer of fascia (a casing of connective tissue that envelops our organs—something most of us knew nothing about before medical school). The consistency of the fascia was like dried-out chicken breast. We covered Joe's face, primarily out of respect but also to help us focus. Even still, my mind would wander. Who *was* he? Did he spend most of his seven decades in Toronto, or did he move around a lot, like I did? And how did he die? When we die, our cells swell with water, making the tissues what we call edematous. Did Joe, swollen in death, look markedly different now than he had when he was alive?

"Want to go next?" Cary asked, looking at me with his scalpel held up. He was a jovial 23-year-old from a farming community in Prince Edward Island, the Atlantic province my family first moved to from the U.K. in the early 1990s. Like many of my fellow medical students, Cary was social, kind, earnest, and also incredibly conscientious and studious. As a class, we looked after one another, and there was an expectation that we all stay well-rounded.

"Sure," I said. I reflexively looked at Joe as if to make eye contact and ensure he was okay with what I was about to do. I sliced into his wrist—a bit too deeply, at first—then maneuvered the scalpel up a bit, cutting just under the epidermis, splitting it like a curtain to unveil the beaded yellow layer underneath that was a mix of fascia and fat. Deeper down was muscle, a pale pink after being devoid of blood. Deeper still lay bone and an intricate network of nerves and vessels webbed throughout.

Cutting into Joe built upon another ritual we had just completed: the receipt of our "bone box." The long rectangular black case, lined with faded grey brushed velvet, contained mostly long bones: the femur, humerus, radius, and ulna. Maybe a rib or sternum—never a skull, and the tiny bones are omitted. Having been passed along since the 1970s, each bone box had been assigned to some 50 previous students. We each neatly wrote our name in Sharpie marker on a piece of masking tape placed on top, covering the others underneath. The person who had the box before me was named Samuel or Samantha—only a fragment of tape remained visible. The idea that the same anonymous discolored femur may have been examined by a student who had since become a world-class orthopedic surgeon was humbling.

We didn't know if each box contained the bones of one person or many. Some were bright white and looked newer, while others had taken on a dull, brownish hue. There were also rumors about where the bones were sourced from.

One time, traveling north on the Toronto subway to visit my parents for the weekend, I brought my bone box to study. We had heard the horror story of a student from the early 90s once leaving his box on transit, only to have its discovery be mistaken for evidence of a crime. On receiving our bone box, the professor made us promise that we'd never lose sight of it.

On that particular Friday, an older gentleman sat across from me, and, observing this long black case on my lap, he asked, "How long have you been playing the saxophone?" I was glad my stop was next.

The mysteries of the bone box represented a line of demarcation we were taught to reinforce, one between doctor and patient. Doctors choose when to be coy with patients and their families and when to express themselves, in part for self-protection but mostly to shield the curious questioner from a world we are taught to believe they are better off not knowing too much about. And so that barrier is erected on the very first day of medical school.

Dissection is a ritualized transgression—in no other context but surgery is it normal to cut into the flesh of a fellow human. This transcendence of social norms serves as a socialization into the medical profession, a normalized hazing, perhaps. But the purposeful anonymity of Joe and other cadavers helped teach us that we needed to compartmentalize. This separation would be a running theme throughout our training, a theme that often leaked into the rest of our lives.

And so, on that late August afternoon, as part of the socialized separation of doctors from the rest of society, I was indoctrinated into thinking of the body as separate from the person. The failure to know anything about Joe's history and his story would run counter to what we would soon be taught: that *story* remains the most crucial element of diagnosis and treatment.

*

I remember the morning of March 6, 2012 as a blur. I had left my clinic at the Toronto Western Hospital to have lunch back at my apartment. My attending (the term we give to a staff physician) knew it was a crucial day—Match Day, when I'd learn where I was going to spend the next three to four years, training to be a pediatrician. I logged onto the residency-matching website.

Congratulations, you have matched to…

I matched to a smaller city in Ontario, where I had attended high school. Even though the specialty was pediatrics, every other part felt wrong, and my body was reacting to the news in a way that felt deeper and more authentic. My chest tightened. I felt nauseous. Tears fell. I had loved medical school, my classmates, and my mentors in Toronto, some of whom I had known for over a decade, as I had also spent my undergrad years at the University of Toronto. Then, an epiphany: maybe it wasn't what I would have chosen, but what if there was something awaiting me, something I would only be able to learn there and nowhere else? Perhaps I'd gain better skills in the smaller program and be better able to focus in a quiet city.

I updated my Facebook status, as my classmates were doing, and emailed several mentors with the news, feigning joy, and received several notes of congratulations back. I didn't eat lunch—my appetite had faded. I returned to the clinic and shared the news. My attending seemed to know, averting her gaze after her "Congratulations" was met by my meek smile.

After work, my class met up at a local bar to celebrate. Everyone was wearing T-shirts with their program name in orange letters. I learned that five classmates hadn't matched at all, and I felt guilty for my disappointment, resolving to be more grateful. After that day, we would remember the Hippocratic Oath we took on the first day of medical school and how it would apply to our future patients.

2.

With its roots in the 5th century B.C., the Hippocratic Oath is one of the oldest known documents, and I had learned it to the point of delivering it by rote. My connection to it was deepened upon learning about the Walker Library of the History of Human Imagination in Ridgefield, Connecticut. Among numerous artifacts representing the history of human discovery was a 1745 work by anatomist Jacques Gautier d'Agoty, "The Flayed Angel," or "Ange Anatomique," that captured my imagination. This life-size portrait of a demure nude woman, whose back is slit open along the spine, with skin and muscles peeled away to expose the underlying bones, helped me feel the vulnerability of the patient as she hands over her care to a healer. Every cell in my body seemed to cry out: *"Do no harm."*

In the ancient Greek world of Hippocrates, illness was classified according to the four humors (phlegm, black bile, blood, and yellow bile), and Hippocrates was first to distinguish between types of disease—such as acute and chronic. The overarching approach of medicine was to facilitate self-healing through remedies as vast as honey, vegetables, oils, and massage. In his most famous document, "On the Physician," Hippocrates described the ideal characteristics of physicians as honest, considerate, and beyond corruption. A key set of lines became the basis of the Hippocratic Oath: "I will never do harm to anyone...I will give no deadly medicine if asked... All that may come to my knowledge in the exercise of my profession or in daily commerce...I will keep to myself, holding such things shameful to be spoken about, and will never reveal."

Looking back further in time, Hippocrates had a connection to the gods that points toward the mysterious nature of healing. Myth tells us that his teacher's teacher, Chiron, was a centaur, meaning he was half human, half horse, but unlike other centaurs, his front legs were human. He was also immortal. Chiron lived at the base of Mount Pelion, located in modern-day Greece, around 510 B.C. Chiron was granted powers for healing and taught by his foster father, Apollo. He subsequently instructed many Greek healers, such as Heracles (Hercules), Achilles, and Asclepius, who would go on to teach Hippocrates. One day, Chiron was at a gathering of centaurs and gods. Hercules was playing with a bow when he accidentally shot Chiron in the knee with a poisoned arrow. Chiron recoiled in pain and swiftly dragged himself from the party to a cave on a faraway mountaintop. Unable to heal himself after nine days, during which he tried every known medicine and herb, Chiron negotiated with Zeus to give up his immortality if it would put an end to his intolerable pain—effectively asking Zeus to allow him to die. He died within a few weeks, suggesting that an immortal would choose death over a lifetime of pain.

The name Asclepius may seem familiar, as the most recognizable medical symbol depicts a snake wrapped around "the staff of Asclepius." Asclepius, an orphan rescued by Apollo, was the traditional Greek god of healing. The snake licked Asclepius clean and taught him knowledge. In ancient Greece, snakes represented healing, wisdom, and resurrection. Asclepius became a wunderkind of sorts and was able to evade death and bring people back from the dead.

*

Western medicine grew from European roots during the Middle Ages, when the first recognized school of medicine was formed in the town of Salerno, Italy. Would-be physicians from all over Europe flocked to Salerno, as did patients who were sick and wanted a novel treatment or cure, earning Salerno the moniker "Town of Hippocrates." The Salernitana school became a template for other medical schools later founded in France, Italy, and Switzerland, and, eventually, North America and around the world.

By the 1500s, barber surgeons in Europe used bloodletting as a core part of healing, with the idea that most maladies were due to too much blood circulating in the body. These surgeons also cauterized wounds and performed limb amputation. In 1536, France's Ambroise Paré, appalled at the lack of pain control options available, created a topical anesthetic made of a combination of turpentine, egg yolk, and rose oil. When it was offered to civilians and soldiers wounded in the siege of Turin of 1640, those who received the balm healed faster and had less pain. Paré was also among the first to tie ligatures during battle for limb injuries so that wounds to arteries didn't result in excessive blood loss.

Since ancient times, cultures from around the world have innovated new curative techniques as Paré did while exploring the mind-body connection and the role of traditional plants, spirituality, and dietary practices. But the most crucial element of medicine may not be the history of medical methods as much as it is the individual history that doctors obtain from their patients.

3.

While my classmates and I might never know how Joe ended up in the basement anatomy lab, we would learn that taking the history of the patient is the most salient element of medicine, both for diagnosis and treatment. As the oft-quoted Canadian physician William Osler once said, "The good physician treats the disease; the great physician treats the patient who has the disease."* As medical students, we spent months refining the art of history-taking. First, we'd ask about the chief complaint. Then, we would climb the rungs of inquiry by asking the history of the present illness (HPI), delving into when the symptoms started, asking about any alleviating or worsening factors, assessing the quality and severity of the pain, and seeking suspicions of what the patient believes the problem to be. We then ask about the patient's past medical history, including previous surgeries and coexisting conditions, family history, social history (which covers things like income and food security, recent family changes, and employment), medications they are taking, known allergies, and their drug and alcohol use. Only then do we start the physical exam.

---

* Osler has also said some less savory things: "The first duties of the physician is to educate the masses not to take medicine," which goes against the idea of prudent use of medication and adherence to such medication. But my personal favorite might be: "One finger in the throat and one in the rectum makes a good diagnostician." It's just a bit cheeky!

My obstetrics and gynecology rotation in medical school taught me the value of fully understanding a patient's history. A patient disclosed she was in an abusive relationship. She had been in to see us for fertility counseling. As she was 42, my attending indicated she was looking at very poor odds of conceiving. Alone with her in the room, I learned why she wanted to get pregnant. It had nothing to do with wanting a child but everything to do with having a son to satisfy her demanding husband. She told me life with him was like walking on eggshells—not knowing what he might say or do next, worried he could walk out at any minute, leaving her financially unstable. Having a baby was her last-ditch effort to save the illusion of their marriage. The patient's symptoms—hypervigilance, sleeplessness, inability to concentrate, and a profound sense of hopelessness—all suggested to my medical student mind that the patient seemed depressed and anxious. Her story led us to focus more on her safety and well-being than on fertility treatments, and eventually, she was able to find the courage to leave her difficult situation.

Storytelling is also important for doctors to process their experiences with life and death, as well as their own evolution. Roger I. Lee, a World War I medic who served as the president of the American Medical Association in 1945, left behind a remarkable understanding of the medical profession and the doctor's role within it in his 1944 essay "Are Doctors People?" published in the *New England Journal of Medicine*. He wrote:

> We must accept the fact that the community, from the days of folklore and the medicine man to the present, conceives the medicine man and the doctor as someone apart from the rest of the tribe or the rest of the community...Doctors are human beings notwithstanding the fact they are not supposed to be tired, to have vacations or to enjoy uninterrupted dinners or gold games.

And he acknowledged the role of the social sciences in medicine:

> Whereas the doctor looks at his patient through a microscope, the social scientists look at illness through a telescope....[with

the giants of] Disease, Idleness, Ignorance, Poverty and Want...
[and] within the fold of this cult, however, poverty is the mother
of disease. The paternity of disease is usually left obscure.

Lee was a pioneer in his recognition of the social aspects of disease that usually
only comes from keen observation and through patterns noticed while taking a
detailed history from patients.

Many doctors now expand on the idea of narrative medicine by writing
fiction and nonfiction for wider audiences. One of the first was Mikhail
Bulgakov's *A Country Doctor's Notebook*, published in 1925, which is an unusual
meld of autobiography and fiction. A young doctor named Mikhail is fresh
out of medical school and asked to serve in a small town in Russia. He
details his feelings of imposter syndrome as he performs procedures he had
only learned about in medical textbooks. It's an early recollection of the
struggles newly trained student doctors face.

Decades after Lee and Bulgakov, the term "narrative medicine" was coined
by Rita Charon, a Harvard-trained physician who holds a Ph.D. in English
Literature and now serves as the Founding Chair and Professor of Medical
Humanities and Ethics at Columbia University Medical School. It effectively
refers to creating narrative—a story—as a way to integrate and understand a
patient-doctor encounter. It can also be a method to improve their own well-
being and process difficult emotions.

There's some evidence that narrative medicine, as it was taught in my
medical school and as employed by physicians, can help decrease feelings of
burnout, anxiety, and depression in practitioners. Expressive writing has been
studied by psychologist James Pennebaker for decades as a way to integrate
challenging experiences, many of which involve our own health. So, while
understanding the patient's story is crucial, doctors must also understand their
own story in relation to the patient and the healthcare context in which they
work. Indeed, there were pressures that would arise in my own narrative that
I had yet to understand that were affecting my health, and if I was going to
give my all to my patients, I needed to become whole. I hoped the experiences
gained in the hospital would help guide me.

4.

When I reflect on the early days of working in an academic medical setting, the initial months passed without much trouble. One of my early clinical experiences, centered on pediatric care, quickly became a personal favorite and I felt I was performing well. However, the dynamics among those working together that year were unique, with varying personalities occasionally creating friction. In time, a shrewlike bespectacled ringleader came to the fore in the group, and some voiced concerns about tensions and frictions she caused. I focused on my work and aimed to stay under the radar.

Weekly staff presentations were held for physicians to present on various topics relevant to medical cases. During these sessions, I noticed that some older staff were particularly quick to critique, often with a sharpness that felt excessive. At first, I was relieved not to have drawn their attention. Early on, I requested a day off to attend a conference, thinking it aligned with the institution's educational policies. To my surprise, the request was initially denied. After some back-and-forth, I received approval, though the response left me uneasy—it carried the implication that this was a one-time exception, with an undertone suggesting, *Don't expect this to happen again.*

When I returned from the conference, the atmosphere had shifted. I found myself increasingly under scrutiny, with my decisions frequently questioned by those above me, especially the one who reluctantly granted the conference approval. The collegial environment I had previously enjoyed seemed to have evaporated, replaced by an air of persistent tension. What had felt manageable before now became overwhelming, and even individuals I had worked well with began to adopt the same critical tone.

The feedback I eventually received was disheartening. Many of the issues raised were things I had not been informed about during the clinical shifts, and some seemed impossible to confirm.

The stress weighed heavily on me, both mentally and physically, making it difficult to perform at my best. Looking back, it became clear that what I had experienced reflected broader patterns found in challenging work environments—where unexpected pushback can escalate into more systemic resistance. Over time, this pattern took a toll on my health in ways I couldn't fully understand at the time.

If Columbia University narrative medicine expert Rita Charon is correct, and humans are natural storytellers, perhaps the act of writing a story is similar to taking the history of a patient: it can be used to connect the dots for healers as well. In her best-selling book *Untamed*, Glennon Doyle poignantly writes that "the moral arc of our life bends toward meaning, especially if we bend it that way with all our damn might." If there was a moral arc to my story, it was up to me to find it—and bend it. And so began my quest for healing.

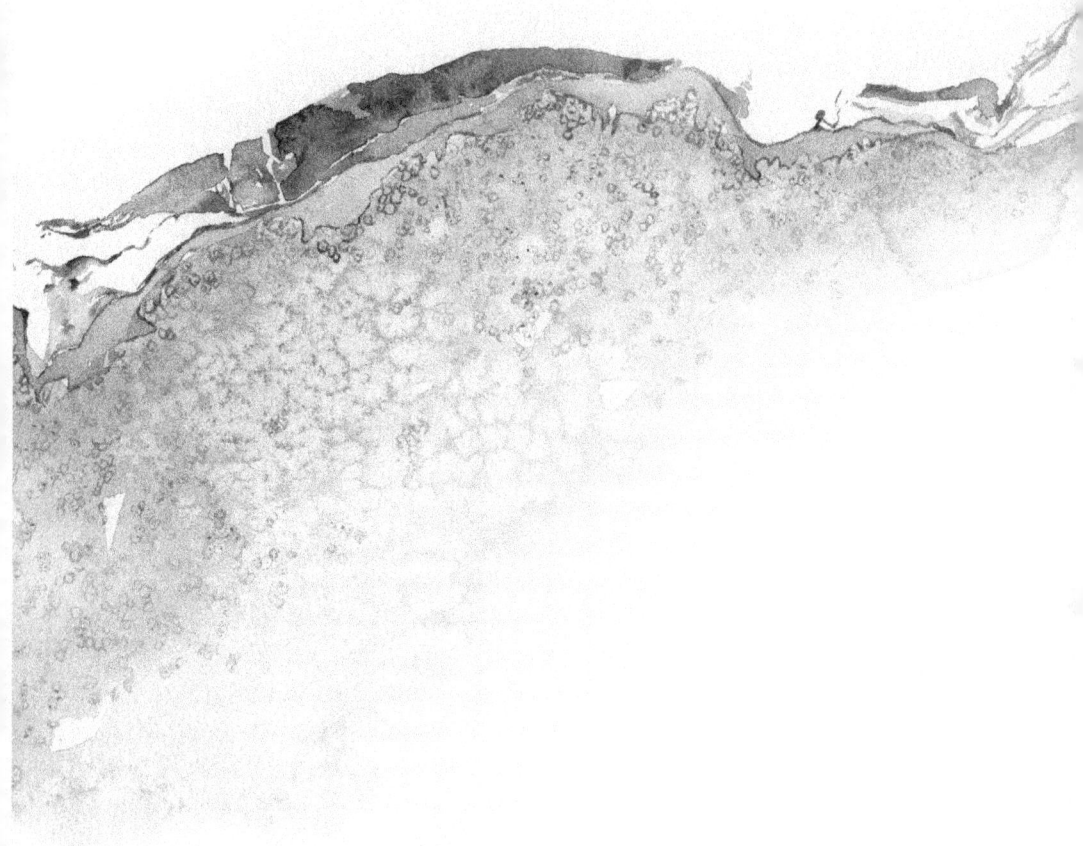

CHAPTER TWO

From Cell to Body

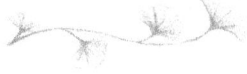

"There is someone who looks after us from behind the curtain.
In truth we are not here, this is our shadow."
— Rumi

1.

The bee was huge, apparently.

I was eight years old, in the third grade, and playing marbles with two friends on the playground over the lunchtime recess at Parkside Elementary School in Summerside, Prince Edward Island. The spring air had a slight chill, which was intermittently whisked away by the beaming sun. My friends and I were crouched down on the pavement. I had won the last round: two giant cat's eyes—the glass spheres with wisps of feathers inside. Our French teacher, Monsieur Chaisson, passed by to let us know there were five minutes left before the bell. As he walked away, he made a joke about the marbles. I actually don't think Monsieur Chaisson had more than a working knowledge of French, but he was one of our favorites because he was always funny.

Suddenly, there was a blood-curdling scream. My friends and I looked up— it was Monsieur Chaisson, running towards us, his hands flapping about. It was an odd sight, reminiscent of the Pied Piper. A trail of students ran behind him. "A bee!" someone shouted as the crowd ran towards us. Reflexively, my friends and I stood up—if we hadn't, we would have been trampled, or worse, maybe

13

killed by this dangerous bee. I pinched up my marbles and stuck them into the pocket of my Oshkosh overalls.

We ran around the side of the school, out past the soccer field. Numbering around 20 and led by Monsieur Chaisson, we began to look like a swarm of bees ourselves. Most of us had recently seen the film *My Girl*, which was released earlier that year. I had rented it for a sleepover, and my friends and I had cried uncontrollably as the movie ended in tragedy, with Macauley Culkin succumbing to his severe anaphylaxis to bee stings. None of us third graders wanted to die like that, nor did Mr. Chaisson. So, we ran. Then suddenly, I felt something jab into the back of my right foot. Someone was literally on my heels.

"Ow!!" I exclaimed before tripping forward onto the pavement. It was Toby, a boy in my class.

"Sorry," he mumbled without stopping. The swarm fanned out so as not to stumble on my crouched figure and joined up again just ahead of me.

I lifted my aching knees up. My left one was lightly scraped. The right, however, looked mangled. A thin patch of brown skin the size of a quarter had lifted off, revealing bright pink tissue underneath, speckles of dark grey gravel framing it on one side. And in the middle, a glistening white spot. Could it have been bone? Before I could peer any closer, the wound gushed bright red blood.

By now, Monsieur Chaisson and the other students were walking back towards me, their weakest link. Embarrassed, I picked myself up. I quickly wiped away my tears. I needed to be tough. I looked down at my right shin, which was now coated with a thick line of dark red blood, staining the edges of my pink crew sock a deep berry red.

"Are you alright, Amitha?" Monsieur Chaisson asked as he approached, the gaggle of students crowded behind him. I saw Toby crouch among them, seemingly afraid to see the damage he might have caused.

"Yes," I lied.

Monsieur Chaisson peered at the damage. "Go to the nurse's office and get bandaged up," he instructed.

I complied and limped into the school.

By the time I arrived, the bleeding had stopped. In its place, a viscous sheet of maroon sat in the middle of my knee. It seemed like a little miracle. That bright pink patch was all but gone. And the sliver of bone, if it *was* indeed bone, was also hidden. It made me wonder whether it was all just an illusion. The nurse arrived and cleaned off the clot with an alcohol swab.

"You don't want it to get infected," she said sternly, as though that had been my master plan. She took one look at my vaccine chart—"OK, it looks like you've had the tetanus shot, so you don't need that again."

I had no clue what she was referring to, but I nodded my head. She pasted a peach-colored band-aid on the wound. It was supposed to be "skin-colored," like the "flesh-colored" colored pencils we used in art class, yet another thing that didn't quite fit with my brown skin. But it served its purpose. Instantly, that injury, the pain, the gush of blood, the peek into what lay underneath, seemed ephemeral. It was the first time I'd seen my body begin to heal from something. Even though the nurse had seemed to disrupt the natural process, I could almost feel it happening under the soft plastic that was stuck to my knee. I walked to class a little relieved: it was as though the injury had never happened.

The band-aid would fall off in the bath a couple of days later, the white cotton displaying only a tiny dark-red dot. My knee was healing. A scab had formed. Over weeks, it would become a keloid—boggy soft tissue that would be fun to touch because it felt so different from the surrounding knee.

Now, thinking back to that moment, I see the idea of having "thick skin" as a way we describe resilience. It never made sense to me: when skin thickens and hypertrophies (or enlarges) in response to injury, as it did when I was eight, it looks stronger but is, in fact, *weaker*. There are no more hair follicles, and the layers of tissue never fully repair. A repeat injury to that tissue is likely to be worse than a similar injury inflicted on the surrounding, healthier skin.

The scar was an imperfect method to reduce further harm from the elements, like taping plastic over a broken window. Our bodies haven't figured out how to heal seamlessly: we always have a reminder through a scar of some kind. Yet, we understand a lot more about healing the body than we do about our minds. Reflecting on my need to heal both my body and mind, I needed to better understand how our bodies heal. So, I thought back again to medical school and what a man named Roger and human physiology had taught me about making myself whole again.

*

Fifteen years after that third-grade scrape, I'd see my first wound from the vantage point of a medical student and marvel in much the same way. I was on a clinical rotation on the 14th Floor "Cardinal Carter West" at St. Michael's Hospital in downtown Toronto. I had quickly fallen in love with internal medicine. The work was challenging and demanded our critical thinking skills.

One evening, a patient called Roger was admitted to Room 7 overnight. Roger was an "NFA" patient; that is, he had "no fixed address." More colloquially, Roger was homeless. He was admitted after he'd managed to crawl into the emergency room on a particularly cold night. It was only November, but some nights, Toronto could hit as low as -4F (-20C) before December. That had been one of those nights. Both of Roger's lower legs were blue and covered with wounds from what appeared to be a mix of cellulitis (inflamed skin) secondary to multiple infections and frostbite. There were areas of hyperpigmentation (dark brown splotches) and other areas of raw pink skin. Our attending, Dr. Serge, had a niche in wound care and asked us to read about the pathophysiology behind the case. Roger was to be my patient.

On day one, I dreaded seeing Roger. He wasn't very talkative, and the room smelled pungently like a cocktail of vomit, body odor, and urine. Many homeless people are stigmatized due to a lack of access to bathing facilities, and it's an awful predicament. Some specialists would wear masks when they saw them to prevent themselves from vomiting. I usually tried to ignore the odors. One gastroenterologist I knew had a habit of dabbing essential oils onto the inside of her mask if she was doing a colonoscopy to buffer the scent of feces—we all had our ways of adapting to unpleasant smells as respectfully as possible. I asked Roger a few questions about his pain and examined his skin with gloves. I wrote my notes silently. I would do the same on the second day. On day three, however, he seemed to warm to me. "I missed seeing my favorite nurse," he exclaimed when I walked in on a Thursday morning.

"I'm actually a medical student," I corrected (I was becoming used to the assumption) with a smile.

"Oh, sorry," he said.

"How are you feeling?" I asked.

"Much better now. They've been putting these small white sheets over my legs now, and they're starting to hurt a lot less. I think that's what's helping," he said—pointing to the trash can, which housed some used rectangular wipes. I wasn't sure what they were, so I flipped back to the notes from his wound-care team. In addition to washing his legs twice a day with warm soap and water, the lead wound-care nurse began to dry them and apply sheets of colloidal silver. I hadn't heard of that before.

"It sounds like they're putting a special medication on your legs," I told Roger, "I don't know much about it, but I'm going to ask. It sounds like it might be silver." Roger looked at me strangely—"No, it doesn't look all that silvery to me," he said, "but whatever you say!" He grinned.

"You seem to be in a really good mood today," I said.

"Well, I'm just glad to be here, I guess, and to rest my legs," he replied.

An orderly interrupted to drop off Roger's breakfast. While he ate, he shared more about his injury. It seemed chronic—it had been years since his skin had been healthy. He had some ulcers on his feet that may have been due to diabetes, but he had access to a foot-care nurse back then, before he was homeless. Roger shared that he used to work as a line cook.

I was perplexed. Roger seemed to have lived a relatively ordinary life up until three years earlier. He had lost his job after an angry outburst with his boss and ended up being unable to pay his rent, so he was evicted. He landed in a shelter but left it for the street. "Shelters are terrible. People in there are animals. I can't tell you how many times I've had my shoes—even my dog—stolen. I'd rather sleep in a bus shelter or park," he said.

Later, I found the wound-care team at the nursing station and asked about the colloidal silver. They told me there was evidence it had anti-viral, anti-bacterial, and anti-fungal properties but was only for external use. Interestingly, what was new was perhaps old again—topical application of substances to the skin has been used for thousands of years.

2.

In Egyptian lore that dates back some 5,000 years, a woman named Gula, who possessed the head of a dog, served as the goddess of healing. During that time, herbal remedies were common: everything from pine sap to fruits like prunes was said to be ingested or applied to the skin. Centuries later, Egyptologist Edwin Smith purchased a papyrus from Luxor in the late 1800s that described ancient Egyptian medical treatments, including sutures for wounds and topical honey for infections. But it also went further: another papyrus, dated some 3,500 years ago, included spells to ward off spirits harnessed through amulets.

Thousands of years later, in ancient Rome, Claudius Galen (126-216 C.E.), whose father dreamt his son was commanded to study medicine by Asclepius, the Greek god of medicine, wrote about the importance of general hygiene (via bathing) in maintaining health—something that applied today with Roger. Dioscorides' book, *De Materia Medica (On Medical Substances)*, was a tome detailing the use of opium, herbs, and alcohol for pain relief during procedures; these treatments had become commonplace. Galen's *On the Properties of Simple Drugs* categorized and described the properties, preparation, and uses of various medicinal substances, impacting the world of pharmacology for centuries. In part due to them, while the Dark Ages birthed many untrained medical providers and charlatans peddling practices like witchcraft, it also ushered in the creation of early hospitals and aspects of the modern-day medical exam, like taking a pulse and noting a patient's breathing. Bloodletting and using leeches were popularized during this time, with the idea that sickness was secondary to too much blood circulating. In fact, doctors back then had been nicknamed "leeches." The role of poetry, prayer, and music also reached prominence.

Ibn Sina, one of the most famous doctors of the Islamic Golden Age, had a particular interest in using metals for healing. Ibn Sina authored two books—*Kitab al-Shifa (The Book of Healing)* as well as the *Al Qanun fi al-Tibb (The Canon of Medicine)*—which detailed both mineral and plant-derived healing methods that would go on to influence medicine for the next 500 years.

In his *Kitab al-Mansouri fi al-Tibb (The Book on Medicine Dedicated to al-Mansur)*, Iranian physician Al-Rhazi described approaches to treatment, such as diet and hygiene, while outlining the components of diagnosis, therapy, and surgery.

Importantly, Al-Rhazi was one of the first to recognize that some diseases did *not* have a cure, and that doctors shouldn't be blamed for this. He relied on herbs, minerals, and mercury-containing drugs and was an early proponent of sutures and casting to heal wounds and bones.

Of the "alchemists," a group credited with the impossible task of changing metals like lead into gold (though they never succeeded), as well as promoting a "universal remedy" to cure all diseases, the most famous was Jabbir ibn Hayyan, a predecessor of Al-Rhazi and Ibn Sina. He would grind mercury, sulfur, and gold to use as ointments and potions. Alchemy was so popular that it would dominate during the time of the Crusades in the 11th and 12th centuries. In Europe, leaders like Albertus Magnus combined it with Christian prayer as a way to "clean the soul and heal," which lost favor after the advent of the scientific method.

Today, there was a sort of "alchemy" in the silver dressing applied to Roger's legs, but it was expensive, so the team could only provide it for another day or so.

Once Monday rolled around, I was excited to give Roger some good news: we had decided during morning rounds that he could leave the hospital the following morning with a prescription for ointments. This news usually left patients relieved, even gleeful. Yet when I explained the discharge plan to Roger, he looked upset.

"But don't I need more time to heal?"

"No," I replied. "Besides, you'll increase your risk of a hospital-acquired infection if you stick around," I advised.

"Oh. Well, I like it here. I like you, and Dr. Serge, and the wound-care team. I don't want to leave," he said.

For Roger, being in the hospital was healing in and of itself—healing to his soul to sleep in a warm room with food delivered three times a day. The fact that people were caring for him went much further than the silver wraps on his legs. But Roger couldn't stay. He was stable, and more acute patients in the emergency room needed to be admitted. We worked with the discharge planning team to try to assist him with a housing liaison, but the reality was he faced a long waitlist for public housing. This wasn't a problem we could solve. It was much bigger than an infection, so we drew a line. Roger would need to go back to a shelter or back to the street. He would probably choose the latter.

My internal medicine rotation was only six weeks, so I didn't see Roger return—if he ever did. I wasn't convinced he ever picked up the prescription ointments. How would he have afforded them? I wondered if part of him was conflicted: if his legs healed, then he wouldn't have a reason to return, no reason to recover those other aspects of himself. But his poverty, combined with an illness that was exacerbated by the same poverty, meant that his wound wouldn't heal in the way that mine did as a child. Then, I wondered if the reason the medical profession turns an earnest blind eye to these impossible situations—the massive social inequities—was because it's the easiest way to cope with our limitations.

Whether it was my knee in the third grade or Roger's more serious leg infection, our bodies undergo a predictable set of steps for self-repair. But to appreciate exactly *how* requires a wander back to Germany in the 1800s to understand the theory that we have cells in the first place, and then, how our cells repair themselves after injury.

3.

In 1839, German physician and researcher Theodor Schwann published a theory in which he made three observations. The first was that the cell is the most basic unit of structure and physiology of living things. The second was that the cell is both a distinct entity and a building block. His third observation was unusual and ultimately wrong: that cells arise out of spontaneous generation, similar to crystals. It would take another sixteen years for the father of modern pathology, Rudolph Virchow, to sort out Schwann's faulty third premise.

Like Schwann, Virchow was based in Germany; however, he was a polymath: a physician, cellular biologist, doctor, writer, and politician. Inspired by a theory from one of his colleagues, Robert Remak (though some have argued Virchow attributed the idea to himself and that Remak was, in fact, his rival), Virchow published a treatise in 1855 entitled "*Omnis cellula e cellula*," Latin for "cells arise from other cells," which became crucial to understanding how cells reproduce to repair tissue after injury, effectively replacing the injured cells.

After Virchow's discovery, the next major mission was to sort out how cells become damaged in the first place. Two of the biggest names in public health and medicine in the 1800s were the microbiologists Louis Pasteur of France and Robert Koch of Germany. Like Remak and Virchow, Pasteur and Koch were rivals, and their work was pivotal to how we understand both disease and healing.

In the 1860s, Pasteur was researching diseases in silkworms, finding that microbes were the source. By preventing silkworms from becoming infected, Pasteur helped revitalize the French silk industry. He spent the following decades studying vaccines and investigating the veterinary disease anthrax, which was also seen as a threat to humans.

Based in Germany, Pasteur's rival, Robert Koch, was 20 years younger and a rising star in both microbiology and medicine. He also studied anthrax and inoculated rodents with diseased spleens of farm animals. Koch then purified the microbes in a laboratory culture. In 1880, after moving to Berlin, he developed his "Koch's postulates"* to summarize how microbes cause disease. Later on, in 1905, his work on isolating the organism responsible for tuberculosis was awarded the Nobel Prize.

Since these pivotal discoveries, scientists have sought to understand *how* cells become damaged in the first place and why this often occurs during cell division. Cellular injury may be due to many things: chemical agents such as chemotherapy (which is therapeutic when applied to cancer cells), heat (for instance, radiation from the sun's ultraviolet light), blunt force that breaks the tissues (like a knife wound), infectious organisms (like viruses), and auto-immune factors which attack the cell as though it were a foreign invader. Many of these processes are reversible, though we're just beginning to understand the mechanism. For instance, a bacteria may attack the heart, but its actions may be reversed through antibiotics. In other cases, the processes are irreversible;

---

* Koch's postulates are: i) The bacteria must be present in every case of the disease. ii) The bacteria must be isolated from the host with the disease and grown in pure culture iii) The specific disease must be reproduced when a pure culture of the bacteria is inoculated into a healthy, susceptible host.

however, the tissue can still heal. And naturally, there are instances where an irreversible process leads to death primarily by apoptosis (programmed cell death, which begins by ions like calcium entering the cell once the membrane is disturbed by an outside factor) or necrosis (which can often happen when blood flow is impeded, cutting off oxygen and glucose to the cell).

Given the many means through which cells can be damaged, there are also ways, albeit fewer, that cells can repair themselves. Often, the body will remove the damaged cell through the spleen (which acts as a filter for damaged cells, along with modulating the number of white cells, red cells, and platelets circulating in the blood). Typically, the body first attempts to fix the cell through DNA repair. For larger tissues, it may regenerate parenchyma cells to help bridge the damage left by the faulty cells or through flexible stromal cells, which support the damaged cells.

*

When it comes to how cells, and then tissues, repair themselves, there are many moving parts, and without an advanced degree in cellular biology it can be challenging to understand how the various elements fit together. To better understand this process, I found a seminal paper by Wallace Marshall, a biochemist and biophysicist at the University of California, San Francisco (UCSF), published in *Science* in 2017. With his colleague Sindy Tang, they compared the cell to a spacecraft. So, when a hole is punched through a cell, the repair must occur by stopping the run-off of cytoplasm (the liquid stuff inside the cell) and then, subsequently, regenerating the damaged parts. They also distinguished between "wound healing" and "regeneration." In the former, it's more like a tap being shut off, where a clot prevents further loss of blood. This is what happened when I injured my knee. On the other hand, when a cell "rebuilds and replaces missing components," it can be classified as regeneration. Wound healing must, however, take place *before* regeneration, which later would be clear when it comes to healing from mental and emotional ailments.

Within the cell resides DNA, which also undergoes its own healing process through DNA repair. Years after the structure of DNA was elucidated by scientists Rosalind Franklin, Francis Crick, and Jim Watson, DNA was found to be inherently unstable and subject to damage by ionizing radiation and the sun's ultraviolet radiation. At the cellular level, DNA damage is the most crucial to understand. DNA repair was discovered by accident by an American scientist named Albert Kelner in what is now known as the Cold Spring Harbor Laboratory in upstate New York. To better understand it, I called Errol Friedberg, a South African-American professor emeritus from the University of Texas Southwestern. He wrote a review about the history of DNA repair, so he simplified the overall mechanism for me: "Two DNA molecules line up next to each other, and the damaged one exchanges its strand so it becomes normal again," Friedberg told me.

More recently, the DNA repair field gained immense ground through a new discovery called CRISPR-Cas9, which was discovered at the same time by two labs: one in Europe and one at the University of California Berkeley. When I spoke with Sam Sternberg in 2015 about it, he was just finishing his post-doctoral work in one of those labs. His supervisor was none other than Jennifer Doudna, one of the co-recipients (with Emmanuelle Charpentier) of the 2020 Nobel Prize in Chemistry. Sternberg now runs his own lab out of Columbia University.

CRISPR stands for "Clustered Regularly Interspaced Short Palindromic Repeats," which are areas of DNA that are widespread in microbes such as bacteria. It was first found in 1987 in *E. coli*, but it took twenty years for scientists to discover protein-coding genes called "Cas" (CRISPR-associated) in milk-fermenting bacteria in 2007. It was then found to produce RNA that could go on to detect viral DNA by pairing with it and cutting that DNA in half, subsequently destroying the virus. The precise molecular components for this DNA cutting reaction were named "CRISPR-Cas9."

"To make a long story short, when it comes to genome repair, with CRISPR-Cas9, scientists would have the power to introduce permanent, precise changes to the genome virtually anywhere they desired," Sternberg told me. "Genes could be turned on or off to determine their functional significance, cancer-causing mutations could be simulated and studied in human cells grown in the lab, and most promisingly, genetic diseases in human patients might be treatable—even curable—by editing away the disease-causative mutations." CRISPR-Cas9 succeeded as a genome editing tool inside human cells almost immediately and is now being used to tackle eliminating certain genetic diseases, such as cystic fibrosis (which is often a result of a singular gene mutation). As Sternberg put it, CRISPR-Cas9 "has incredible potential to alleviate human suffering for a number of genetic diseases."

Once the foundation of cellular repair was established, the field of "regenerative medicine" was born. Coined in 1992, the field was used as part of the work by Leland Kaiser, who envisioned the use of technology to regenerate organ systems. In 2010, President Barack Obama relaxed the regulations on stem cell work, which helped facilitate stem cell treatment for spinal cord injury by the Geron Corporation. And the rest, you might say, is history.

Now that we know how cells heal and regenerate, how can we apply this micro-level understanding of healing all the way up to animals and, eventually, humans? Wound healing may be better appreciated through model organisms, specifically those that regenerate in ways humans cannot. In regeneration, which takes place after healing, the cell must rebuild that which has been damaged within. The key may lie in a humble amphibian native to Mexico.

4.

The axolotl is probably the king of regeneration. Known colloquially as the "Mexican salamander," it's native to Lake Xochimilco in Mexico. It's one of the only salamanders that lives totally in water and retains its gills. One March morning, I found myself at the Royal Ontario Museum (known affectionately as the "ROM") in Toronto, making my way up to the Keenan Family Gallery of Hands-on Biodiversity located on the second floor. Hidden in the corner were some mossy frogs, cockroaches, and scorpions (all in tanks). In one tank were the axolotls—two of them: a dark green, almost black, female swimming playfully amongst the rocks and plastic seaweed and a rather shy translucent-white male axolotl with bright red fins around its ears. The white one was similar to the model organism used by scientists for decades to study regeneration. Two male high schoolers walked by as I peered into the tank, watching to see if the male axolotl would come out of the small cave in which he had found himself.

"What's that?" One of the boys asked me.

I began to rattle off some interesting facts about the axolotl that I had recently read as part of my research for this book. Immediately, both boys seemed a little shocked and, perhaps, a little intrigued. A volunteer walked over to ask if I was an expert.

"No," I said sheepishly, realizing I likely sounded like someone who had an overly restrictive interest in this odd creature. "I'm just working on a project about them," I said as I quietly made my way out.

Like the comic book hero, Wolverine, the axolotl has unique self-healing capabilities: it can regenerate many of its body parts. If, for instance, there's a spinal cord lesion, it can fully regenerate the spinal cord and regain its motor and sensory control. In 1968, a controversial paper in *Science* titled "Transplantation of Axolotl Heads" showed that an axolotl head could be transplanted onto the torso of another, and both organisms still somehow lived. Advancements in medical ethics, even those including animals, preclude those types of experiments now, but axolotls are still studied in labs across Europe and North America. Axolotls have become popular pets, even though they are officially on the endangered list. Domestication requires special permits, however, and illegal selling still occurs.

I knew I needed to learn from an expert first-hand, so I made my way into Ramsay Wright Laboratories on St. George Street, a few blocks down from the ROM, to speak to a young scientist in regeneration research, Joshua Currie. On the first floor, a crowd of undergraduates were in the student lounge, cramming for a biology exam, quizzing each other on terms and comparing lab notes. It had been over twelve years since I set foot in Ramsay Wright—I had an organic chemistry tutorial there as an undergraduate. It was my toughest class. The building still had the same faint, musty smell. Currie, having recently moved from Dresden, Germany, was just setting up his lab and hadn't yet hired graduate students. His office was bare other than an aloe plant on the windowsill and an iMac perched on a small desk near the window.

"The difference, even from geckos, is that with the axolotl, architecture is preserved. And we have a common ancestry, but as humans, we lost the regeneration capability on the way," Currie told me. Currently, Currie, now based at Wake Forest University in North Carolina, is focusing on understanding the "where, when, and how" of regeneration, specifically where signaling molecules are active and when they are expressed.

"Right now, there are studies where stem cells are injected directly into patients, but they don't integrate into the tissues or contribute directly to healing. So, there is a big gap between how animals regenerate and how we could use this to elicit a similar response in humans, where there is an inflammatory response that leads down the regeneration pathway as opposed to the scarring pathway," Currie told me.

Led by a scientist named Karen Echeverri, research from Ireland found that the gene c-Fos is upregulated in the glial cells (cells that coat the nerves) after spinal cord injury, and when paired with the gene JunB in the axolotl, they regained functional spinal cord. However, in humans, the pairing is with a different gene called c-Jun, which leads to scar formation.

"It's all about who you partner with directly after injury and how that drives you toward either regeneration or forming scar tissue. It's kind of like in life, who you partner with can have a really positive or negative effect," Echeverri explained in an interview. Unlike the axolotl, humans generate scar tissue instead of new spinal cords, which is why, when humans sever their spinal cords, they usually remain paralyzed. For Currie, the ultimate goal is to one day put forth a "recipe" to divert scarring towards regenerative healing. This work will one day form a foundation for how we may be able to heal the most stubborn tissue of the spinal cord, but applying this knowledge to humans is tricky.

In early 2019, a controversial study using stem cells to treat spinal cord injuries was announced, yet the work around this hadn't actually been published. A journalist's article in *Nature*, however, reported that the study involved 113 participants who received stem cells that were obtained from their own bone marrow, and all but one regained some of their movement and sensation. Other journalists expressed concerns regarding the trial not being double-blinded and the unusually small sample size, which greatly affected the quality of the trial. As well, the mode of action of how an intravenous therapy would work wasn't clear. That said, every day, it seems new innovations are attempting to help us regenerate and heal, but we're still a long way off from getting anywhere close to being as proficient as the humble axolotl.

*

In my own quest for healing, I tried to discern where my symptoms were coming from and knew I wasn't dealing with a wound I could visibly see. Instead, I started with an afternoon assessment interview with a psychologist, Dr. Morgan, where she gathered a history from me for two hours. I arrived a few minutes late, having scrambled to leave the hospital on time and running into various last-minute requests to follow up lab work and complete my patient notes.

When I sat down with Dr. Morgan, I went into detail about when my symptoms started. The following day involved about seven hours of neuropsychological testing. I took a memory test where I had to draw photos from memory after looking at them for a few minutes. Then, there was a "faces test" to understand expressions of empathy, followed by a traditional IQ test and a test of my grip strength. I was exhausted by the end. After the arduous day, Dr. Morgan sat me down across from her large glass desk. She said she would have the results within a few weeks, but immediately, she seemed concerned.

"Right now, based on what I'm seeing—something is very wrong," Dr. Morgan said. "I'll put it this way: someone with these results would never have gotten through medical school, let alone met the requirements for admission. Your memory especially…it suggests…" she trailed off. She reiterated that she would get the results to me soon.

A few days later, I went to see the hospital's wellness officer, Dr. Tepper. Rolling up her sleeves that exposed a tattoo of a calla lily, Dr. Tepper asked me to tell her what was going on. As I did with Dr. Morgan, I explained when my symptoms started, that everything seemed to change after I returned from a course, and how the more senior physician behaved afterward, which began a downward spiral of treatment that seemed deliberately misaligned with my performance. Things had seemed fine before—not perfect but not toxic. Dr. Tepper then leaned in and gave me an empathic warning to be on guard and protect myself, suggesting she knew what I was experiencing firsthand. I felt a mix of relief that I was understood, but fear at what may lie ahead.

5.

The first time I saw my mother cry was in 1989. We were living in Stoke-on-Trent, England, where my father was a senior house officer in obstetrics at a local hospital. My mother, an anesthesiologist, was home taking care of my brother, sister, and me. It was early in the morning, and she was about to help us brush our teeth. The phone rang, and we all gathered in the living room, where the phone rested. She picked it up, spoke a few words in Tamil, and fell silent. The tube of toothpaste dropped out of her hand, and she leaned against the fireplace mantle. She began sobbing, hung up, and sat down on a nearby chair. Not knowing what happened, I asked. The words were hard to comprehend between her gasps, but she said that my uncle (whom we called "Mama" in Tamil)—her younger brother—had lost his foot to a landmine in Sri Lanka. It was my first real taste of the troubles in the country my parents had left years before I was born.

In July 1983, Sri Lanka was thrown into decades of civil war between the minority Tamil population, of which my family is a part, and the majority Singhalese population. The government had historically been comprised of Singhalese, who were predominantly Buddhist. Tamils are predominantly Hindu. However, there are Christians—mostly Catholic—from both ethnic groups, as well as a small proportion of Muslim Sri Lankans. My father left Sri Lanka in 1979, before the war began, and my mother joined him in 1981. They settled in the United Kingdom, where I was born a few years later. Both had completed their medical training—my father at Madras Medical College in India and my mother at the University of Colombo in Sri Lanka—but had to re-qualify for British licensure, a process that would take several years. When the war broke out, a flood of refugees, primarily the Tamil minority, left for countries like the U.K., U.S., Canada, Australia, and Germany. Though the war ended in 2011, tensions are still palpable in parts of Sri Lanka today.

Just as Sri Lanka had been torn by civil war, Mama never fully recovered from losing his foot. His ankle was covered in skin, and he simply attached a brown plastic prosthetic foot. A jovial and optimistic man by nature, it didn't dampen his goals and his work as an engineer, though my mother would wonder if his disability was part of why he never married. Decades after his accident, the world of prostheses and biosimilar devices for amputees is filled with possibilities. Research on regeneration, as well, has set the foundation for a future where those like my uncle may one day not need to rely on prostheses at all.

Incorporating synthetic materials has played a role in modulating wound healing. At Northwestern University in Chicago, in partnership with the University of California, San Diego (UC San Diego), scientists have designed a way to insert a bioactivated, biodegradable nanomaterial that alters the body's natural inflammatory response into a signal that allows healing instead of scarring following a heart attack, overcoming the signaling pathway Echeverri described. The research team believes it will be several years before they can introduce the nanomaterial intervention in clinical trials, but it could be applied to heart disease, peripheral artery disease, and even metastatic cancer, given the similarities in the inflammatory response.

Three-dimensional (3-D) printing has also advanced how well our cells and tissues heal. In March 2019, scientists from the Wake Forest Institute for Regenerative Medicine (WFIRM) presented their "mobile skin bioprinting system," which allows two layers of skin to be "printed" right onto the wound. The idea is that this bioprinter, filled with healthy cells—specifically dermal fibroblasts and epidermal keratinocytes obtained by biopsy from the patient's normal tissues—could be wheeled to the bedside in a burn unit or a trauma bay. Fibroblasts make extracellular matrix and collagen, while the keratinocytes form a barrier function in the epidermis. The cells are added into a water-based gel and inserted into the bioprinter.

"If you deliver the patient's own cells, they do actively contribute to wound healing by organizing up front to start the healing process much faster," said James Yoo, M.D., Ph.D., who led the research team and co-authored the paper, when interviewed about his work. "While there are other types of wound healing products available to treat wounds and help them close, those products don't actually contribute directly to the creation of skin."

*

Max Ortiz Catalan is originally from just outside of Mexico City and is now based out of Chalmers University in Gothenburg, on Sweden's west coast. Chalmers boasts an impressive repertoire of research and, for the last decade, has recruited heavily for scientists in the healthcare and medical fields. Ortiz Catalan sees healing with technology as totally separate from regeneration, and his obsession is phantom pain: the pain that amputees feel in limbs they no longer have.

I first learned about phantom pain in medical school; mirror therapy was the standard of care and remains so today. Mirror therapy involves having a patient look at their existing limb in a mirror while visualizing their other limb as functional and present (though it is a mirror image of the existing limb). Then, by viewing the phantom limb "move" (as a reflection of the real limb), the pain disappears. This treatment has been around for decades, with little in the way of innovation, so when I came across Ortiz Catalan's research, which uses virtual reality (VR) and augmented reality (AR) instead of mirrors, I was impressed. VR and AR are effectively more advanced mirror therapy.

In 2016, Ortiz Catalan's group published a seminal article in the *Lancet* titled "Phantom Motor Execution Facilitated by Machine Learning and Augmented Reality as Treatment for Phantom Limb Pain: A Single Group, Clinical Trial in Patients with Chronic Intractable Phantom Limb Pain." The 14 patients (all but one based in Sweden) were guided through 12 AR and VR sessions that incorporated gaming to "retrain" this phantom limb. The patients were monitored for symptoms and requirements for pain medication. For all patients, the average pain decrease was close to half, and there was an impact on other aspects, such as how often their sleep was interrupted due to pain (sleep deprivation, in general, can make us more attuned to pain). The improvements lasted for up to six months.

So how does it work? Imagine a patient looking at themselves in a mirror and seeing space where their phantom limb exists. This is their reality. Now imagine the same patient in an AR or VR context, where they can now "see" a limb instead of space. They can then manipulate this limb by moving it around, using it to pick up objects, and so forth in the AR and VR world.

"We demonstrated that if an amputee can see and manipulate a 'virtual' limb—which is projected over their limb stump—in space, over time, the brain retrains these areas," Ortiz Catalan told me. "Through this retraining, the brain reorganizes itself to focus on motor control and less on pain firing."

Over time, actively "using" this limb, the brain down-regulates the pain signals and up-regulates the signals used for movement. Eventually, the pain is almost undetectable, as it would be for a healthy working limb. After that pilot study, Ortiz Catalan and his team expanded the work to include other centers around the world as part of a multicenter trial, shifting the existing paradigm. Mirror therapy is thought to work through the visual system—our minds "see" a real limb instead of the space where a limb has been amputated and attempt to move it, which then decreases the pain signals fired to that area.

Publishing his work in 2020, Ortiz Catalan's group discovered something else: the treatment works without needing the visual system. Instead, it's the sense of *movement* itself (and firing in the motor cortex) that retrains the brain. Whether one sees the movement or not is irrelevant, though "seeing" helps facilitate the movement.

"It's not because you can *see* it that you feel better; it's because you are *moving* it that you feel better. The visual feedback allows you to see what you're doing, and it's helpful, but in the paper, it's clear that if someone is blind and has an amputation, they can still establish that control and, perhaps through other feedback that is tactile or auditory, they compensate, but it's the movement that decreases the pain response," he told me. This suggests that even mirror therapy, which was thought to rely on the visual system, likely works due to the sense of movement.

What motivated Ortiz Catalan to question the role of mirror therapy and the basis for how it works in the first place? To answer that, we must head back to his origin story. Born in the small Mexican town of Toluca (which happens to be about an hour's drive from Lake Xochimilco, home of the axolotl!) to a sociologist father and an educator mother, he began tinkering with computers in high school, after an uncle offered to teach him how to build his own. It was far less expensive than buying a brand-new one off the shelf.

In university, he was torn between engineering and psychology, choosing the former. It was the first year a new field called mechatronic engineering was offered, which combined computer science, industrial engineering, and mechanical engineering. Ortiz Catalan then went to France for a study year abroad, which instilled a sense of adventure and where he learned to navigate a different language and culture. Returning to Mexico the following year, he completed a degree and worked in a factory, running the electrical unit. But he wasn't fulfilled.

"The salary was good. The job was...you know, what can I say, 'good?' But I had read *The Brief History of Time* by Stephen Hawking and realized I wanted to do a master's which would allow me to blend science and psychology and engineering in a new way. The program in Sweden [at Chalmers] came up in complex adaptive systems, which was a new science, so I took it," he told me.

Complex adaptive systems are perhaps most helpfully illustrated by the example of the butterfly effect—in which a small change in one system can set off another event like a tornado in another distant but connected system. It also includes chaos theory and artificial neural nets.

In Gothenburg, the founder of a prosthetics company caught Ortiz Catalan's attention, and he decided to do a master's project focused on developing neural interfaces that could be implanted into the body to control movement. The group offered to pay for his Ph.D. if he stayed, so he did. Ortiz Catalan attributes his unusual background, curiosity, and ability to find connections between different fields as keys to pushing the field forward.

"Something I've been told a lot is that I can connect the dots," he told me. "I happened to have the right background in electrical engineering and in computer algorithms, but also understood the implant design part so I could put it all together." Ortiz Catalan was referring to piecing together a puzzle that eventually made sense and fueled his purpose. I was about to do the same myself.

6.

I reflected on my conversation with the wellness officer, who mentioned that others had also come to her for support, sharing similar concerns about their experiences. At one point, she paused and briefly mentioned that she had once worked in a similar environment at the same hospital as I but had eventually moved on. She didn't elaborate, leaving me uncertain about what she was trying to convey. I found myself questioning the situation—was I just encountering isolated challenges with a few difficult individuals, or was there something more systemic at play? And if others had faced similar issues, why hadn't these patterns been formally addressed?

Thus far, whether it was the injury in the third grade or Roger's devastating skin condition, I understood how physical injuries healed. It's what medical school and the biomedical model used as a framework. A rare Mexican salamander and new technologies, from CRISPR-Cas9 to 3-D printing to augmented and virtual reality, could amplify how we physically heal. Our cells and the tissues they form enter into an elaborate choreography for healing. Too often, the evidence is invisible, so the only way the injury is memorialized is through our own memories. Sometimes, a visible scar is easily overlooked by others, but to us, it represents a battle wound of sorts: thick skin in theory but softer in reality.

Yet, this framework focused on the regeneration of new tissue in response to physical wounds, and while helpful in understanding how my body might undo the damage stress had on my cholesterol, it was of no use to understanding the psychological stresses that were causing my mind to falter. Something else was needed that went beyond the flesh and the damage done to it. Clearly, as smart as my cells were, they could not offer me every type of healing. As insightful as my self-awareness was, it had limits. The concerns raised by those I sought guidance from were valid. Yet, despite my years of medical education, I struggled to find a way to set healing in motion—both for my mind and, potentially, my body. The path to recovery felt elusive, just beyond my control, leaving me searching for ways to restore my well-being and regain a sense of balance.

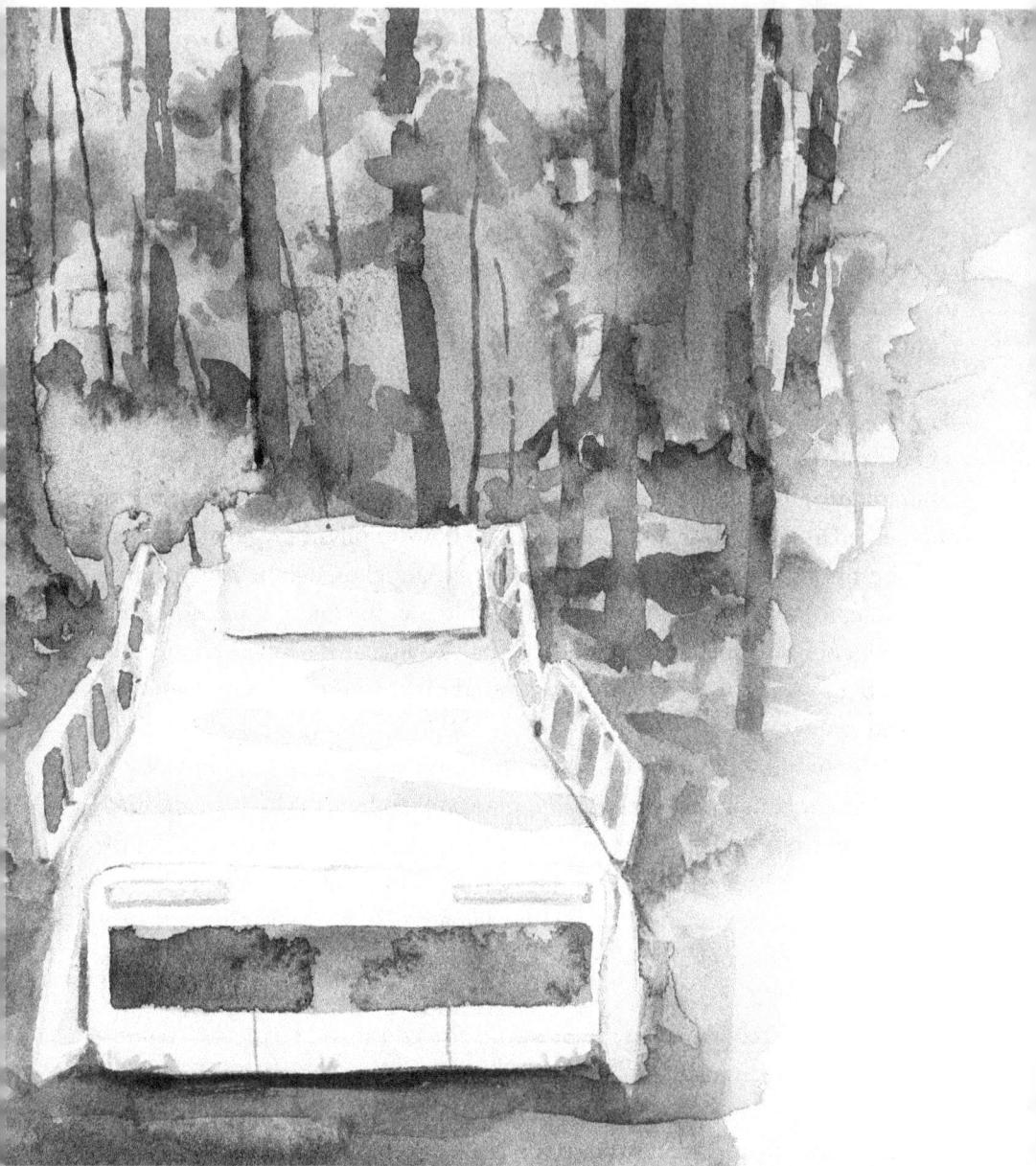

CHAPTER THREE

Surroundings

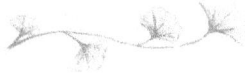

"If you watch how nature deals with adversity, continually renewing itself, you can't help but learn."

— Bernie Siegel

1.

Abald African-American man pointed me towards a hallway as a little girl went by, pushing someone I took to be her sister in a wheelchair, with an I.V. pole trailing. Their mother was just steps behind. In all directions, I saw adults and children, lots and lots of children bustling about. I made my way toward an atrium drenched in soft springtime light. A large grey whale hung from the ceiling. In the middle stood a large plastic oak tree, from which hung five white birdhouses. Down one hallway, blue plastic birds appeared midflight. Every few feet stood a model animal: a squirrel, a bear, or a fox. Bright motifs of flowers, butterflies, and other forest-like images decorated the windows. No wall was bare. We weren't in an amusement park. We were in the Nationwide Children's Hospital in Columbus, Ohio. The winner of countless design awards for the previous three years, it ranked within the top 10 for children's hospitals in the United States. And this was just the atrium.

Upstairs, the pediatric Clinical Teaching Unit (CTU) echoed the same lively design principles. Each individual patient room measured about 300 square feet with enough space for a parent to spend the night. Small magnets that clung to the magnetic wall paint allowed for the easy display of get-well cards

35

and drawings. Patients could even customize the lighting in their rooms. I had just come in from walking in the hospital garden with a patient and his family, whom I was interviewing for a magazine story about a devastating genetic disease. We had covered only a little of the six acres of greenspace surrounding the hospital. The grounds included a garden, walking paths, and nooks where patients could read.

Admittedly, after a 12-hour drive from where I resided in Canada, I was surprised to feel rejuvenated by being in a hospital because what I found was a far cry from the dark and confining cement building where I had been working. I had come to Columbus to interview a pediatric neurologist, but what made the greater impression on me was the benefit of being in that bright, airy space. The children's hospital to which I was assigned was designed in the 1970s and had very few windows or sources of natural light. Even some of the patient rooms had no windows. Harsh fluorescent light dominated. The ceilings were unusually low as well, which added to the sense of confinement. And the noise: monitors, pagers, phones, pagers, and overhead announcements—did I mention those antiquated pagers?

The idea that our physical environment can impact how we heal isn't new. As Paul Barach, a physician-scientist, wrote in a 2008 paper: "One of the greatest ironies of modern medicine is that the very environments created to heal are the cause of countless injuries, illnesses, and death to the vulnerable population they were created to serve." *

*

In the hospital, it's not unusual to see teenagers in "crisis," the term doctors often use to describe mental health breakdowns. Often, they're seen in the emergency room, which can be noisy and, with no semblance of privacy, is

---

* We'll learn more about the placebo effect in a later chapter, but some researchers, such as Jonas Rehn and Kai Schuster out of Germany, suggest that the placebo effect may also be part of why hospital design seems to have a healing effect. In their 2017 study (Rehn and Schuster. Clinic Design as Placebo: using design to promote healing and support treatments. *Behavioral Sciences* 2017), they found that patients self-rated behavior change as more likely if they were provided care in a more modern clinic space. This is termed the "design placebo."

not particularly conducive to emotional safety, an element crucial to trust and, thus, treatment. However, one night while on call in the children's hospital, I attended to a patient on the 6th floor—the psychiatric ward.

A teenager, whom we'll call Mac, had been brought in after taking a combination of pills, including painkillers and antidepressants. Although many people assume the first step in such cases is to "pump the stomach," that isn't usually the approach. Instead, we consult poison control and use specific calculations to determine if the substances are likely to clear naturally through the liver and kidneys. That night, Mac was placed in a private room, but they had already tried to leave against medical advice—referred to as "AMA."

"Hey, Mac," I began, sitting down in the plastic chair across from them. "It sounds like the nurses are worried because you tried to leave. What's going on?"

"Yeah, I think I'm ready to go home," Mac replied, giving me a curious look. Adolescents often navigate a complex space between following rules and testing their boundaries, and Mac seemed no different.

They wore a black T-shirt emblazoned with the name of a local band. Their arms were decorated with pen drawings, some overlaid on older scars that had started to fade. It wasn't unusual for teens struggling with anxiety or depression to turn to self-harm or express themselves through doodles on their skin. Mac's drawings were a collection of abstract shapes, symbols, and animals, suggesting a complicated inner world.

Earlier, while reviewing their chart, I had noted that this wasn't Mac's first encounter with the hospital. They had dealt with bullying and challenges in school, which had left a lasting impact on their self-esteem. Mac had also faced several mental health crises before, with multiple suicide attempts. Each time, they had been admitted and later discharged—only to return to a world filled with social pressures and uncertainty.

"How about we reassess in the morning?" I suggested gently.

"I just feel trapped here!" Mac raised their voice, frustration cracking through. Then, as if embarrassed, they looked down and began picking at their fingernails.

The room around us was stark and utilitarian. A small bed was tucked against the wall, where Mac sat with one leg crossed and the other dangling off the edge. The large window offered a view of the night, though it provided little comfort at this hour. Apart from a small desk and the chair I occupied, the room was bare, designed to eliminate anything that could be used for self-harm. For safety reasons, Mac's personal belongings had been left with the nurse.

"I get that," I said. "I'd probably feel the same way. Let's see if the nurse will let you walk in the hallway for a bit. Then we can try to get some rest."

"Okay!" Mac grinned, a small but welcome shift in the moment. I knew the doors were locked, so the walk wouldn't offer the escape Mac seemed to want, but it might help ease their anxiety for a little while.

I wondered if more light or warmth might have helped—a splash of color, a comforting poster, or a familiar blanket from home. Hospitals are often built with safety in mind, but not necessarily with healing at heart. What Mac seemed to need most, however, was human connection—a reminder that they were not alone. And that, at least, I could offer.

2.

Imagining the space in which a child with cancer may receive chemotherapy treatment, a visual of a children's hospital often comes to mind, perhaps with walls painted in fun colors. There may be some stickers and posters. If the child is lucky, there may be a window allowing some natural light, perhaps a decent view. Usually, there is a TV. How well do these strategies keep the average child engaged, comfortable, and feeling well during their treatment?

Children's Hospital of Orange County, through the work of a company named Reimagine Well, dared to think about the issue differently. At that hospital, children needing chemotherapy are brought into a special infusion room called an Infusionarium™. The Infusionarium contains "immersive healing experiences" directed by patient surveys, enabling them to be virtually transported to any location in the world that they believe would best support their healing. The program began with the outpatient infusion center and then expanded into the inpatient infusion floor. Today, the Infusionarium experience has been added to all smart TVs on the inpatient oncology floor of the hospital.

"They can choose between swimming with dolphins in the Caribbean or going on an African Safari, flying without wings…even heading to outer space," co-founder Roger Holzberg told me. The result is that children report feeling less pain during chemotherapy. They are also calmer and actually *look forward* to the hospital visit, which children usually dread. Clinicians classify this approach as "distraction therapy" (which has been well-researched as a pain and anxiety reduction technique)* and report significant drops in the need for side-effects medications.

Holzberg, 66, is a former Disney Imagineer—a term used for a group of visionaries, designers, and engineers who envision Disney theme parks—and a cancer survivor himself, who saw that hours-long chemotherapy could be made into an "adventure." More recently, Reimagine Well has worked with hospitals in Miami, Wisconsin, and Nebraska to gamify treatments—everything from radiation to brain scans—for children to reduce the need for sedation. In other situations, it does the opposite by inducing calmness and comfort through X-Box interactions, which superimpose the layout of the procedure room and encourage the child to search for Easter eggs as a way to induce relaxation and reduce anxiety before being taken to the procedure room. The most significant decrease in sedation has been noted in children under five.

In 2018, Holzberg began teaching a curriculum called "Experience Design in Healthcare" at the California Institute of the Arts. But before starting, he made one thing clear to the Dean of the Institute: "I would only teach if I could let each class operate as a studio to provide *real* solutions to *real* problems in *real* hospitals," Holzberg recalls. "In other words, teaching for the sake of teaching was nothing I ever aspired to do, but solutioning *real* problems is absolutely a passion of mine." What followed was a formal partnership between Reimagine Well and the CalArts experience-design program.

---

* The foundational Proof of Concept (PoC) study took place at Nebraska Medicine. Using a radiotherapy trainer, with education by a child life specialist, the need for sedation was significantly decreased. Prior to this program almost all children under 10 were fully sedated. Previously all children under 5 years of age received anesthesia, but during the PoC study period, the mean age was lowered to 2.6 years.

Holzberg and his class now have several other partnerships, including with Henry Mayo Hospital in California. The palliative care team at Henry Mayo posed a new challenge, as it is an *adult* hospital environment, and adults are particularly hard to please, no less comfort and reassure. Holzberg's challenge is to bring creativity into palliative care, where—unlike treating children with cancer—there is no anticipation of a positive outcome. "We had a social worker share that, at the end of life, families often come together in a hospital room and just sit and stare at one another, and nobody knows what to say. I thought: There's got to be a better way to approach that part of the 'human journey' and to reduce anxiety and bring people together during that time. So, we developed a program that includes experiential learning and activities that calm families and builds legacies for the patients," Holzberg said. And this includes design elements.

Two of these elements include immersive environments. The first is a Tranquility Room for patients and families. This offers a unique space to be in as their family member is dying. In the other space, Holzberg and his students have created a "Resiliency Room," where the clinical team can spend 20-30 minutes after a tough shift to reset. "The idea is that they could choose between going on a virtual Safari in Africa or doing a mindfulness meditation with a meditation master, or even visiting the World of the Future…just to relax and recharge so they are better able to go back into the work environment," Holzberg told me.

But how did Holzberg come to realize that the environments in hospitals were ripe for disruption without the need to involve brick and mortar? When he was eight years old, attending the World's Fair in Flushing Meadows, New York, he saw the first audio-animatronic figure: "Great Moments with Mr. Lincoln."

"I nearly tore my dad's jacket sleeve off when I asked: 'How did that happen?' And his response stuck with me: 'A man named Walt Disney invented that.' That was the beginning, and since then, I have been drawn to what's known as 'experience design,'" Holzberg told me. He initially worked in special effects and production design, writing IMAX films, and he was later recruited by the Disney Imagineering division to work on the Millennium Celebration and led the creative teams on the "100 Years of Magic" portfolio in all Disney World theme parks. Just after 9/11, when there were fewer travelers, Holzberg pitched the idea of creating a "virtual" Magic Kingdom, which drew five-plus-million children around the U.S. to create their own personalized adventure experiences. That's when the seed of combining the virtual and the dimensional—side by side—was planted.

Another unexpected moment led Holzberg to see healthcare—and healing—differently. In 2004, he noticed he was gaining weight and feeling less energetic in the afternoons. His doctor took an MRI of his neck: it was thyroid cancer. This shifted his perspective again.

"You see a physician across from you speaking a language you don't understand. I call it the 'terror moment,' when you're in shock, and you don't make the most rational decisions since you are operating out of fear…you're staring at your own mortality," Holzberg told me. Undergoing radiation treatment, he realized his experience in the hospital was exactly the opposite of what it was like at Disney. "The walls in the hospital hadn't been painted since the 1980s, and this was the most *un*-healing experience I could imagine. I came from a place where the *architecture of reassurance* is what we practiced in Disney parks worldwide. It didn't even smell right! It hit me like a ton of bricks that the patient experience, even though I didn't know that term yet, was something to be worked on."

The experience inspired him to apply his creative talents to cancer as the first consulting Creative Director for the National Cancer Institute (NCI) before co-founding Reimagine Well as a way to combine the best of what he'd learned during his fifteen years at Disney with the gaps he had experienced in healthcare design.

"When John Hench, the lead architectural designer of Disneyland, coined the phrase the 'architecture of reassurance,' he did it for a reason. Disney parks are designed to be a safe place for families to play. At Reimagine Well, we try to create an 'architecture of *healing*,' creating a safe and special place for patients and families to heal. My years at Disney informed what I did to create an emotionally engaging space for people to play. I realized the same tools could be used for patients and families to experience the patient journey," Holzberg said.

Whether through efforts at Nationwide Children's Hospital, the lack of adaptation at my own hospital, or Holzberg's initiatives for adults, it's clear that our physical environments greatly impact how ill we feel and can be designed to promote healing. As I left the Columbus hospital, I could only imagine the difference the environment here in Columbus made for the young patients trying to heal in such a positive space—and the difference it made for the healers themselves. Could this environmental tone and impact explain some of what I had experienced myself? To better understand, I needed to dive deeper into what the science suggests about whether our physical environments can meaningfully improve how we heal.

3.

Springtime in Stockholm, Sweden, is windy. Still, the sun beats down, and since Sweden touts itself as the largest archipelago in the world, sailboats and yachts crisscross in every body of water. Every building seems to incorporate some form of greenspace—a garden or small park, for instance. The city is organized on a grid, making it easy to explore on foot. As you might expect in a country whose capital is so thoughtfully designed for living well, Sweden has one of the best healthcare systems in the world. And this is where American hospital architect Roger Ulrich, probably the most influential living person in hospital design, spends half of his time.

As a practice that was distinct from other forms of architecture, hospital design gained attention in the early 1980s. But the idea that surrounding patients with nature as well as art and music to restore harmony and healing when other treatments weren't available dates back as far as ancient Greece, with the inclusion of greenery or, more commonly, bringing in musicians to play for ill aristocrats.

In modern times, the movement to consider how the design of our physical spaces impacts our health arguably started with the 19th-century nurse Florence Nightingale. In 1860, she wrote that the benefits of placing patients in rooms with a window and sunlight were "quite perceptible in promoting recovery." Nightingale was among the first to attribute differences in mortality to hospital design. Today, the concept of using design elements specifically to promote health is dubbed "salutogenic architecture" (a term popularized in the mid-1990s), which runs against the chaos of ill health. A sense of meaning and purpose in the space is also intended to prevent illness.

In the 1970s, Ulrich examined this idea head-on. He analyzed records of 46 patients in a suburban Pennsylvania hospital who had a window in their hospital recovery room after having their gallbladder surgically removed. Half of the patients had a view of trees. The other half had a view of a brick wall. Ulrich measured how long each group stayed in hospital. In a paper published in *Science* in April 1984, aptly entitled "View Through a Window May Influence Recovery from Surgery," Ulrich described his surprising findings. Patients with a tree view had a statistically significantly lower length of stay, just under eight days, in contrast to the average of nine days in hospital for those who spent their recoveries looking at a wall. But that wasn't all he found. Those with a tree view needed fewer painkillers and had lower rates of post-surgical complications. In other words, Ulrich's study was one of the first to suggest that, yes, hospital design can indeed play a direct role in healing.

After that study, Ulrich created a Theory of Supportive Design, contributed to a new movement in healthcare architecture called "Evidence-Based Design," and has led or partnered on hundreds of studies looking at the effect of design on health. He has worked as a consultant for various hospitals as well, such as the Lurie Children's Hospital in Chicago, which has some elements that are similar to Nationwide, as well as Stanford's new Lucille Packard Children's Hospital.

Ulrich is over six feet tall, with black-streaked grey hair and hooded eyes. He became energetic in discussing his work with me. "It's a no-brainer that design is important for health. We can look at the Massachusetts General Hospital tragedy in the early 1990s for a clue," Ulrich told me.

He was referring to a devastating outbreak at Massachusetts General Hospital in the early 1990s of *Aspergillus*, a type of fungus that spread when a patient with the disease received the same air as a patient without the disease. According to a commissioned but unpublished report Ulrich contributed to, several in-hospital deaths secondary to this outbreak followed. Since then, that hospital and many others have re-established new design codes, specifically underscoring the importance of air quality and the need to have separate ventilation systems in each room. Now, in the United States, the Centers for Disease Prevention and Control have strict regulations for hospital ventilation systems, specifically that air should be refreshed in the patient's room at least 12 times an hour.

I reflected on the time I spent working in the academic healthcare setting. It wasn't unusual for multiple patients to share a room, even though research suggests that private rooms can better support recovery and well-being. This design choice, however, was part of a larger balancing act—constraints in funding and space often lead to trade-offs that prioritize capacity over individual comfort. It's a reality faced by many healthcare facilities striving to meet growing patient needs with limited resources. Arguably, it would be better to have two patients in a room as opposed to one patient in a room and another stuck in the emergency room or not admitted at all. But it's not just funding and space limitations that hamper great design for healing; it's the inability to evolve in response to changing expectations from patients as well as new evidence from health design research. For Mac, it potentially impacted their ability to heal through the inability to create an environment conducive to healing.

Ulrich grew up as a curious boy on a farm in rural Michigan. Nature was front and center, and he believes it influenced his approach to designing for health. I asked if, hypothetically, we could create a hospital right now, what might be the key elements to ensure it was supportive of healing? For him, three answers came easily: natural light, allowing for social support through flexible visitation policies, and something he had plenty of growing up in the country: quiet.

*

When most people think of Dyson, they think of the famous vacuum cleaner brand. Well, Sir James Dyson also funded a unique hospital called the Dyson Centre for Neonatal Care, located in Bath, England, which incorporates light-colored wood and greenery, a pebbled garden, and a serious investment in soundproof materials. The result is a facility said to be eight decibels quieter than the neonatal intensive care unit (NICU) it replaced. Ulrich penned an essay in the *Lancet* in 2006 about evidence-based healthcare architecture, in which he highlighted the damage done by noisy healthcare environments:

> Noise has been associated with sleep loss and fragmentation, high blood pressure and heart rates, worse rates of recovery from myocardial infarction, and decreased oxygen saturation in infants in neonatal intensive care. For staff, noise is a stressful latent environmental condition that increases fatigue and job strain, and in some clinical situations heightens risk of error. Health-care building projects should therefore accord high priority to creating much quieter environments.

Indeed, noise can be destructive, and that's why many hospitals are seeking to reduce it. In many inpatient NICUs, electronic "ears" that light up like traffic lights identify the current noise level. Red means excessively noisy. Green means quiet. Orange means "warning" on the way to red. Noise results in hyperarousal, where the body takes on a fight or flight state, with heart rate and blood pressure rising. This affects how well patients heal. The infants admitted to the NICU center in Bath, for instance, slept longer than in other nurseries. The same design team in Bath is now creating a cancer center focused on similar design principles.

Thoughtful design also makes an impact on how the hospital staff functions. Design principles, specifically layout and flow or accessibility, can result in improved teamwork and communication. I expanded upon this concept in an article for *The New York Times* on "Design Thinking," which laid out how design is used to improve challenges and the patient experience in hospitals. In that article, I discussed all the forms design thinking can take—from architecture to innovation. Indeed, Dyson was onto something, but it's unclear if these ideas have been translated into practical steps in hospitals.

*

If you need a rundown on how evidence-based design works in practice, Terry Peters is the person you want by your side. A young architect based at Ryerson University in Toronto with expertise in health design, she is the ideal person with whom to explore the insides of Bridgepoint Active Health Center, a facility recently built according to the evidence-based design principles pioneered by Ulrich. With Peters as an interpretive guide, I felt I could get a little deeper into the innovative concepts at work in the building.

As we toured Bridgepoint one afternoon, Peters pointed to all of the design elements that were thoughtfully chosen to assist in healing. For instance, 90% of patient spaces get at least three hours of daylight each day, regardless of the time of year. The center, aimed at caring for elderly patients, is focused primarily on rehabilitation. Not surprisingly, then, one of Bridgepoint's key objectives is to get patients up and moving, and its rehabilitation pool looks over a neighboring park, enticing patients to get in their aquatic reps if only to enjoy the verdant view.

Views are important all over this facility. Each patient room has both a horizontal and vertical window; as patients recover and move from being supine on a bed to standing up and walking again, there is a different vantage point to be enjoyed. As well, many of the windows offer an alcove for a patient to step into so they feel closer to the outside. There are also many of what Peters calls "meaningful views"—views that include items of interest in the foreground, middle ground, and distance. In addition, the walls of Bridgepoint are accented with calming colors: light green to represent the park on one end and light blue to represent the end of the hospital that looks toward a lake. Natural light flows throughout, and walls and ceilings are made from wood and cork materials. Furniture is ergonomic, and colors such as sage green and sky blue help lend a calm, almost spa-like sense to the place.

Bridgepoint also has special rooms for light therapy for delirium, an assessment kitchen to ensure patients are able to use the oven and fridge after their "new normal," and even a walking labyrinth that helps facilitate mindful walks. Having come from a very stressful environment, I could sense the calm among the healthcare workers, from the rehabilitation specialists to the nurses and the doctors. Something was clearly going right here. The research suggests that patients at Bridgepoint *believe* they recover faster, and even when symptoms of depression and well-being didn't change, patients' *perceptions* of their mental health improved.

Bridgepoint's innovations are being echoed by similar initiatives around the world. For instance, the Evington Centre dementia care ward, part of the Leicestershire NHS Trust in England, has avoided using shiny floors because they appear wet and could cause agitation or anxiety in their patients. As well, bathrooms are painted in contrasting colors instead of the more usual all-white to avoid confusion around distinguishing a toilet from a nearby wall. As a result, patients at Evington require less psychotropic medication.

The Scandinavian "Outdoor Care Retreat," located in Oslo, Norway, has elements such as skylights for sunlight to flow into it and oak walls that make the place smell a bit like a sauna. The cabins are typically booked by patients from the nearby hospital, and the entire retreat is integrated within Oslo University's main hospital. Each cabin has a main room for sleeping and resting, another for "conversation and treatment," and a bathroom. Colorful pillows are meant for lying on the floor while you peer up through a large skylight that exposes the tree canopy outside.

More recently, under the direction of Canadian architect Moshe Safdie, a new hospital in Cartagena, Colombia, aims to bring the "outside in" through the thoughtful use of light, space, materials, and color—effectively creating a healing space that resembles a spa or wellness organization as opposed to a traditional hospital.

But these hospitals and healing centers require significant financial investment to build healing-friendly spaces. This is where a new organization called the International Well Building Institute™ comes in. In 2014, they created the WELL Building Standard™ to rate buildings based on their ability to facilitate health and wellness. In 2019, the institute was featured by *Fast*

Company as one of the most innovative wellness companies for that year. The standards were developed through a peer-review process, and now buildings can apply to be certified as "WELL" based on a set of strict criteria. Peters is herself now credentialed as a "WELL" building assessor.

For the many hospitals that do not have the luxury of affording drastic changes to improve their physical environments, a garden is one relatively inexpensive way to include some of the innovations Ulrich has been proposing. The Prouty Garden at the Children's Hospital in Boston is a great example, with walkways and a modest fountain. A YouTube video from 2011 featured a young heart transplant patient named Aidan Schwalbe who appears delighted by the garden; the impact it had on his mental well-being (and possibly his physical health after his transplant) was clear, at least for that moment. And where limited space won't allow gardens, even small potted plants have benefitted patients' well-being. In New York City, NYU Langone Medical Center has started bringing plants into the hospital for long-term care patients. Only blocks away, horticultural therapy at the Rusk Rehabilitation Center has patients tend mini-gardens and learn about plants—from flower arranging to planting. These initiatives reinforce findings from a 2019 study led by Ulrich, which discovered that creating a garden inside the hospital can help families of patients in the ICU deal with stress.*

Whether it was the Nationwide Children's Hospital, Bridgepoint, Dyson, the Oslo retreat hospital, or Safdie's vision for a new sort of hospital entirely, one thing was clear: the physical design of hospitals matters in terms of how well we heal. But the mention of gardens specifically intrigued me: if placing a dose of nature inside the hospital helps, is there a healing effect to being in nature itself?

---

* Scales, like the Present Functioning Visual Analogy Sales (PFVAS), can be used to assess the impact of such gardens: before and after each visit for instance researchers can measure the improvement in the "sadness" scale among those visiting the garden.

4.

On a damp Saturday morning, I drove to the small town of Carp, Ontario. I parked at what looked to be the entrance to a forest surrounded by a large lake. Most of the people I saw around me were wearing long sleeves and hats with mosquito netting. Once I got out of the car, it became clear why the other attendees of the Carp Ridge EcoWellness resort were dressed this way. The mosquitoes were horrible.

I'd come to Carp to partake in the increasingly popular practice of forest therapy, which originates in the Japanese tradition "Shinrin Yoku" (literally "forest bathing"). There are over 500 forest guides across North America trained according to standards set by the Association of Nature and Forest Therapy (ANFT), based in the United States.

Over the past two decades, there's been a renewed interest in how nature influences our well-being: everything from Richard Louv's books—*The Nature Principle* and *Last Child in the Woods*— to Florence Williams' *The Nature Fix*, which includes an entire section on forest bathing. One doctor at UCSF Benioff Children's Hospital in Oakland, Dr. Nooshin Razani, a pediatric infectious disease expert and director of the Center for Nature and Health, has gone so far as to offer "park prescriptions" as part of a national movement to bring a piece of nature to children—for healing as well as prevention. Her program, linked to the East Bay Park District, intends to improve accessibility to nature for children from low-income areas. One Saturday a month, she leads a group of up to 50 people through a forest on the outskirts of Oakland. These parks are lush, typically housing huge redwood trees and lakes. The groups consist of one of her patients (aged between a few months and 18 years) and at least one family member, though often several will join. Even her physician colleagues, from family doctors to surgeons, have attended. The pediatrics residency program at UCSF Benioff Children's Hospital in Oakland has recently expanded to offer inhabitants from the surrounding neighborhood a chance to experience Razani's initiative.

"It's a low-cost activity, and I consider it a 'community-based self-healing tool' that's available to all of us…sometimes the doctors need it just as much as the patients," Razani told me.

But can nature, by itself, heal?

In Carp, I was to spend the next few hours in the care of one of those guides, a middle-aged woman named Kiki.

Once the day's attendees had gathered, facilitators split us into eight groups. Kiki led my group of six into the woods and sat us down next to an oak tree. We formed a small circle beside it, and she asked us to share memories of childhood moments spent in nature that still fill us with joy. I described walking with my mother to collect acorns and chestnuts, reminded by the presence of seeds scattered across the forest floor around me now. Others were reminded of walks taken in the wild when they were Boy Scouts or Girl Guides.

"What do you hear, smell, see?" Kiki asked, encouraging us to use all five senses to become deeply immersed in the experience. We were deep in a forest, surrounded by old-growth trees. A few squirrels scurried by, and the forest floor was covered in leaves and acorns. I took in the scent of pine and the fresh rain-soaked grass. Three birds—chickadees if I had to guess—chirped on a tree branch nearby, with others—crows and geese—in the distance. An older lady told the group that she was undergoing a difficult and stressful period in her life and that being amongst the trees felt "healing," which made me wonder if her feelings were supported by science.

As we got up for our walk, some of the other group members commented on the sounds of the forest, such as insects, birds, and the rustling of leaves, that we became more attuned to with silence. The mosquitoes had become quite vicious, and I began to find it hard to "be present" while warding them off. Somehow, they had seemed immune to the DEET I had slathered myself with.

Towards the end of our slow stroll, which took almost two hours, Kiki led us to the side of the lake to partake in a tea ceremony. Our miniature ceramic mugs were filled with hot tea where white pine needles had been steeped. I left feeling relaxed and more at peace, with a more centered mind, albeit with at least two dozen mosquito bites.

*

In 2017, I traveled to Japan to meet with Dr. Hirotaka Ochiai, a surgeon based at Tokyo Medical Center, and her husband, Toshiya Ochiai, who was at the time the CEO of the Japan-based International Society of Nature and Forest Medicine. They offer forest therapy to ambulatory patients in one of Tokyo's largest hospitals. Dr. Ochiai is trained in forest therapy, and she currently conducts most of her sessions (with volunteer participants, not patients) within a forest in Nagano, about three hours from Tokyo, with the help of a local guide. The Ochiais are not alone as physicians embracing this therapeutic practice. According to the Association of Nature and Forest Therapy in the U.S., physicians from top institutions across the U.S. and Canada have expressed interest in training as therapists.

"The hypersonic natural world can be soothing, and things are always moving even while we are still…it can be very calming," Ochiai told me.

Research—mostly conducted in Japan and Korea—shows that time in nature, specifically in lush forests, can decrease stress and blood pressure, lower cortisol, and improve heart-rate variability (the variation of time between each heartbeat, which may reflect high stress when variability isn't constant) while boosting one's mood. A meta-analysis in 2010, which was focused on exercising in nature, found improvements to self-esteem, particularly in younger participants, and that overall effects on mood were heightened when there was water nearby; even a small bubbling stream had an impact.

Theories abound as to why time spent in forests can provide health benefits. Some have suggested that the chemicals emitted from trees (phytoncides) have a physiological effect on our stress levels, while others suggest the sounds (birds chirping, rustling leaves) can lend us a sense of calm, something music streaming companies like Spotify have harnessed. Yet the evidence is, admittedly, scant to support these theories, and some research points to very limited effects.

For instance, a cross-sectional study from Korea found no change in blood pressure with forest bathing, and a systematic review from 2010 found that while there may be benefits to mood and energy, the effects on attention, blood pressure, and cortisol may not be statistically significant. A 2017 systematic review found that while forest therapy is promising for depression, the studies involved lacked robust methodology. Evidence *does* suggest that being in nature can generally be helpful to the brain. Richard Louv's term "nature deficit disorder," which more formally is termed "Attention Restoration Theory," refers to how nature can restore executive function in the brain in the same areas that may be affected by mindfulness meditation.

Ultimately, to me, forest bathing seemed like a reasonable approach to combine mindfulness and exposure to nature in a way that had the potential to heal from both physical and emotional wounds. Whether the long-term impact was sustainable is unclear, but for now, it was a method that helped me pause and regain my strength so that I could decide what I needed next for my healing.

Japanese forests, as well as cities, are home to a tree that perhaps best embodies healing: the Gingko. Indeed, the Gingko has bounced back from its share of troubles, most alarmingly, the bombing of Hiroshima. On August 6, 1945, the atomic bomb was dropped on Hiroshima, causing massive destruction and loss of life. Despite the devastation, several Ginkgo Biloba trees near the blast's epicenter survived. After the Hiroshima bombing, which scorched people, buildings, and trees, thousands of Gingkos mysteriously survived by regenerating from the inside. While the bark was burnt, the inside was not. These trees sprouted new leaves within a few months, demonstrating an extraordinary ability to endure and regenerate. It's known for its exceptional durability and longevity. Indeed, Ginkgo trees have a strong regenerative capacity. Even when damaged, they can regrow from their roots or trunk. It is one of the oldest tree species on Earth, dating back over 200 million years, earning it the nickname "living fossil."

In Peter Crane's 2015 book, *Gingko, The Tree That Time Forgot*, he underscores that the species almost went extinct at the end of the last ice age but eventually made its way to Japan in the 13th century, where it flourished. As Crane explains to Emma Butel in a 2018 interview for *Inverse* magazine: "Somewhere underneath all of the destruction, a tiny cylinder of living cells had to have survived…the extreme organization of its cell tissues created a compartment that was immune to destruction."

Gingko blooms in the spring, reminding us of their survival. As such, Gingko, for me, became a metaphor for healing from within—of healing from the most profound of devastations. As Oliver Sacks wrote in *The New Yorker* in 2014, not long before his death, each Gingko tree also miraculously sheds all of its leaves almost on the same day. There's clearly a special consciousness that resides in the Gingko. Soon, I'd understand even more about how to embody this symbol of healing.

5.

The report from Dr. Morgan, the psychologist I had consulted, arrived quickly, just as she had promised. I read it carefully, taking in her observations. She had been right—particularly about the areas where I struggled with memory and concentration. My cognitive function, she noted, resembled patterns sometimes seen in individuals experiencing significant mental strain. Her conclusion was that, given my strong academic performance in medical school and other clinical experiences, the challenges I was facing were likely a reflection of stress that had gone unnoticed and unaddressed for longer than I had realized.

The alternative explanation for these test results was something more sinister: my brain could be degenerating. As I was a female in my late 20s, presenting with low mood as well, she worried these results could signal multiple sclerosis (MS), a disease in which lesions pop up in the brain as an autoimmune response with no known cause. Over time, MS can attack the white matter in the brain and spinal cord, debilitating someone physically to the point where they'd eventually need a wheelchair. She recommended I get an MRI of my brain.

I made my way to Princess Margaret Hospital in Toronto two months after Dr. Morgan's report had recommended the MRI. This scan could change everything. A few years earlier, a male colleague in the same program I was enrolled in had died because of a brain tumor. He was well-liked and respected, and the staff still talked about him. Maybe this is how it ends for me, I thought, as I dressed in a blue gown that would allow the enormous machine to read my insides like an open book. Maybe all this craziness was just a weird detour into getting an MRI that could save my life. So, with that possibility in mind, I got in and let the banging and clicking in the machine happen. My heart began to beat faster. Could something be awry? Did the technician see something while I was in the scanner? Might she have called in a colleague?

When it was over, I stepped out of the scanner and put my shoes on. As I was leaving, I tried to gather from the technician's face if she had seen a huge abnormal blob or not. She was keeping too neutral a bearing for me to tell. "Did you see anything?" I asked, then added, "I'm a doctor, so I'm just curious," hoping it would convince her to budge. She paused, then said, "Legally, I can't share anything. I'm sorry." Of course, I knew that but had momentarily forgotten I was the patient, not the doctor.

It would become a pattern: hurry up and wait. I dwelled on the many scans I had seen while on duty—from huge masses to shrunken white matter tissue due to infection. It ran the gamut. Then, I blocked it out. This wasn't helping. I needed to figure out my next step.

A few weeks later, my family doctor called. The MRI results were in—all clear. No sign of multiple sclerosis or another neurodegenerative disorder. I was back to square one. What the hell was happening?

I emailed Dr. Tepper with an update but got a bounce-back: the hospital wellness officer had left her position.

6.

Baltimore is dubbed "Charm City," almost ironically. Certainly, when I lived there during my master's training at Johns Hopkins University, I found pockets of what we might typically label as charming—around the harbor, for instance, which had cobblestone streets. Yet it was tough to see that the area around the Public Health School, where I was studying, had become gentrified with wealthy professors and government workers commuting to D.C.

My apartment in Baltimore was a far cry from the forest in Japan. It was a building in the Mount Vernon area, which was greener than most parts of the city. It used to house the Standard Oil Company. But there were consequences to these troubled areas as well. At least twice, I was followed, and once, a driver ordered me into his car (I didn't get in). Other times, young children would be approached by local police and questioned for playing near public property. The bizarre city planning made it difficult to walk anywhere, but one day, I thought it would be a good idea to try.

It was only a 20-minute walk from my apartment to school. I was attending the prestigious Johns Hopkins Bloomberg School of Public Health in the Global Disease Epidemiology and Control Master's Program. I excelled in my coursework and won prizes and grants. Things were just flowing. So, I began my walk from The Standard to North Wolfe Street under bridges and along the busy streets. As I neared the school, I passed by a particularly run-down neighborhood. Even though it was a school day, young Black children were playing in the yards of their low-income housing. The sidewalk was littered with broken beer bottles, yet chubby toddlers walked about barefoot. My chest tightened with a sense of guilt.

Many of the houses were boarded up, which gave an air of temporariness. A classmate explained that they were boarded up to prevent "crack addicts from squatting" or gang members from gathering. I made my way to the entrance of Hopkins and looked a few blocks ahead, where the previous week, my classmates and I had explored a local food hangout. It ended up being a small food court that served fried chicken, grits, cheap cheeseburgers, and greasy pizza. It was heart disease and diabetes embodied, with the only edible alternative offerings being bags of chips and soda at the local corner store. In other words, the area was both a "food swamp," the term used for areas with copious fast-food options and convenience stores, and a "food desert," the term used for an area with little to no access to nutritious food.

Another time, when tutoring local elementary schoolers in math, I asked if they had their textbooks. "No," they said. I asked why, expecting maybe they'd forgotten them. "Our teacher thinks we'll steal them," one girl had said. The irony of studying the social determinants of health in that multimillion-dollar building with state-of-the-art facilities, which sat side-by-side with one of the poorest and most disenfranchised neighborhoods in the country, was never lost on me. The evidence suggests neighborhoods, like poorly designed hospitals, can indeed make you sick. But can they also help you heal?

A 2018 article published in *Lancet Planetary Health* reported on a cross-sectional study of 122,993 participants with major depressive disorder in the United Kingdom. The researchers described the protective effect of residential greenness on depression, which was even greater among women, those under

60, and residents in poorer neighborhoods. The fact that Baltimore is not a walkable city may make residents more prone to chronic disease. The most famous study to evaluate social and physical environments in neighborhoods was perhaps the Jackson Heart Study led by Samson Gebreab. The researchers analyzed data from more than 3,500 non-diabetic patients and found that over 14% had a diagnosis of Type 2 diabetes after a follow-up period of seven years. They then compared where these participants lived versus those who had not received a diagnosis of diabetes. It seems that neighborhoods with a lower density of "unfavorable" food shops (like convenience stores) have a significantly lower incidence of diabetes. Notably, in this study, social cohesion, something we discuss in the next chapter, also decreased the risk.

On the other hand, the 2015 Boston Area Community Health (BACH) Survey led by Rebecca Piccolo of the New England Research Institute, which looked at the increased risk of Type 2 diabetes among African-American and Hispanic study participants, found that once the factors of age, race, and gender were controlled for, the neighborhood effects were actually small. However, the lack of neighborhood safety—which could affect walkability and physical activity—may have contributed to an increased risk of diabetes. As such, the authors suggested that focusing on strengthening community ties (social cohesion) and attracting healthful food stores (addressing food deserts and food swamps) would be key prevention mechanisms.

Years later, while working in the *ABC News* Medical Unit in New York City, I was given one of my toughest assignments yet: to make some sense of the crisis involving migrant children on the Mexico-U.S. border who were being forcibly separated from their parents. A photo that captured a tragedy had sparked public and media interest: a 2-year-old Honduran girl named Yanela Denise Valera, wearing a bright pink long-sleeved shirt, jean shorts, and magenta shoes, stood crying and terrified as her mother, Sandra Sanchez, was arrested after crossing the Rio Grande in a raft. To make it worse, the American border patrol guard had arrested the mother while she was breastfeeding her child. The photo was captured on June 11, 2018 by Pulitzer Prize-winner John Moore. Not only was it a clear manifestation of an immense time of injustice, but it exemplified how a dangerous physical environment, especially leaving one for another, can affect health and well-being.

So, when we think about youth and the role of neighborhoods (or the social environment—including country of birth—more generally), we cannot overlook the adverse childhood experiences (ACEs). While at *ABC News*, I interviewed the director of Harvard's Center on the Developing Child, Dr. Jack Shonkoff, about ACEs, specifically the toxic stress faced in such dire circumstances. Sometimes, despite the best evidence and advocacy, escaping one environment for another for the sake of one's well-being is an incredibly tall task, and this is most clearly seen in our neighborhoods.

"Early experiences [such as forcible separation] get into our bodies and affect brain, immune, cardiovascular, and metabolic systems. It has a multi-system effect, from disrupting brain architecture, which impacts learning and emotional development, to affecting how well our immune systems fight infections," Shonkoff told me. He referred to it partly in the context of migrant children—but among non-migrants factors like exposure to gun violence, living in a single-parent home, constant threat of violence, financial and food insecurity, and even school-related stress (like the child who said she couldn't bring home textbooks) all have an impact.

The landmark 1998 ACE study in the *American Journal of Preventative Medicine* by Felitti and colleagues used a questionnaire that had been mailed to over 13,000 adults to look at seven categories of ACEs: psychological, physical, or sexual abuse; violence against the mother; living with substance abuse in the home; mental or suicidal issues in the home; and imprisonment. Over 50% of those who responded had experiences in at least one category, and 25% had experiences in more than one. Also, there was a graded relationship among those with experiences in more than four categories: they had a four-to-twelve-fold increase in health risks. ACEs affect children throughout childhood but also extend into adulthood and can have an immense impact on their mental as well as physical well-being.

Other research has found that ACEs increase the risk of violence, substance use, and mental illness. ACEs also affect healing. Studies have reported associations with telomere (the protein caps on the end of chromosomes that shorten with age, stress, smoking, and so on), length, and harder-to-heal conditions, such as trauma, among those children with ACEs compared to those who have no history of them. As such, making neighborhoods more livable and conducive to health and healing must also address these stressors that affect children early in life.

But here's the good news: fixing the built environment of neighborhoods can improve healing. We know that removing fast-food access and increasing park space may have a direct impact on insulin resistance and Type 2 diabetes. A Cleveland intervention called "Healthy Eating & Active Living" (HEAL), which used neighborhood-based lifestyle interventions, including improving food affordability and access through neighborhood gardens, community kitchens, and free exercise classes, engaged the community to improve their social and physical environment. A similar Baltimore-based program, the "B'More Healthy Communities for Kids" (BHCK), is a multi-level intervention program (meaning several initiatives introduced at once), aimed at low-income African-American youth aged 10-14 and their families. It created changes at a systems level (not just aimed at the individual) through building partnerships with policymakers, restaurants, and corner stores. I would have loved to have seen these changes happen in Baltimore when I lived there, but it's heartening that changes are underway.

7.

The cold linoleum smells of sour industrial cleaner. It's a familiar odor in the hospital, one that used to sting my nostrils when a patient room was freshly mopped. I make my way into the basement room, towards my locker. It had been painted a salmon color and is chipped. I hadn't noticed that before my impending separation from this place; the immediacy of escape brings everything into full focus.

I fumbled with the combination lock. It rarely opened on the first try, requiring more precision than seemed reasonable for something so analog. The door creaked open, and my nylon coat hung limply inside. My brown Birkenstocks were neatly tucked to the left, a rare occurrence since I had arrived early that morning. As I reached for my things, I noticed tiny blue plastic beads scattered across the bottom of the locker. I had almost forgotten—weeks earlier, the handmade lanyard I bought from a gift shop at a Toronto hospital had broken. The cashier had told me the lanyards were crafted by local artisans as a small way to support healthcare workers. It had felt meaningful at the time, but now, in this setting, it felt like a relic from a different chapter.

When the lanyard snapped, I had hurriedly collected the beads, dropping them into the locker without much thought. I had considered replacing it with a new lanyard bearing the logo of the hospital where I now worked, but I chose not to. I didn't feel connected to that place, and I certainly didn't want to carry a reminder of the difficult experiences I had encountered there.

Lisa, a trusted mentor, stood quietly beside me as I gathered my things. Though the weather outside was warm, I put on my jacket—I needed the extra pockets for the bags and books I carried. As I closed the locker door, a glimmer caught my eye. Nestled among the remaining beads was a small silver charm, a piece of the broken lanyard I hadn't noticed before. It read, "Follow your dreams."

"How fitting," Lisa said with a smile as she glanced at the charm in my hand. For a brief moment, I felt reassured, as if all the challenges I had faced were part of a larger story—one that I couldn't fully understand just yet. It wasn't a failure; it was a choice to step away from an environment that no longer felt right. As we walked out, I passed a couple of colleagues who greeted me warmly, unaware of the significance of the moment. To them, it was just another day. But for me, it was a quiet, symbolic ending—a reminder that while one person's turning point might go unnoticed by others, it can still mark the beginning of something new.

8.

Though I was not yet a published writer, I had read with hope Oliver Sacks' posthumous essay in *The New York Times* titled "The Healing Power of Gardens," an excerpt from his last published book of essays, *Everything in its Place*. The opening paragraph stuck out to me:

As a writer, I find gardens essential to the creative process; as a physician, I take my patients to gardens whenever possible. All of us have had the experience of wandering through a lush garden or a timeless desert, walking by a river or an ocean, or climbing a mountain and finding ourselves simultaneously calmed and reinvigorated, engaged in mind, refreshed in body and spirit. The importance of these physiological states on individual and community health is fundamental and wide-ranging.

Years later, Sacks' editor, Peter, at *The New York Times* would be one of mine as well. But at that moment, I only knew that the physical environment at my old hospital likely contributed in a small way to my poor well-being and, perhaps, to burnout among the individuals who chose to bully others over whom they may hold power. Roger Holzberg helped show me that the physical environment impacts how healthcare professionals are able to do their best work and also how patients are able to experience their healing. The Infusionarium™ especially serves to normalize unpleasant and exhausting experiences like chemotherapy by allowing for a minor emotional and mental escape. It's a way to augment one's imagination, and I could begin to do that in my own mind by re-imagining what a healthier future path might be like, to see the light at the end of this twisted tunnel. Roger Ulrich provided the pioneering foundation for how design can heal, and Terri Peters was handed that baton as one of this generation's trailblazing architects.

Mac, as a patient, embodied a sense of confinement that felt all too familiar. Though our circumstances were different, we were both navigating environments that felt restrictive—each of us in search of some sense of relief. I offered Mac a small moment of respite, knowing that I too would need to find ways to care for myself. In that moment, I realized that while I couldn't control every situation, I did have some agency over where and how I spent my time. Whether through walks in a quiet forest or simply being more intentional in shaping my daily surroundings, I could choose environments that fostered healing and renewal.

And I embraced the lesson learned from the almighty Gingko: as much as I felt that I was being destroyed from the outside, I would always have the life force inside me. It would give me purpose and direction, as well as the motivation to keep moving forward even when the situation felt impossible. One thing became painfully clear above all—my surroundings were the major factor behind my poor health, and it went beyond just the brick-and-mortar. Our social bonds create a safety net for healing, a buffer even during difficult times. That connection, at a time when a former surgeon-general pointed to the "loneliness epidemic," is crucial. I had no idea that the relationships we foster can actually help both our minds and bodies heal, and I began to learn that while visiting a planned community just outside of Atlanta, Georgia, and a remote village on a Japanese island.

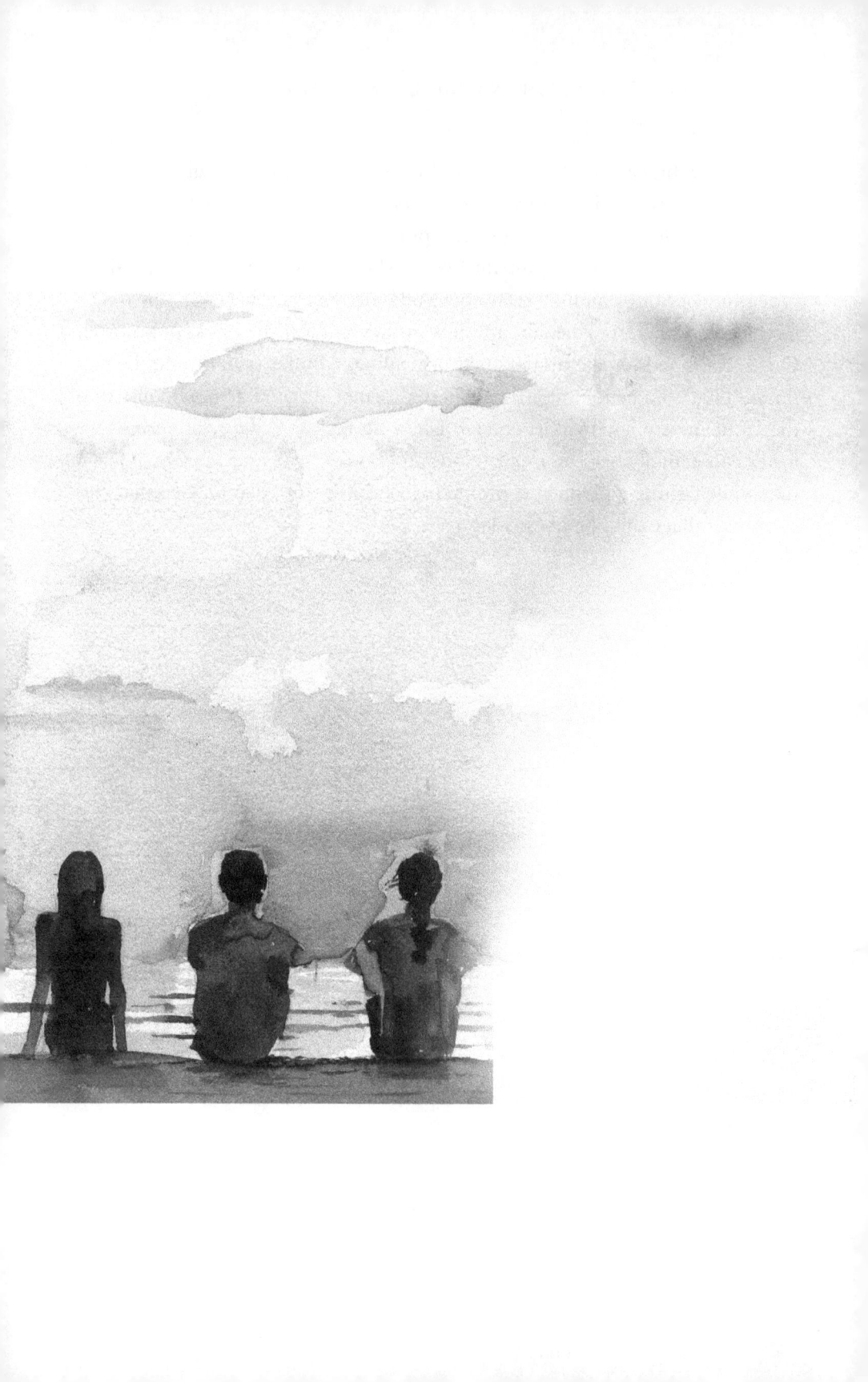

CHAPTER FOUR

Network Effects

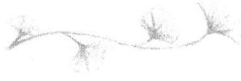

"When a flower doesn't bloom, you fix the environment in which the flower grows, not the flower."

— Alexander den Heijer

1.

Known as the "longevity village," Ogimi sits on the northwestern coast of Okinawa Island in Japan. There are very few cars; instead, bubbling brooks abound. The region is bordered by lush, subtropical forest and a stretch of sandy beach that runs along the main highway. Inland presents a mix of dirt roads, rice fields, small farms, and traditional homes called "minka." Wooden patios encircle these homes, which have sliding doors with sheer paneling and fragrant tatami flooring. There are very few restaurants and only one major market. Ogimi earned its "longevity" title because, historically, it has lodged the most centenarians per square mile anywhere on Earth. Why would that be? It seems the outstandingly long, healthy life-span of its residents is in part due to the town's regularly scheduled social interactions via "moais" (pronounced as "mo-eyes"). This local term refers to its tight-knit community village networks. I was invited to sit in on a gathering of such a network arranged by the Japanese National Council of Social Welfare, where I met 90-year-old Fumi Teruya.

Teruya was a slight woman, perhaps 4 foot 8 and 90 pounds, with fine features and weathered tanned skin. Her thinning dove-grey hair was cut short. Her dentures were immaculate, as was her style of dressing. She was wearing a yellow cardigan with three buttons fastened atop a blouse with a scalloped collar, finishing her outfit with dark green slacks and black shoes that would be more suitable for an office than for a community gathering. We first met after she played a Japanese game similar to croquet called "gateball" at a local park (where groups would meet several times a week to play and socialize, much like a recreational softball league would in North America), and later at the Taiho Community Center, where centenarians meet once a week for planned activities and for checkups of vital signs like their blood pressure.

I joined for one round of a seated bowling-like activity before having a longer chat with Teruya. She explained that every morning she swept the deck of her home, which allowed her to get daily exercise and rely on a routine. But it also allowed her to catch up with village neighbors, who would stop to chat when they saw Teruya on her deck during their morning walks. The latter element, spontaneous and welcome social connection, was key to her well-being. In addition, friends regularly came over to cook lunch with her, and she spent evenings singing or chatting with her neighbors. Teruya believed that those doses—short and long—of community connection helped keep her happy and youthful. And it was clear that social connection was not merely organized visits with friends: it was *built into* the routines of Ogimi residents—be it through gateball games, community center visits, or tending to her house.

When I observed the other residents of Ogimi, centenarians and noncentenarians alike, their diet was largely plant-based with soy and fish. They seemed active, social, and youthful compared to people in North America or Western Europe. It reflected the other blue zones, which have demonstrated everything from lower incidence of heart disease, dementia, and cancer.

The strength and fitness of Teruya and her neighbors impressed me, but it was not a surprise. Broadly speaking, East Asia has played an immense role in our understanding of complementary healing. From China came a theory of the body as a system of energy flow and its obstructions; these roots go back over 4,000 years. Traditional Chinese medicine (TCM) is a therapeutic system described in the ancient text Huang-di Nei'Jing (written by the emperor Huangdi around 2600 B.C.) as balancing the role of yin qi (female energy) and yang qi (male energy). Acupuncture, a central aspect of TCM, aims to correct for stagnant qi (lifeforce energy), which was to be responsible for most ailments. China also developed modes of pain relief that were the precursors of those still in use today. Physician Zhang Zhongjing (150-219 C.E.) wrote a treatise that included a hundred herb-based remedies for everything from fever to animal bites. He wrote of a Chinese surgeon named Hua T'o, who is understood to have invented the anesthetic "mafeisan," which is comprised of opium, cannabis, and other elements. Other traditional therapies from Chinese medicine, such as wormwood (derived from the Artemisia plant), were beginning to be used for acupuncture and moxibustion (burning on the back to improve qi flow) at this time. Japan has a similar approach, but it is termed "Kampo," adapted from when TCM was introduced in the 5th century.

*

About 7,000 miles from Ogimi sits Serenbe, a small community 30 minutes south of Atlanta, Georgia. It was there where I met Michael Taylor, a "reformed lawyer" from New York City, for lunch on a veranda with white wicker chairs and sweet iced tea. It's hard to ignore the historical contrast. A century ago, the grounds near Serenbe could have accommodated slave plantations marked by large homes with matching verandas and wicker chairs. The enslaved may also have relied on their ability to form social connections as a way of surviving the most horrific circumstances. But today, this was only an eerie reminder of the dual histories of the South—an area renowned for hospitality and being welcoming, with a fraught history of just the opposite. Georgia had recently "turned blue," after all, and so change was evident.

Growing up in Washington, D.C., Taylor moved to New York City in 2005 to attend college. He finished law school and started a career in corporate law in Manhattan in 2014. However, over the years, school and work took a toll, and he began to feel disconnected from himself.

"I don't think we were meant to sit in offices with three monitors and update documents for 12 hours a day," he told me. "I didn't feel connected. I didn't feel like I was doing anything except for stressing out about commas. I felt like a corporate drone."

Taylor is a Jewish man with a ruddy complexion and light brown hair. With his baritone voice, he is the encapsulation of "jolly," smiling even as he describes a very real bout of anxiety. "I'm classic middle child. Kind of a work-hard, play-hard, funny guy who was very social. But eventually, in the city, I stopped spending time with friends. I didn't have a formal diagnosis—but it was more than just run-of-the-mill Jewish anxiety and angst, and I knew I needed to work with someone to sort through it," he told me.

A friend of his from college had moved to Serenbe, a wellness community covering several thousand acres on the edge of Atlanta. Founded in 2004, its miles of trails wind through forests and meadows to connect homes and restaurants, artists' studios, and businesses. In 2005, Taylor began visiting for one weekend a year, as a break. "I found Serenbe helpful in terms of ego release…it gave me a new appreciation of self and my relationship to the world," he recalls. The effect on Taylor seems in line with Serenbe's purpose, as the community took its name from joining the words serenity and being.

With time, Michael looked forward to that one weekend a year until he finally hit a wall with his career. His anxiety had become so overwhelming that, in 2015, he left New York and moved to Serenbe, accompanied by a rescue dog named Myra, a Bichon-Spaniel mix. He also changed careers—selling real estate around Serenbe. And, as all good stories go, he found love, meeting his wife there, too. They welcomed their first child in early 2020 and welcomed their second in late 2021.

"Compared to 2014, my sense of well-being is so much better. I was kind of in a dark hole. I had felt alone, and now I feel connected to nature, the universe, and other people. My parents noticed a difference. And the thing is—what I always tell people is that I really didn't know how shitty I was feeling until I began to feel better. I guess it takes light to know darkness, as they say," Taylor told me.

After our lunch, I met with Steve Nygren, who founded Serenbe with his wife, Marie Lupo Nygren. As the story goes, they were first enthralled with the landscape in 1991 during a visit from Atlanta with their young girls. Fast forward to 2004, by which time they had a small house there, and their love for the land turned into a more serious commitment. Steve, 73, is a tall and genteel Southern man of Swedish heritage with snowy white hair. Marie, 68, on the other hand, is a modern-day bohemian who could be mistaken for a yoga instructor, with streaks of white in her dark grey hair. Steve had spent years in the hospitality business, owning Pleasant Peasants restaurant in Atlanta, among others. During a golf-cart tour of Serenbe led by Steve, I asked about the motivation behind his new venture.

"There was a slow shift in my value system," he answered. The mansion in Atlanta and the lifestyle that went along with it had lost their appeal. "We had everything money could buy, but as a family, we could hardly wait to get to the shack and connect to nature. So, one January morning, I made the decision to sell my company, which was 34 restaurants in the state, and restore an old farmhouse."

The Nygrens' story doesn't end with an isolated home in the countryside, of course. When a plan surfaced to bulldoze 40,000 acres of the surrounding landscape for commercial developments, they felt compelled to stand up. The answer? Buy it and protect 70% while building on the remainder.

After spending some vacation time with a friend in England and learning more about the English countryside and sacred geometry involved in the English village system, they used these principles to create a larger planned community with a central core. During his time in Europe, Nygren also learned more about how end-of-life care was delivered, which was unlike the isolation and sterility of many care facilities in North America. European institutions more typically harness social connections to increase quality of life as opposed to merely extending longevity. With their eldest daughter in high school, the Nygrens built a bigger house, followed by hundreds of others over the span of months. Today, over 650 residents call Serenbe home, and it's comprised of three hamlets and houses a 25-acre organic farm. Each of the three hamlets is dedicated to a different theme. Range focuses on farm-to-table food (and houses the farm and organic garden that serves the community and three restaurants on the property). Mado focuses on health and wellness, and Selborne focuses on the arts and culture. But it's the harnessing of the physical environment to improve *social* connection that makes Serenbe stand out.

"The houses are built into a forest garden instead of having landscaping around each house. The houses built on one side of a street step up off the curb, whereas the others step down towards a ravine or forest. There's also a gentle introduction to a center of commerce—small shops, for instance—that are part of the hamlet," Nygren told me excitedly. "We've added slow curves to the roads, so it feels more natural, as opposed to being on a grid. And each time you see a streetlight, it's a signal to a path into the forest, so it's easier to walk as opposed to getting in something with wheels."

Biophilic design, or city planning that aspires to connect residents through nature and community, remains a core tenet at Serenbe. Design that facilitates social connection is the most prominent aspect. For instance, residents don't have their own mailboxes but instead use a common mail center, so neighbors have a reason to bump into one another. All homes have a front porch so everyone can see their neighbors, similar to what we saw in Ogimi, with Teruya's porch that she would sweep every morning. There's also a mix between single-family housing and multifamily apartments. A Montessori school that goes up to the third grade is located in the middle of the neighborhood, and a charter high school sits right outside the property. Trash cans (which are hidden below ground) blend into the sidewalk. Activities like book clubs and wine meetups happen weekly, but I also met a woman who spoke about the community members coming together to help her cook and take care of her children after a cancer diagnosis.

There is no formal vetting process for who gets to live in Serenbe, but residents seem to self-select—those willing to pay a bit more to support community initiatives in the arts and other gatherings and those willing to commute into Atlanta. Many are entrepreneurs who have the flexibility to work at least partly at home. The types of businesses that have sprung up also tell a story: a forest labyrinth, a wellness center (offering classes in everything from goat yoga to guided meditation), a cold-pressed juice shop, and a fitness center. The highlight of Serenbe, though, is its sprawling organic farm in the neighborhood dubbed Range, and most people in Serenbe use the community farm. The residents are professionals: teachers, actors, doctors, and lawyers. This provides a nudge for neighbors to mingle as they walk over to buy their vegetables. A medicinal garden on the property does the same.

Every year, Serenbe hosts two conferences: a biophilic leadership summit in April (with city planners from places like San Francisco attending) and a Fall developer conference for the wider public. Nygren shares that he's working with other developers around the U.S. to consult on similar planned communities—from upstate New York to Florida to Ohio and North Carolina—and has founded his own consulting firm called "Nygren Placemaking" for this purpose. At least one such plan in the Midwest was a massive failure. "They had everything but a Steve Nygren," one Serenbe resident told me; Nygren had earned the nickname of "Willy Wonka of Serenbe" for a reason: he's a visionary but also someone who is able to lead a collective and get things done.* The takeaway is that this very approach can be applied to both neighborhood design and hospital design, something Nygren cemented for me.

"The two important components I see are the connection to nature and the connection to each other," he said to me. When I asked Nygren about what, in his early life, motivated him to create Serenbe, he had an interesting answer. He grew up in a multigenerational household as an only child with an alcoholic father and mother who constantly worried about their finances. "I felt a lot of loneliness as an only child. I knew I was not going to stay on the farm or be sucked into that life but had to get away and find something else. I believed destiny was mine to make. Otherwise, I'd get trapped in that default destiny. I had good examples of what that looked like, and I vowed to carve my own path," he told me. Later, he followed his curiosity to ultimately lead him to re-envision what "community" looks and feels like, undoubtedly informed by his childhood, which was wrought with the opposite: loneliness and a yearning to belong.

Indeed, Serenbe, which as of 2024 is home to 1,400 residents, has taken some of what we have learned from Ogimi village in Okinawa and brought it to rural Georgia, but it took someone like Steve Nygren and a passion for connection seeded as a child to make it a reality. Yet, loneliness is one thing; social connections may help prevent and "treat" loneliness, clearly, and both Michael Taylor and Fumi Teruya spoke to the benefits of community connection. But does the evidence suggest that our social networks can go further to actually promote healing? This led to my conversation with the two scholars behind the Okinawa longevity research.

2.

Researcher Makoto Suzuki, M.D., Ph.D., of the Okinawa Research Center for Longevity Science (ORCLS) has been studying local centenarians like Fumi

---

* Nygren is acutely aware of the potential health benefits, and so it's no surprise that in 2020 and 2021, demand for housing in Serenbe ballooned by over 200 percent, secondary to an exodus due to the COVID-19 pandemic, and the demand continues to outstrip supply.

Teruya since 1976. "*Moais* involve ritualized connections that are both reliable and close-knit, which involve those with a common interest but not usually a common professional identity," Suzuki said. "In my own *moai*, we have 10 members, and I'm the only doctor. A time is decided, a venue is decided, and the rules are decided as well," Suzuki told me. Suzuki's ORCLS research partner since the late 1990s and co-author of *The Okinawa Program*, Craig Wilcox, added, "A *moai* is more than just a friend group. It's often village-based and consists of rituals and institutions that keep people connected."

We know that loneliness can be harmful to our health. Vivek Murthy covered the devastating consequences of isolation on our health in his 2020 book, *Together*, but first brought this connection to public attention—effectively comparing loneliness to cigarette smoking—when he served as President Barack Obama's surgeon general. But the benefits of social relationships go beyond preventing disease. A strong social network may boost longevity and help with healing. A study from 2020, led by New Zealand-based researcher Yoram Barak, reported that living until 100 without chronic disease is linked to high levels of social engagement. Subjective well-being, according to self-report and overall happiness, is also linked to social relationships, which is probably common sense to most of us.

Social engagement generally has health-promoting effects. However, as shown in a systematic review from 2019, which found an inconsistent relationship between social activity and cognitive function, the kind of social engagement that takes place may affect the degree of benefit it provides.

*

While researchers have hypothesized that social networks impact physical and mental health via the brain or anti-inflammatory processes, the exact mechanism by which strong social networks impact healing remains a mystery. A famous study from 1996, called "Social and Emotional Support and Its Implication for Health," compared the healing process after surgery in patients who had a roommate in the hospital and those who didn't. This study found that patients without a roommate were slower to recover, which suggests that the social connection that comes with companionship may help wounds heal faster. In medical settings, this benefit needs to be balanced with the increased risk of acquiring hospital-induced infection from closer proximity to others.

Indeed, having friends and loved ones help with post-surgical care is likely a factor in faster, perhaps more thorough, healing, and this was found in another study of how social support may also be helpful in healing diabetic foot ulcers. Is there a mediating effect of being plugged into a social network and bouncing back physically? Might the impact of hormones such as oxytocin contribute to this resilience?

One of the most interesting studies to consider the social effects of healing came out of Auckland in 2017, co-authored by University of Auckland researcher Elizabeth Broadbent, who has been studying this association for 15 years. She and her team looked at social closeness and how well skin recovered after it was punctured. They found that social interaction did have a beneficial effect and was also accompanied by a self-reported decrease in stress.

"We wondered if the *type* of social support was what mattered. So, for instance, when people come in and think they are at a job interview and believe it would be less stressful if they knew the people in the room, well, that isn't helpful for wound healing because [that same person] could heighten anxiety levels. We looked instead at wound healing while two participants unknown to each other were paired while going through the same procedure. The other half of the group went through the procedure alone," Broadbent told me. "What happened then, with the group that was paired, was 'social induction,' meaning they got to know each other through a task. This allows the forming of a relationship with someone over a shorter period of time."

Broadbent has been studying the role of stress and wound healing for 15 years, and in addition to social support, has looked at the role of things like expressive writing (where patients write down their thoughts and feelings in order to process an event). Her research also found that the protective effects of marriage, specifically as a social support initiative, are mainly valuable for men. "It may be because women are traditionally more nurturing," Broadbent told me. In reality, the explanation may be more complicated. I thought back to some of my own relationships and feeling more nurtured by my partner. Maybe there is a gender element, but the association isn't universal.

*

Integrating what I had learned, I knew I needed my social support—the friends I had neglected or withdrawn from during the stress at the hospital. So, I sought out Nazanin, a dermatologist I had known for years when we met in our first year of university in my undergraduate physics class, and Victoria, a pharmacist I had also met that year. Others, friends and acquaintances from medical school, had somehow gotten wind of my debacle, and reached out with comfort and stories of others' struggles in the same institution, and I was reminded of how special our class was. Another former classmate, Dara, met me for coffee and tried to advise me. "It's really hard to see you like this. This isn't you," she said, "Can you maybe switch to [a post] closer to Toronto?" I shook my head, knowing how difficult making that switch would be. Dara saw how I had lost weight and seemed to have lost a lot of confidence. We had shared the same passion for global health and were outspoken and driven. These qualities during medical school in Toronto had been supported, but in my hospital in a totally different city, they were punished. I hugged her. Friendship is healing, too.

To better understand this cause-effect relationship between social support and resiliency, we can look at sociology. In 1991, two sociologists named Richard Nisbett and Lee Ross wrote what's perhaps the seminal social psychology textbook called *The Person and the Situation*, arguing that most of our behavior—what we deem as "our personality"—is actually shaped by our environments. Such influence pervades us for the better or worse. Nordic countries such as Denmark, Finland, and Sweden have three elements that are associated with a high level of happiness among their residents: equality, social trust, and having a welfare state. The World Happiness Report of 2020 described it more specifically as the sense of where the government provides a secure foundation for its citizens.

During my undergraduate sociology of medicine course, an entire lecture and textbook chapter was devoted to the ways medical students are indoctrinated into the profession. Years later, now facing what I faced, I finally connected indoctrination to my experience in this one specific academic hospital environment. In medical school, I had been elected to the student council, felt connected to my classmates, and was supported by mentors and peers. I thrived. Then, all of a sudden, I had landed in a place that was the opposite of healthy and not merely overly mechanized. I found myself in an unhealthy environment that went beyond the norms of a hospital.

Herbert Freudenberger, who coined the term "burnout" in 1974 to mean the end result of severe and ongoing stress combined with having "high ideals," applied it to the "helping" professions such as doctors and nurses. Eight years later, he even wrote a book called *Situational Anxiety*, which described how anxiety is often dependent on the situation. It's effectively a variation of what Ross and Nisbett would later describe. Then, in 2019, journalist Johann Hari published *Lost Connections*, a memoir of sorts, where he interrogates the root of depression, inspired by his own lived experience. He reached a personal conclusion that echoed that of Nisbett and Ross: that his depression was largely an environmental issue as opposed to solely a chemical imbalance in the brain. This is effectively how Michael Taylor experienced his childhood anxiety and also perfectly explained my own anxiety and depression—after all, they were *workplace-induced*. Indeed, depression can have multiple contributing factors: social circumstances, physical environment, a difficult workplace, and, in rare cases, purely a biochemical shift in the brain. I was experiencing a normal response to an abnormal situation, not vice versa: this pattern is most often clear among patients experiencing physical trauma, and can be deadly.

3.

As a newly minted doctor, I entered the small room in the emergency department with a hint of dread. I'd been called to consult on a 2-month-old infant, Baby J, admitted for what was called "Trauma X" or possible "non-accidental injury"—"NAI" for short. It meant that the initial admitting emergency physicians were concerned about the possibility of child abuse.

The parents appeared young, likely in their early twenties. The father, restless and distracted, paced the room with his eyes glued to his phone. The mother sat quietly on the edge of a lounge chair, her hair pulled back into a loose ponytail, her posture suggesting both exhaustion and anxiety. There was an air of uncertainty between them, the kind that often accompanies long hours spent waiting for news—hovering between hope and fear, unsure of what would come next. I introduced myself. "Hi, my name's Amitha, and I'm one of the doctors here tonight. How are you?"

"We've been better," the man said, briefly looking up.

The mother spoke quickly. "I have no idea why, but he just didn't want to feed," she said. She then went on to describe how she breastfed initially but then stopped because it was hurting too much, so she switched to formula.

I nodded my head. "Why don't we start at the beginning?" I offered.

In situations like these, as part of taking the child's history, doctors ask about the infant's birth and then move forward toward the present condition or start with the present and move backward. I chose the latter, as the most important information was around the circumstances of his injury—and this would be part of a medical record that could potentially be presented or referred to in the legal system. It needed to be as accurate as possible; if we were interrupted or if Baby J's parents became tired, we needed, at the very least, to be able to accurately describe the circumstances.

"When was the last time you felt like Baby J was himself?" Not wanting to feed, after all, could be due to many things, including sepsis or a severe infection of the body that can spread and shut down all of its organs and ultimately lead to death. I had to push aside the findings of torn blood vessels at the back of the eye (termed retinal hemorrhages) that were shared with me. Bias in clinical judgement is a major issue, and already I could feel my mind reminding me of Occam's razor: the most unified explanation, which is often the simplest, is the most likely to be correct. Even if Baby J had been abused, a fair documentation of the history and physical exam was a must—but I needed also to note anything unusual in the parents' behavior.

The father was pacing. When Baby J cried, his mother didn't soothe him. They spoke about the child like he was a burden. They made no statements suggesting concern and didn't ask if Baby J would be okay. They focused instead on when they would be allowed to leave. I asked if they had an explanation for Baby J's injuries. Abusive parents might say their child rolled off a bed, for instance, usually a telling sign when infants have not yet reached the rolling stage of development. But according to these parents, Baby J's injuries "just appeared."

When I examined Baby J, he took to my arms comfortingly, but his eyes wouldn't focus, and he felt slightly floppy. This could mean many things, including brain damage. My examination was thorough and included diagrams locating the bruises I found on his body; they were mostly on his chest, abdomen, and legs. He didn't cry or turn to his mother or father to exhibit preference while held by a stranger: all would be typical for an infant his age. I wrote my notes up in detail, including what I had noticed in the nonverbal and verbal cues from the parents. Then, I told the parents that I would review the plan with my team and order some tests. And no, I couldn't tell them when they could leave yet. It was 2:00 am.

The tests began. There is an entire "NAI workup" that includes scans of the brain to look for fractures and bruising. There are special images taken of the back of the eye, called the retina, a thin membrane that focuses light which only ophthalmologists (eye specialists) can assess well. If the retina's blood vessels are torn, which can happen if the infant is shaken, they result in retinal hemorrhages. Then, there are a series of X-rays that we call the "bone series" that scan the entire child's body for new fractures as well as older "healed" fractures, which can point to a pattern. There is also blood work—specifically that which helps us rule out other causes of bruising. Very rare genetic diseases such as osteogenesis imperfecta (OI), or "brittle bone disease," can cause bruising and fractures in children as well as in adults, so ruling that out is key (though I had seen an instance of both things—child abuse faced by a child with OI presenting at the same time).* The in-hospital Child Neglect Service (CNS) would then determine, based on the testing, whether they should intervene.

Sure enough, with Baby J, the ophthalmologists found diffuse retinal hemorrhages, suggesting he could have been shaken so severely that his blood vessels popped. Baby J was now likely to be partially blind. Imaging results revealed multiple fractures in the patient's thigh, upper arm, and ribs. Several of the rib fractures showed signs of healing, indicating older injuries. The scans also identified a recent skull fracture. Surprisingly, the child had visited the emergency department a few months earlier with a single fracture that had been classified as accidental at the time.

---

* I wrote about this case in 2018 for *Discover* magazine https://www.discovermagazine.com/health/eye-of-the-beholder

My more experienced staff colleague, Dr. Perry, explained the case was transitioned to the appropriate specialty service for further evaluation, with child protection services becoming involved to assess the family's situation. It was noted that the family had received support from extended relatives, and the situation had been under observation by the community child-welfare agency for some time.

"So this means that Baby J will be fostered, right?" I asked. "I mean, this is the second time, and he could die if there's another time." Dr. Perry shook her head. Foster care isn't an easy route either. Often, the best outcomes occur with close monitoring and reliable support from extended family.

It just didn't seem fair. One junior member of the CNS service had taken issue with my documentation being "too detailed." I had worked with CNS services before, with other attendings, and as a medical student in another institution, and was taught to document objectively with as much detail as possible, as the medical file was a legal document. The same member of CNS happened to be the person responsible for not following up after Baby J's initial fracture months ago, so I was reassured by Dr. Perry that my detailed documentation was likely helpful and necessary. Clearly, though, I wasn't understanding something here. Perhaps it was a concern over mislabeling the case as abuse. But when a young child's life was at risk, why *wouldn't* we be more cautious?

I went home at 9:00 am, having been up for twenty-eight hours straight. The lack of sleep didn't exhaust me as much as the emotion; I felt overwhelmed by the need to stay calm with Baby J's parents, who clearly needed some compassion as they weren't handling parenting very well— but who also didn't appear to have the best interests of their child in mind. Added to that was the sheer futility of being stuck in a position where I could only report what I saw but couldn't advocate (and if my detailed notes were considered advocacy, I would get a slap on the wrist). Later that day, the case was brought to my attention as part of the care team's ongoing coordination. The plan involved returning the child to the family, with closer oversight by the child protection agency and increased involvement from a relative. As I listened to the plan, a sense of unease settled over me. I couldn't shake the fear that the next time I heard about this child, it might be tragic news.

To remedy Baby J's injuries, lasering of his retina back together and casting of his broken bones was not enough. He needed to be lifted up and out of that inhospitable and abusive social environment to a place and family that could love him and protect him, where he could thrive and grow into a happy toddler and, hopefully, a well-adjusted adult who had just been through several tough months as a baby.

I could help treat Baby J, but I couldn't heal him. If an abusive environment was impacting my spirit and mind and leaving me—with my healthy upbringing, education, and family support—feeling mired in an abyss of toxicity with so few options out, what kind of future was this baby facing? I vowed that, while I couldn't heal Baby J, maybe this experience could propel me forward as an advocate for others in my position, as well as other children who may benefit from an advocate. My core goal would be to emphasize how the impact of our environments can sometimes prevent us from thriving. I decided that the advocacy would need to start tomorrow after the tears ran out and I finally had some much-needed sleep.

*

Three years later, I was driving across the border towards Maryland while researching the same magazine piece that had first taken me to Nationwide Children's Hospital. The story involved another young boy, but this time, the battle was against an incurable childhood condition called Batten Disease (known colloquially as "childhood dementia"), subtype CLN2. My interest had been sparked months before by a review article written by a German physician named Alfried Kohlschütter, in which he described various forms of Batten Disease. The only form of "developmental regression" we were taught in medical school was Rett's Syndrome, which predominantly affects girls and impacts how the brain develops. Later, I learned about Childhood Disintegrative Disorder (CDD), which involves developmental delays and a form of psychosis (so it impacts the mind). Batten Disease was different. It's a neurological disease with no clear cause but devastating impacts secondary to a buildup of a form of waste in the brain. And the FDA was in the midst of reviewing applications for a new enzyme-replacement treatment.

It was Kohlschüetter who, via email, had introduced me to Dr. Emily de los Reyes, based at Nationwide Children's Hospital in Columbus. She then put me in touch with one of her patients, Conner, who lived outside of Baltimore. My aim was to get to know Conner and how the disease was affecting him and his family and share how access to this new treatment could halt its progression. But what struck me most was how Conner's mother, Holly Beish, described how much of the support she and the family needed was coming from an unlikely place: social media.

Typically, we don't associate online communication with anything healthy, but in this instance, it had helped Holly advocate for her son's difficult case and build a sense of community around her family. She had created the Facebook group "Fighting for Conner and Batten Disease Awareness" when her son was newly diagnosed. And while there's no question that it ultimately took enzyme replacement therapy to stop the disease from progressing as rapidly, I was there to investigate how part of Conner's healing took place within the Beish home through connections with other families touched by this rare disease. Their case showed me that the relationship between social media and our mental health isn't as clear-cut as we usually think.

In the Fall of 2017, psychologist Janet Twenge wrote an article for *The Atlantic* entitled "Have Smartphones Destroyed a Generation?" in which she described the crisis of prevalent anxiety and depression among teenagers and how social media has effectively caused this crisis. Twenge cited research, mostly her own, as well as anecdotal evidence from her own observations (she mentions that in 2012, she noticed an abrupt shift in teen behaviors and emotional states), yet most of the article struck me as conjecture: conjecture I initially agreed with, to be sure, as the relationship *feels*, intuitively, correct. However, while there are correlations, certainly, with social media use and the presence of anxiety and depression in adolescents, it's hard to tease out the exact impact. In 2019, a piece published in the *Scientific American* entitled, aptly, "Social Media Has Not Destroyed a Generation," suggested just the opposite of what Twenge asserted, that social media wasn't solely to blame and the relationship between social media and poor mental health may be significant only in heavy social media users—those who spent over three hours a day on those platforms.

Three years later, in 2020, a documentary called *The Social Dilemma* dove further into how social media networks can more broadly change users' behavior to be more conducive to addiction, as well as depression. Later, a damning *Wall Street Journal* investigation report about Facebook and what internal researchers knew about the harms to adolescents suggested the picture is complex (Facebook, for their part, responded with a counterargument from their Head of Research). We do know that there are crucial design elements in social media platforms that fuel addictive behavior and dopamine surges, and these elements are intentional, as they drive users to advertising. Jonathan Haidt's 2024 book, *The Anxious Generation*, dives into the impact on adolescents specifically, taking a more thorough journalistic approach to the issue.

What insights can we glean from researchers' indecision about the effects of social media? We might understand the quandary by observing what we're doing with the platforms on which we spend so much of our time. When we participate as voyeurs, comparing ourselves implicitly or explicitly to others, then this *comparison* may lend itself to poor emotional health. Of course, that's no different from looking through a fashion magazine and wishing to be taller, shorter, curvier, skinnier, darker-skinned, lighter-skinned, more muscular, less muscular, and so forth. The distinction is that social media offers us thousands more points of stimuli of comparison—particularly around activities and accomplishments.

That said, when the connection is less voyeuristic and more focused on *authentic* connection, primarily through a shared interest or life challenge, the opposite might result: the emotional uplifting characteristic of a healthy friendship. The research is also becoming clearer around the *quality* of social media interaction and the time spent. In general, high-quality interactions with individuals who are also friends offline or those who engage back (reciprocity) in a positive way, combined with reduced time on a given app (less than three hours per day), may allow for the benefits of community connection without the downsides of toxicity or worsening feelings of loneliness. This balance is what I saw support the Beishes.

Even years after I worked on that story, I was getting updates from their Facebook group. Conner remained stable, but the disease was still terminal. Did social media directly contribute to Conner's healing? No. But what *has* healed is the family's initial loss of connection. Upon initially receiving Conner's diagnosis, Holly and her husband had felt utterly alone with a disease none of their family members or friends could understand. Now, the Beishes are more plugged into other families and have the opportunity to share and receive knowledge and wisdom with those around the world. The help they give others helps give them a sense of purpose and meaning while also keeping themselves up to date on the latest clinical trials and treatments, for Conner's sake. So, in this way, social media *can* be a tool for healing, as it creates communities that can be conducive to support, much as our real-life social surroundings might. We still must remain actively aware of the drawbacks, especially as it relates to pathology such as addiction.

5.

Evaluating my own use of social media, I realized I needed to reconnect in the most offline way possible: yoga teacher training. There was a course later that Spring offered by a reputable school, but it was all the way in Baja California, Mexico. There was also a mindfulness meditation retreat that had filled up in upstate New York but was offered in Denmark.

Just as I was preparing to embark on back-to-back resets, an old college friend, Chris, replied to a LinkedIn request I had sent inquiring about potential consulting work with the United Nations agency he worked for. He had some job ideas that could potentially tide me over. For the moment, I needed to navigate my way out of this brutal situation—striving for fairness and contending with the impact on my mental and physical health—and return back onto solid ground. I let him know that I was hoping to delve deeper into my yoga and meditation practices with this trip to Denmark and then Mexico, so I would be offline for most of the next two months. Then, the morning of my flight, I saw that Chris had messaged me late in the evening, Geneva time, and the message was surprisingly flattering.

I hadn't seen Chris in years, and we had only exchanged a few messages by that point. This was a bit bold. A few hours later, he sent another message, apologizing for being so forward; he'd been out at a bar with some friends. I just responded with a smiling emoji. I didn't feel like discussing it. I had enough to occupy my mind, and his forwardness felt endearing at a time when I was willing to soak up any ray of positivity. Besides, Chris offered a little morsel of mystery on top of the support I was surrounding myself with from my close friends and family.

Indeed, the lessons from Fumi Teruya, Michael Taylor, Baby J, and the Beishes all pointed clearly to one thing: the people with whom we surround ourselves, whether our immediate family, the communities in which we live, or the purposeful connections we cultivate in person or online, can be massively influential to our health and well-being, and thus can be massively transformative in our healing. With Teruya, it was implementing something small into her daily routine, like sweeping her deck as a way to encounter others in her community. For me, it would be ensuring my days were filled with at least one opportunity to connect with someone meaningfully. With Baby J, it was clear how an abusive environment can lead to harm. While my situation couldn't be compared to the abuse of an infant, the power of one harmful situation on physical and emotional health is still clear. Michael Taylor's experience more closely represented mine, as a professional who ultimately chose to leave an environment that was eroding his mental health and who took a leap of faith that ultimately led him in the right direction, professionally and personally. His community, Serenbe, effectively helped heal him. And last, the lesson Holly Beish and so many mothers of children with special needs teach us daily: that sometimes we aren't aware of our own power to overcome the most unexpected and devastating realities and that seeking community online when offline community is limited, can be what makes the most meaningful difference.

Each one of these stories underscores what Nisbett and Ross put forth in the early 1990s: that it's most often our "situations" that influence our behavior. Now, it becomes clear that navigating *out of* harmful situations impacts how well we are able to heal physically and emotionally. So, with that, I boarded my flight with the intent to dive deeply into yoga and mindfulness meditation and the communities of support it offered with the goal of rehabilitating my injured soul and body.

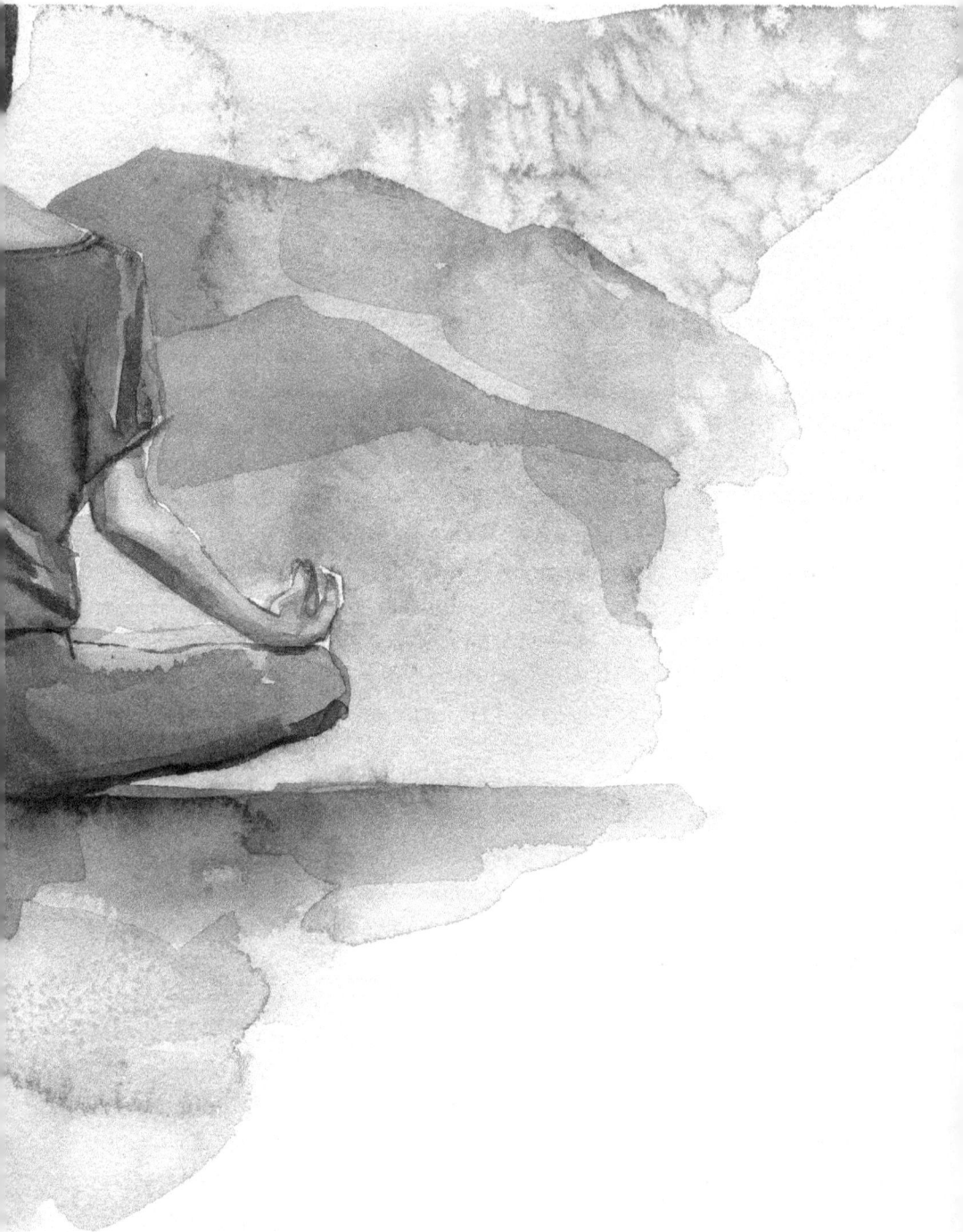

CHAPTER FIVE

Mind Medicine

"Life shrinks or expands in proportion to one's courage."
—Anaïs Nin

1.

I wasn't alone in my reasons for coming to Denmark; many at the retreat were drawn there to help them face their own healing challenges. We were in Aarhus, a picturesque town on the country's east coast that is redolent of old Danish charm. A short hike through fields of wildflowers could find me standing at the edge of the world, on cliffs overlooking nothing but the sprawling Kattegat Sea. That time of year, in June, the days are the longest, with the sun rising around 4:30 am and setting around 9:30 pm. I was there to learn a technique called mindfulness-based stress reduction, or "MBSR," from its creator, Jon Kabat-Zinn.

Some at the retreat were long-time followers of Kabat-Zinn and his books. His twice-yearly retreats at the Omega Institute in Rhinebeck, New York, typically fill up within minutes of being posted. Kabat-Zinn himself has a unique story. Having studied under a Nobel laureate in physics at the Massachusetts Institute of Technology (MIT) in the 1970s, he shifted trajectory after a fateful trip to Japan. He became immersed there in Zen Buddhism so that he could focus on studying the mind and the benefits of meditation, particularly for those dealing with stress and anxiety. Back then his methods were denounced; in the 1970s and 1980s, meditation was not as popular in the West as it is today.

He was labeled a quack at worst and out of touch at best. Now, however, he's one of the most sought-after speakers in North America, regularly selling out venues as large as the Lincoln Center in New York.

Kabat-Zinn's calm voice is at once Zen-like and hardcore Manhattanite. It's also my favorite voice to listen to when doing a guided meditation as an app or CD, and that week, in Aarhus, he was leading a 10-day meditation retreat for over 300 people. I felt lucky to be one of them.

We all filed into a large gymnasium, took a seat or lay on our chosen yoga mats. There were meditation cushions for most of us, fancy wooden meditation seats for a few, and for a handful, simply a plain old chair.

"So now we're going to start with assuming a position that suggests dignity, sitting upright, knees ideally below the hips in a cross-legged position, eyes slightly open or softly closed, focusing on a spot just beyond your cushion. Knowing there's nowhere you need to be but here. And that, right here, in this moment, there's more right with you than wrong with you, as long as you're breathing," Kabat-Zinn began.

It was exactly what I needed to hear. It was time, it seemed, to go inward for answers, or at the very least—as I had been advised months earlier—for joy and peace. I wanted assurance that I was spending my time wisely. Was there scientific evidence that shows meditation can heal the mind?

2.

The Denmark retreat was co-taught with Kabat-Zinn's long-term MBSR partner, Dr. Saki Santorelli. For several decades they had been running an 8-week MBSR program at the University of Massachusetts and surrounding hospitals for patients with chronic pain, and Kabat-Zinn had been publishing his studies in this field.

His first paper on the impact of MBSR on chronic pain was published in 1985 in the *Journal of Behavioral Medicine*. In that study, in which 90 patients were trained at the University of Massachusetts 10-week Stress Reduction and Relaxation Program, reductions were seen not just in pain but also in mood issues like anxiety and depression. The participants also needed less pain medication and were more active. These improvements were maintained for 15 months. However, when they were asked about pain in the "present moment," their perceived pain stayed at the same level as previous (no changes in baseline), suggesting that they only experienced pain when they were hyperaware of their body.

After that study, Kabat-Zinn and his colleagues soon began to offer MBSR to medical students and doctors associated with the University of Massachusetts as well. One of Santorelli's and Kabat-Zinn's first studies together looked at the potential benefits of MBSR for anxiety. There, 22 participants who met the diagnostic criteria for an anxiety disorder received weekly MBSR training for one month and then monthly for three months. They found that anxiety as well as depression scores were reduced and remained reduced at follow-up after three years, regardless of whether they continued their practice. It appears that the impact of an 8-week MBSR course can mimic the brain function seen in those who have been meditating for years. Changes are seen in the amygdala specifically.

The research on MBSR, as a standardized technique, has exploded over the past two decades. Many high-quality, systematic reviews of smaller trials have been released. That said, there is no gold-standard Cochrane Systematic Review, which pools and analyzes statistical results, assessing the efficacy of "mindfulness-based approaches," a term that includes structured interventions like MBSR as well as less formalized meditation techniques.

One of the most authoritative reviews so far was published in 2014 in the *Journal of the American Medical Association (JAMA),* which found moderate evidence that psychosocial stress, in general, may be reduced when utilizing mindfulness practices. Across 47 trials, mindfulness meditation showed improvement in levels of anxiety, depression, and chronic pain at the 3-6 month mark; however, general stress and mental health-related quality of life weren't impacted much, and neither were sleep, weight, attention, or mood in general. The review didn't explain the reasons why these latter elements were not impacted and also didn't appear to find that these programs were more helpful than any active treatment—for instance, with medication. It certainly appeared that anxiety sufferers still needed other therapies.

Research by Erica Sibinga, based at Johns Hopkins University, has applied MBSR to youth anxiety. But it wasn't until 2016 that she published the results of a randomized controlled trial (RCT) focused on teaching MBSR to eighth-grade students in Baltimore, Maryland. In that trial, 300 students across two Baltimore public schools were randomized to either MBSR or a basic health education program. After the training, the students receiving MBSR training had lower levels of depression, rumination (the psychiatric definition for continuously thinking about dark thoughts), and self-hostility. Subsequent studies found that MBSR can also help improve youth anxiety. In 2011, Sibinga found that MBSR could assist HIV-infected and at-risk youth to decrease hospital admissions while improving interpersonal relationships, school achievement, and physical health.

Mindfulness-based meditation, more broadly, even if it isn't as structured as MBSR, has been linked to many health benefits, everything from improving the immune system to blood pressure. But a key review from 2012 found very limited evidence for several conditions, such as diabetes or cardiovascular disease—both of which include stress as a risk factor. Indeed, it seems that, much like Kabat-Zinn and Santorelli have described, the evidence is strongest for chronic pain, fibromyalgia, and chronic low back pain. Yet, the most cutting-edge research now looks to see if mindfulness can be used in one of the most hard-to-treat psychiatric conditions: schizophrenia.

*

My mother's older sister was a brilliant young woman who was always at the top of her class in their village in Jaffna, Sri Lanka. But once my aunt reached her late teens, she began having what psychiatrists refer to as "negative symptoms"—withdrawal, depression, and blunted emotional responses. As this was in the late 1960s, there was little awareness around mental health disorders, especially in South Asia. Over time, she began hearing voices and having unusual, aggressive responses to everyday requests, such as closing a door. It became clear that she had some sort of psychotic disorder.

My grandfather was advised to admit her to an institution when she was in her early 20s, but during the drive to the facility, the family changed their minds. My aunt would stay at home. Years later, she received a diagnosis of schizophrenia and was managed with antipsychotic medication. She never ended up going to university or using her brilliant brain in the way the family had expected she would—life instead sent her on a detour. Yet, she remained one of the most kind-hearted people you'd ever meet. While medication was undoubtedly crucial to managing my aunt's symptoms, I had wondered for years if other forms of therapy—specifically one that incorporated meditation techniques—might have helped her *heal* the parts of her brain that were impacted.

In 2017, a group of researchers from both The Hong Kong Polytechnic University Faculty of Health and Social Sciences and the School of Health & Social Care at Edinburgh Napier University sought to explore the potential healing power of meditation on schizophrenia. Their randomized controlled trial of mindfulness-based psychoeducation for those with schizophrenia, of the 600 participants in Scotland and Hong Kong, found that those in the mindfulness group has a statistically significant different rehospitalization rate. Remission was around 7% for the mindfulness group, whereas it was over 25% for the other group.

A 2019 systematic review and meta-analysis of 16 studies, which included 1,268 people with schizophrenia who practiced mindful meditation, showed that *hospitalization*s for schizophrenia decreased, though symptoms were not as impacted. But in 2020, a group of researchers from Berlin summarized the evidence for mindfulness-based interventions for schizophrenia and found that there was no evidence of a worsening of psychotic symptoms. Indeed, most studies reported an overall improvement in mood, cognition, and other symptoms that impact daily life.

*

Meditation is not without its controversies. In some cases, it can actually be triggering and, thus, harmful. Some individuals with PTSD, for example, can be flooded with traumatic imagery and re-traumatization in general when sitting in silence. In 2019, a paper by the University of Pennsylvania's Willoughby Britton explored in more detail the potential harms of mindfulness, where she suggested that the benefits likely follow an inverted U-shaped curve: there are benefits to a point—at which time there could be harms such as dissociation, increased distress, substance abuse, negative attention bias, and even anxiety, depression, and pain (the same things mindfulness seeks to improve).

There have been some case reports of psychosis induced by mindfulness meditation, and though extremely rare, this side effect featured prominently in a 2021 article in *Harper's* Magazine that suggested mindfulness efforts could lead to psychosis in some people. On occasion, the *type* of meditation can be controversial.

Years after my time in Denmark, I met an actor who spoke highly of Transcendental Meditation, known as "TM," as it had helped him navigate alcohol addiction. At his suggestion, I attended an information session held in a small wood-paneled room in Manhattan's financial district. The facilitator described the benefits of TM, which ranged from blood pressure reduction to longevity. As the technique was described, reactions in the room were split between those who leaned in with incredible interest, as though under a spell, and others who seemed less convinced. Posters of celebrities, like Oprah, lined the walls with quotes about how valuable TM was to them. Later I learned most of these celebrities no longer practiced TM.

The main way that TM differs from other meditation techniques is both the inclusion of a "personalized mantra" given to the practitioner by the teacher and the fact that it can be financially prohibitive to learn. The evidence behind TM isn't as clear-cut as the facilitator in that room made it seem. It may improve anxiety, according to a 2006 Cochrane review, but it may not be substantially different from other relaxation therapies; heterogeneity within studies remains an issue, which means it's hard to compare them side by side. Notably, a Cochrane review on TM for cardiovascular disease prevention by Louise Hartley and colleagues from RTI Health Solutions was withdrawn after questions were raised about the study analysis.

The controversy with TM in popular culture and media is more around the need to pay large sums of money for a unique mantra, as well as unusual techniques, like one a friend shared: the promotion of something called "yogic flying." "If you practice TM long enough, you really can fly," some have said. Claims like this led to a lawsuit in 1986; films like *David Wants to Fly*, a 2010 documentary aiming to expose the dark side of the cult-like movement, and the memoir *Greetings from Utopia Park: Surviving a Transcendent Childhood* by Claire Hoffman, published in 2016. But I didn't know any of this in that Manhattan room. I just knew that something didn't feel aligned. After a required meeting with a TM recruiter to gauge my commitment enrolling in the course, I left. It wasn't for me, but I knew the technique was very helpful to so many: so much of healing involves choosing those approaches that simply work for us, balancing the potential risks and benefits.

Ultimately, I needed to decide on whether a mindfulness-based meditation practice would help me cope with the stress I was enduring. Clearly, meditation is a technique that can heal and has evidence for healing the mind and, to some degree, the body. But not all forms are necessarily beneficial or even without risk.

Towards the end of the MBSR retreat, Kabat-Zinn shared with me some of his insights about the medical field—a system for healing that, in his view, was broken. "You represent the next generation who are positioned to change it," he said. I wasn't sure if my role in changing it was through mindfulness meditation, which would allow me to be present to my patients, or something bigger. But in that moment, and possibly as a result of two weeks of MBSR, I felt like my emotional healing from the distress of my experience was underway.

3.

"Code White."

I was on call in the hospital when the alarm came over the loudspeaker. A code white is the signal for a violent patient, one that could pose a danger to staff and other patients. I ran up to the ward, where three nurses were huddled in a patient's room. One of them was trying to restrain a highly agitated boy, who, at a glance, seemed to be in his late teens. His worried parents stood nearby. Usually, a security guard would be present for these calls, but I didn't see one.

The patient, whom I'll call Alex, had been admitted a couple of days earlier, presenting with confusion and erratic behavior that raised concerns about a possible neurological condition, including a brain infection. The previous night, they had become agitated, prompting the team to administer medication to help manage the symptoms. A nurse asked if I thought the same medication should be given again, but I wanted to assess Alex myself before making any decisions.

When I reached the bedside, Alex's breathing was rapid, and they looked visibly distressed, sweat dampening their hairline. What I observed seemed more like acute anxiety than anything neurological. After a brief examination, which Alex surprisingly allowed, I asked everyone except their parents and a nurse to leave the room. I decided to try a calming technique I had learned recently. I asked Alex to think of a time when they felt peaceful and happy. After a moment, Alex mentioned a family vacation on the water. I invited them to close their eyes and visualize the sights, sounds, and sensations of that moment. Gradually, their breathing slowed, and they appeared more at ease. When I asked if they needed anything to help them sleep, Alex shook their head. They soon drifted off into a restful sleep.

Later, Alex's parent mentioned that similar relaxation techniques had been effective at home before, though no one at the hospital had thought to ask what might help. When I checked on Alex the next day, a nurse was still stationed at the bedside, as Alex remained listed as a high-risk patient. Alex seemed disoriented, mumbling incomprehensibly. I asked the nurse for a moment alone with Alex, and she stepped out of the room.

I sat beside Alex and looked at them carefully. Something about the situation didn't feel right.

"I don't think you're experiencing a mental health crisis," I said gently. "It seems like there's more going on, and you feel trapped in a situation where it's hard to find a way out."

Alex's expression shifted—they seemed startled, then relieved. Their shoulders relaxed as they exhaled deeply. After a moment of silence, Alex began to speak. "The other night, my dad walked in on me using my laptop. I was... watching something I didn't want him to see. It freaked him out, and I panicked. I just started saying things that didn't make sense so they'd think I was having a breakdown. Now my parents believe I've lost it," Alex confessed, their voice trembling.

Alex continued, sharing that they had been struggling to make sense of their identity. They had friends and interests that made them feel like they should fit a certain mold, but something inside them felt different. They were grappling with feelings that they weren't ready to explore openly, especially given their family's conservative views.

The team had ordered additional diagnostic tests for the next day, including a spinal tap to rule out infection and further brain imaging. Earlier tests had noted a minor abnormality, though it was believed to be a normal variation. The concern was that something more serious might have been missed. Though Alex had already begun a course of antibiotics as a precaution, I doubted that the workup was necessary.

"Alex, you know there are some risks involved with the procedures planned for tomorrow," I said carefully. Alex nodded—they were old enough to make decisions about their care.

"I'll make sure the team knows what's going on," I reassured Alex, "but we'll keep your privacy intact. And for what it's worth, you're not alone in figuring things out. Many people your age feel confused about who they are, and that's okay."

Alex gave a small, cautious smile. "Really?"

"Yes," I replied. "And you don't have to figure it all out today. There's no rush to share anything with your family until you're ready."

We agreed that the details we discussed would be documented confidentially, accessible only to the care team. As I left the room, Alex quickly resumed their disoriented demeanor, slipping back into character as if flipping a switch. I couldn't help but think they might have a future in theater.

I found a quiet spot to document our conversation, marking the entry for limited access to protect Alex's privacy. In my assessment, the symptoms aligned more with anxiety than an organic neurological condition, and I recommended psychiatry involvement.

When I shared my concerns with the senior physician, she angrily dismissed my input, remaining focused on a potential neurological issue. Despite earlier scans suggesting nothing serious, the workup continued. Eventually, the results confirmed there was no infection, and the brain abnormality was deemed a normal anatomical variation. Alex was eventually referred to psychiatry and received support for managing anxiety.

Reflecting on the experience, I realized how crucial it is to listen deeply—not just to symptoms but to the context in which they arise. Alex's case reminded me that while simple explanations can sometimes offer clarity, they can also lead to harmful oversimplifications. In this instance, it wasn't a diagnostic test that made the biggest difference—it was creating a space for Alex to speak openly and feel seen. This experience reinforced for me that compassionate listening is just as important as any medical intervention.

The more senior physician hadn't taken the time to step back and calmly review the full scope of information in Alex's case. No one else had engaged with Alex at length or with empathy to understand the context behind the sudden shift in their behavior. Alex's story reminded me of the paradox inherent in Occam's Razor: while the simplest explanation is often correct—such as a physiological issue causing behavioral changes—relying too heavily on that simplicity in complex cases can lead to unnecessary risks. In Alex's case, this meant a cascade of interventions like invasive procedures and preemptive treatments that could have been avoided with a more careful evaluation.

Creating space for Alex to speak openly was likely the most healing part of their care. But I still wondered—was it the calming technique I had used that enabled Alex to share their truth, or was it simply the presence of someone willing to listen and pay close attention to their suffering? The answer would ultimately come to me years later, in an auditorium in Plymouth, Minnesota.

4.

Sitting onstage, a stocky gentleman with a sing-song voice convinced me that my fingers were magnetic. In front of 80 other physicians, nurses, and psychologists, Dr. Daniel Kohen of the University of Massachusetts was leading me through a classic hypnosis exercise as part of the National Pediatric Hypnosis Training Institute conference. It involved raising my clasped hands in the air, my index fingers held parallel to one another and pointed upwards.

"Now, focus on that space. By doing so, you will notice that your fingers will eventually touch," Kohen said.

My vision became blurry as I noticed, with surprise, that my fingers eventually *did* touch, even though I had tried to keep them apart. My contrarian ways had failed in the face of muscle fatigue.

"If you close your eyes," Kohen continued, "you might then notice that your arms will eventually want to make their way onto your lap."

In my trance—and that's exactly what Kohen had induced—I could hear his voice fade further into the distance. "Once your arms are on your lap, you will feel very relaxed, and this is something that can be available to you whenever you need it." Eventually, there was a silence from him, punctuated by an occasional "that's right" and "that's good."

"In a moment, you will open your eyes and come back to the room," he said.

I reluctantly opened my eyes, exiting a fuzzy space between consciousness and sleep. It felt as if at least twenty minutes had passed. It had been only five. I blinked several times and eventually focused on Kohen—who, in this moment, with his long snowy beard and hair tied back into a low bun, made me think of a modern-day wizard. What had just happened? This wasn't the "pocket-watch" type of hypnosis, so classic in cartoons or stage entertainment.

"How did that feel?" Kohen asked. I responded that I was shocked that my fingers would eventually touch despite my trying to resist. The only thing that surprised me more was seeing that in a room full of eager and engaged healthcare professionals, no one was smirking or rolling their eyes. Instead, they were taking notes.

Indeed, the large size of the crowd and its attentiveness was a testament to the growing popularity of clinical hypnosis and guided imagery workshops and the possibility that these strategies might actually work when relaxation, pain alleviation, or anxiety relief is the goal. But what does the evidence say? And is it enough to appease skeptics?

In 2014, Kohen published a review of clinical hypnosis in pediatrics and the positive effects on everything from headaches to pain and sleep. Hypnosis may also be used as an immune system suppressor in cases where autoimmunity is present, and as a pain modulator in breast cancer patients before and during surgery.

An expert in hypnosis for mental health, Dr. David Spiegel from Stanford University, describes hypnosis as a "state of highly focused attention [combined with] dissociation of competing thoughts and sensations toward the periphery of awareness and enhanced response to social cues." Spiegel has found that hypnosis works on specific brain areas that deal with attention and emotional control. People vary in their ability to be hypnotized, as suggestibility is a key component. There are specific areas of the brain—the dorsolateral prefrontal cortex and the dorsal anterior cingulate cortex, specifically—which may be downregulated during hypnosis to alleviate anxiety or pain. Indeed, the evidence suggests that medical hypnosis can help in the clinical context, specifically if it's led by an experienced facilitator.

*

Before his death in November 2020, Alex Trebek, long-time host of the popular television quiz show *Jeopardy*, credited his "optimistic mindset" with why he believed he would recover from stage-four pancreatic cancer. Though Trebek's mindset didn't save him from the devastating illness, researchers have not dismissed the possibility that he may have been onto something—and they have looked into the effects of mindset on illness with interesting results.

In 2019, researchers published in *The Journal of Allergy and Clinical Immunology: In Practice* results of a trial of oral immunotherapy for peanut allergy in children and teens, where psychological symptoms and bloodwork were obtained. During an explanation of some non-life-threatening symptoms that could result from the immunotherapy, half of the patients were told these were side effects, whereas the other half were told these symptoms signaled desensitization (that the treatment was working). After analyzing the data, the researchers found that the latter group was less anxious, less likely to miss doses of the immunotherapy, and, particularly interesting, they had higher protective antibodies (IgG4). Other studies have explored how patients feeling trust in the healthcare practitioner can show improved immune markers, such as CD4 cell count in HIV patients, common cold symptoms, and glycemic control in diabetes.

An analysis published in 2017 in the *British Medical Journal* expanded on this idea, looking more generally at how a patient's mindset could influence his or her health outcomes. The authors, all from Stanford University (including physician-author Abraham Verghese), wrote that "medical diagnoses and treatments are never isolated from patient mindsets and social context." The Stanford group found that these factors could be responsible for as much as 60% – 90% of clinical improvement, and they argued that randomized clinical trials often ignore these variables. As such, the idea of a "placebo effect" stems from much more than a sugar pill but can encompass a whole range of factors that can influence how patients view their treatment.

So, the question becomes whether the social and psychosocial aspects—namely, trust and mindset—can be harnessed to help patients heal. The Stanford team called for medical training programs to begin recognizing and appreciating these elements in order to influence the clinical encounters of future physicians. They also pressed for incorporating these factors into ongoing research and health systems reform, moving away from an emphasis on the traditional biomedical model of healing, which puts a heavy emphasis on matching symptoms to treatments such as medication or surgery, as opposed to addressing social and psychological factors.

In a commentary penned in 2006 and published in the *Journal of the American College of Cardiology*, Roy Ziegelstein, a cardiologist based at Johns Hopkins University Medical Center, found an inverse relationship between the very negative mindset associated with depression and adherence to cardiac medications. By addressing the patient's depression, adherence to the medication improves. Because of my experience in talking with Alex to find the root cause of their problem, I asked Ziegelstein how his research impacts the patient-doctor encounter. He believes that the shift towards patient-centered medicine, or placing the patient's needs before the competing demands from insurers and health systems, can foster better healing relationships between physicians and patients.

"There's no doubt that the mindset of a patient—of which trust in their doctor is one key part—can affect how they experience their care and treatment. The person's perception, and all of the behaviors that go along with it, can have a powerful effect on an outcome," Ziegelstein told me. Does the way in which "mind-body medicine" may work lead us to question how we understand the placebo effect?

5.

When researching the placebo effect, the name Ted Kaptchuk comes up time and again. Kaptchuk directs Harvard's Program in Placebo Studies at Beth

Israel Deaconess Medical Center in Boston. Trained in Chinese Medicine and acupuncture, he's not a typical Harvard academic. Nonetheless, with his colleagues, his multi-disciplinary research has revolutionized what is known about placebos. Specifically, his research findings, summarized in a 2008 *British Medical Journal* article and a 2015 article in *Trends in Molecular Medicine*, have shown that the placebo effect can be dose-dependent, that devices (such as acupuncture) may have a larger placebo effect compared with pills, and that some of us may be more genetically predisposed to this effect.

However, a review on sham spinal surgery is what may best help us understand the power of placebo. In 2017, a group of researchers from Iowa, Nevada, and Spain assessed a series of orthopedics trials that compared surgery with "sham surgery" (meaning the patient heads into the operating room, receives anesthesia, and is told they had surgery when, in fact, they didn't). That systematic review included six randomized control trials of procedures as diverse as knee arthroscopy, epicondylitis, and vertebroplasty, with 277 subjects, and found that sham surgery was just as effective as actual surgery in terms of reducing pain and disability.

Kaptchuk and others have commented on the ethics of such trials. Years earlier, in 2003, he had conducted his own trial, in which 262 irritable bowel syndrome (IBS) patients were assigned to one of three groups: the first were told to continue their regular routines for their IBS, the second received sham acupuncture with physician interaction limited to five minutes, and the third group received acupuncture with an augmented interaction with the physician of up to 45 minutes during which the physician asked the patient a series of questions aimed at building rapport and conveying empathy. The latter group did the best—improvements of up to 60%. Clearly, of the many contributors to the placebo effect, a meaningful interaction with the healthcare provider makes a powerful difference. More recently, in 2020, Kaptchuk's team found that providing a placebo to a patient can reduce opioid usage by 30% in post-lower back surgery pain management and that MRI may uncover brain areas involved in the placebo effect.

In an interview for NPR's "The Hidden Brain," Kaptchuk was careful to also point out that florid deception is not necessary (which he also wrote about) as the placebo effect can still work, even among patients who are told they are receiving the placebo.

"Everyone believed that deception or concealment is necessary for people to respond to placebo because the idea was, well, you fake people, you trick them; placebo's kind of this trickery," he said. This was backed by studies where "open-label" placebos (i.e., where the participant knew it was a placebo) were prescribed for everything from irritable bowel syndrome, chronic pain, and migraine to fatigue in cancer patients and menopausal hot flashes—and the placebo effect was still seen. In 2018, a group that included Kaptchuk convened to create a consensus report on placebo research. They agreed on one major thing: to inform patients better about placebo and nocebo effects.

So, asking whether mind-body approaches are placebo-like or not may be the incorrect question. Placebos work through the impact on the mind, demonstrating that our minds can, to an extent, create our reality, whether it's around pain perception or, even potentially, our immune system response. With Alex Trebek, even though he succumbed to his cancer, his outlook may have helped him feel healed in some respects — through an acceptance of his reality and peace that he reportedly exuded during his last days. Mindfulness-based approaches enhance a self-regulation function that soothes our responses to pain and suffering, allowing us to create a longer interval between stimulus and response. By definition, *this* is healing.

6.

Baja California is Mexico's most northern state. It's infamous for the popular tourist destination of Tijuana, which is right at the U.S.-Mexico border. About 320 kilometers south is a town called Todos Santos, and 10 kilometers northwest of that is a small village that doesn't even have its own name. It's become a hub for Yandara Yoga, an American-owned yoga teacher-training company. The timing worked out for me, so I applied, was accepted, and took the next flight out for nine days of no internet, full-immersion yoga, sunshine, and whatever else might fortify me.

Yoga is a word derived from the Sanskrit word "Yuj," meaning "yolk" or "join," so it effectively means "union" of the mind and body. Since researchers place the origins of yoga between 5-10,000 years ago, it is ironic that bringing the mind back into a body-focused system is only now a movement in the current Western healthcare system.

The local airport was sweltering and bustling. I strapped on my travel backpack with my yoga mat under one arm. Exchanging pleasantries with two other young women with yoga gear, we learned we were headed to the same place and boarded a public bus. The trek was frightening, as the driver took us down a narrow highway wedged between cliffs on one side and a massive drop on the other—at top speed. When the bus finally made its stop, we bounded out excitedly into the bright noon sunlight, relieved to have made it safely. I would learn when I met the other 15 women instructors, that we had all come both to teach this healing practice to others while healing ourselves.

One teacher was a 40-something divorcée from New Orleans who had recently left her abusive husband and needed a skill through which to rebuild her life. Another was a 50-something mother who sought a way to heal her spirit so she could be more present for her husband and six children after the tragic deaths of her brother and father. Then, there was Karine, a former navy officer who suffered from recurring nightmares that she was about to die. She became my closest friend during the training.

We would wake up at 5 am, do yoga from 5:30 am to 7 am, have yoga instruction, breakfast in silence, more yoga teaching until lunch, then free time until the afternoon yoga class, followed by more yoga teaching, dinner and an evening Satsang (spiritual teaching with music and chanting) before bed. With no internet and no phones permitted, our free time was restricted to reviewing the yoga lesson, sitting with our own thoughts, and bonding over the life challenges that brought us there. Karine kept reminding us of a saying from Alcoholics Anonymous: "If you want to avoid burnout, quit living your life like you're on fire." My experience in that one academic hospital was like being in the midst of a raging fire: stay and die a slow death from the smoke or fight it head-on and risk being burned alive.

Karine was from Nova Scotia, a tell-it-like-it-is, can-do woman who pursued a career in the Canadian Navy because she wanted to serve her country. We immediately hit it off. Like the rest of us, Karine was at a crossroads. She was recently in recovery for alcoholism. Life with her well-built Navy husband seemed perfect, except they had been struggling to conceive. "I feel like something is just wrong with me...with my body. It's not doing what it's supposed to do," she told me one evening on a beach walk.

At Yandara, Karine was working on a better sleep routine, eating more healthfully, and above all, addressing the stress she had built up in the Navy—all things she believed were impacting her ability to conceive. But the stress, Karine realized, could really be traced to so many issues sitting on top of one another. She was adopted but didn't know the circumstances of it until years later. Her birth mother had alcoholism, so Karine was born with mild fetal alcohol spectrum disorder, meaning that she struggled with emotional regulation and would often have angry outbursts. Her upbringing otherwise was healthy and secure, with an adoptive mother who loved her very much and her biological father, who stayed involved until he passed away when Karine was ten.

Along with hundreds of other Navy officers from Canada and around the world, Karine was dispatched to Haiti during the 2010 earthquake to provide humanitarian support and assist with rebuilding efforts. She was shocked to arrive in a place of such devastation. Buildings had crumbled, families were separated, and dead bodies were strewn on the streets. Crowds of Haitians lined up for jugs of water, food rations, and medical care. "It was just overwhelming," she told me. Rescue workers weren't sure where to begin. Where does *anyone* begin when an entire country has been brought to its knees?

One incident stuck out specifically. A young Haitian boy, maybe two or three years old, stood barefoot in the rubble that used to be the orphanage where he lived. His name was Nixon, and he wore only a soiled diaper. He was not crying or reaching out; he just stood there, stunned. Karine carried him out to a nearby camp. When it was time to board the bus heading back to the Navy quarters, she had a breakdown. "First, I couldn't breathe, then I couldn't stop crying," she said. She was evacuated out of Port-au-Prince the following day and saw a crisis psychiatrist. Karine's diagnosis: acute trauma, later manifesting formally as PTSD.

But there was also a personal connection she unearthed later.

"After I spoke with my mom and described that scene with the boy, she told me that it was similar to how they found me as an infant, with my birth mother having abandoned my brother and me to go on a drinking date," Karine recalled. "We'd been left alone for hours. My younger brother had a soiled diaper. So, I resonated with that boy in a way I didn't even realize at the time. Nixon held up a mirror that allowed me to recognize my own experience."

Karine employed numerous means to avoid a relapse into alcoholism, such as talk therapy and anti-anxiety medications. Eye Movement Desensitization and Reprocessing (EMDR) therapy was especially helpful. As evidence for other forms of PTSD suggests, the eyes and the mind are connected. The eyes, I learned in anatomy class, are really just an extension of our brains, made of the same embryonic tissue and exhibiting the same tissue layers. Karine's personal experience affirmed the research stating that meditation can be harmful for those with PTSD.

"Meditation…I just couldn't do it. It just made the thoughts worse, like I couldn't escape," Karine said. But yoga, which is effectively meditation through action, where the focus is on the breath while moving the body and holding positions, was a way to get re-centered and calm her erratic nervous system. "Regular practice allowed me to channel the anxiety in a different way. That's why I was drawn to it," Karine said, "and why going deeply into it over those few weeks meant so much." A few months after we left, Karine would share that she left her emotionally abusive marriage after uncovering a web of lies (including infidelity) by her former husband. So, in a sense, her dreams made sense. A death was near—her old life was making way for the new. A year later, she met someone else, and they conceived a child almost immediately.

It seems a stretch to credit yoga alone with such a reversal of fortune in anyone's health. But as a practice meant to mend the gaps that so often form among mind, spirit, and body, yoga is frequently credited with working wonders for people hoping to heal from an unexpected and unpleasant detour in life—a community I was now a part of. That promise of what might be possible through yoga is part of its popularity, but is there science to support the claims made of its healing effects?

*

In recent years, several academics have explored the impact of yoga on healing, from the impact on reducing depressive symptoms in adults and children to blood pressure improvement. A Cochrane review of yoga for breast cancer patients found it reduced fatigue and improved health-related quality of life compared to education or psychosocial interviews, but that similar results were achieved with any regular exercise.

There is also moderate evidence for yoga benefits in kids with Attention-Deficit/ Hyperactivity Disorder (ADHD)—such as improvements in attentiveness and impulsivity. But as with research in mindfulness, the limitations are widespread. It's difficult to study yoga in a controlled way, given the variability of practice. Related to that difficulty is the challenge of comparing studies as in a meta-analysis or review. There is evidence for breathwork, for instance, but breathwork is also taught in diving and in the military, so teasing this out from any other effects of yoga is problematic.

I realized yoga and medicine were similar in many ways—both are governed by "do no harm" ("ahimsa" in yoga; the Hippocratic Oath in medicine) and involve understanding the union of mind and body. As I prepared to leave Yandara, I felt more at peace with my situation. I knew I could handle it. I spent the last evening with the other newly trained yoginis in the ocean, under the full moon: a community I felt truly connected to due to our shared desire for healing, knowing we would all be re-entering our lives back home. I would cherish those weeks together for years.

7.

Upon returning to the hospital, I sought guidance from Dr. Bends, the psychiatrist described in the introduction, to better understand the challenges I was experiencing with focus and emotional regulation. Dr. Bends worked extensively with healthcare professionals and provided valuable insights. Through careful evaluation, he identified the underlying issue as work-related anxiety and depression.

In a detailed report, Dr. Bends outlined the cognitive difficulties I was facing—trouble concentrating, irritability, and hypervigilance. He noted that these symptoms were closely tied to the specific conditions of my work environment, which placed significant demands on individuals, including extended hours, frequent overnight duties and various forms of workplace bullying that include florid harassment and incivility on top of excessive and unfair scrutiny. His recommendation was clear: it was important for my well-being to consider moving to a healthier professional setting, one more conducive to long-term personal and professional growth.

Anxiety and depression can also induce an inflammatory response that can impact other aspects of physical health—especially heart health. My high cholesterol was due to many factors certainly, but the stress was a likely contributor, for reasons that include the impact the stress hormone cortisol, as well as epinephrine (adrenaline), has on cholesterol. These hormones can increase cholesterol directly or indirectly through the increase in fatty substances called triglycerides.*

I also consulted with a physician from a broader program focused on physician health, who reviewed Dr. Bends' findings and conducted his own thorough evaluation. In his detailed report, he concluded that my symptoms were tied to the stress I had experienced in my work environment, compounded by the intense scrutiny I had faced. Like the other professionals I had consulted, he

---

* Mental health plays a critical role in cardiovascular health. Chronic stress, anxiety, and depression can negatively impact cardiovascular disease (CVD) and elevate ApoB levels, which are a marker of cardiovascular risk. Stress can lead to unfavorable lipid balance by promoting unhealthy behaviors (like poor diet and smoking), increasing inflammation, and worsening metabolic health (Assadi 2017: https://www.ncbi.nlm.nih.gov/pmc/articles/PMC5419930/).

recommended transitioning to a healthier setting, confident that I would thrive in a less toxic, more supportive environment. His validation was reassuring, and his report provided valuable support in helping me move toward a new chapter in my career.

Meeting Alex taught me the importance of how reframing one's reality—through the connection made with a healthcare provider who genuinely sees you—can be a pivotal step toward healing. Research professor and bestselling author Brené Brown has reported that leaders, in order to lead effectively, must care for those they lead. If a leader approaches others with envy, animosity, or anger, it becomes nearly impossible to lead with integrity. In my interaction with Alex, I saw this concept in action. By being present and empathetic, I was able to create a space where Alex felt truly seen. This connection allowed Alex to confront a personal truth that had felt overwhelming and dangerous—a truth that had driven them to endure unnecessary risks within a healthcare system that prioritized physical scans over meaningful engagement with the mind.

Now that I understood what was happening in both my mind and body, I focused on getting myself ready for what might come next and occupied myself with other meaningful pursuits. The latter was inspired in large part by the book *Man's Search for Meaning* by Viktor Frankl. Frankl, also a physician, found himself in the most horrific environment—a Holocaust concentration camp in the late 1930s. If Frankl was able to reframe his situation and tell himself that he would get out and that his time in the concentration camp was part of a larger purpose for his life, then certainly I could handle everything I was facing.

His book only further underscored for me the mind's power as a vessel for healing. We know that often we must change our environments to feel better and be more whole. But Frankl shows us that when external change *isn't* a choice, our mind can become our escape and our salvation. Inspired by Frankl's wisdom and my own appreciation for the mind-body connection, I realized there was only one solution to my problem: change my situation before it *changed me*.

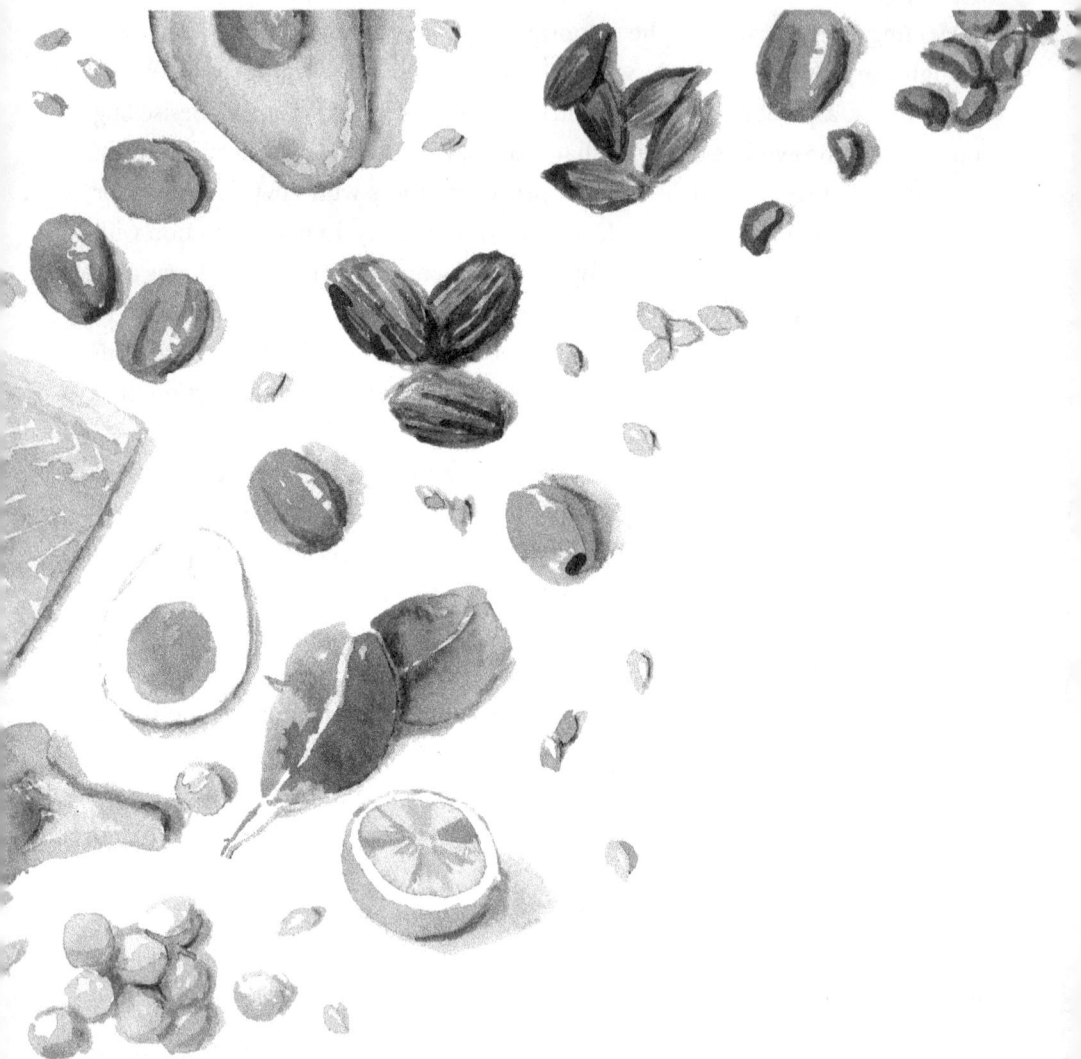

CHAPTER SIX

Nourished

"I imagine one of the reasons people cling to their hates so stubbornly is because they sense, once hate is gone, they will be forced to deal with pain."
— James Baldwin, *Notes of a Native Son*

1.

Surgeons have the best knife skills. They spend years honing their technique in operating rooms (OR), learning to slice through tissue while avoiding precious blood vessels and nerves, and, when it comes to the more advanced surgeons, cut in ways that minimize scarring—a huge step up from our amateur dissections of Joe, the cadaver. Surgery can seem an art more than a science, and one surgeon suggested to me that it is, in many ways, more like sculpting than "medicine, which relies mostly on the mind."

"Few things are as satisfying as cutting something out and knowing the patient never has to worry about it," he told me.

I thought back wistfully to a culinary medicine course I'd signed up for in Napa Valley, California, where I witnessed a surgeon, who hailed from Alaska, meticulously dice an onion. By contrast, my roughly chopped onions left something to be desired. Or perhaps they were just "artisanal," I told myself.

I was there to learn with 100 other physicians and surgeons, some still in training but most well established in their careers, about bringing cooking, as well as basic dietary advice, into the patient encounter. The old stereotype of the overweight internist recommending that their obese patient "just eat better," then returning to the box of donuts on their own desk, is based in reality. Whether it was on the ward, ER, or the staff lounge, high glycemic index foods were everywhere. They provide quick jolts of energy and a dopamine hit when you're swamped with stressful encounters and don't have enough time to grab a healthier option, something that doesn't fare well while managing cholesterol and lipid issues.

In medical school, nutrition was perhaps just two hours of our curriculum and restricted primarily to the biochemistry of various compounds. It was pitiful, but with everything we needed to learn to prepare for our clerkship years (the last two years of medical school, when we are in the hospital), how would there be time to learn about nutrition? After all, isn't that where dieticians come in? What nobody considered was that training in nutrition might help us better prepare for our clerkships, and it would also make us more effective as healers.

The Napa program is run by a physician named David Eisenberg, who is based at Harvard Medical School. He has seen interest in the field of culinary medicine grow over the past decade. Culinary medicine is defined as a field that blends the art of cooking with medical science. It's well established that medical school fails to provide doctors with sufficient skills and knowledge to counsel patients on nutrition. And even those medical specialties in which nutrition plays a large role in management of disease, like gastroenterology and cardiology, don't provide more than cursory nutrition training. Thankfully, the culinary medicine movement is closing that gap by teaching doctors how nutrition can be used to improve health outcomes for a whole host of diseases—everything from diabetes to heart disease to obesity. The field is gaining ground and respectability.

Research shows that training physicians in nutrition is good for patients—for instance, we know that what doctors believe about diseases like obesity influences how they counsel their patients. With obesity, there can be bias towards seeing it as the patient's fault—i.e., the patient eats too much and lacks self-control.

What literature on weight now suggests is that it's largely secondary to a biological setpoint and less about willpower. Setpoint theory holds that a pre-set weight baseline is hardwired into our DNA, so how much our weight changes from that set point can be limited. Diet and access to healthful foods play a role in ensuring we stay within our setpoints.

Even knowing how to cook can impact how effective a doctor's nutrition counseling is. This then trickles down to patients making better dietary choices. For instance, one study found that participating in a culinary medicine training program led to doctors being more confident in cooking and in assessing and advising patients on dietary habits.

*

At my alma mater, the University of Toronto, Dr. David Jenkins, who invented the glycemic index, has taken the lead in teaching medical students about healthful eating and how to understand nutritional labels. Jenkins himself had a unique foray into medicine, which influenced his interest in how nutrition can heal us. As a child growing up in England, he was labeled as less studious at the various private schools he attended in Sussex and Essex. His father was a surgeon, his mother a homemaker, and his grandmother nurtured young David's curiosity. At the age of 12, his family moved to Sydney, Australia, where a high school tutor suggested he apply to do scientific research after he graduated. "My father had always said there were a lot of things that medicine hadn't quite sorted out yet," he recalled. Jenkins' father, by the way, had switched to psychiatry from surgery—almost unheard of at the time, which suggests that an interest in the whole person was perhaps ingrained in this family of healers.

Later enrolled at Oxford, Jenkins met a professor who offered him a job to assist with his research. "The professor saw it as a challenge for him to teach me—a young boy who didn't know much about science or mechanisms," recalled Jenkins. "And then one day, he walked me over to the medical school, and I started taking classes." As a medical student, Jenkins noticed, "Diet seemed to have a large effect on health, so why not explore that?"

In 1981, Jenkins published a landmark paper in the *American Journal of Clinical Nutrition* describing the glycemic index for the first time. In that study, Jenkins and his group fed volunteers who had fasted for several hours 62 different foods and measured their blood glucose over a two-hour period. They shared the data as a percentage of the area under the glucose response curve, effectively comparing it to the same amount of carbohydrate if it was taken as a simple sugar.

Surprisingly, some vegetables spiked quickly—specifically carrots, followed by common packaged breakfast cereals and white rice. Dried legumes had the smallest rise in sugar. Notably, fat and protein sources resulted in a negligible increase. Jenkins has published widely since then—most prominently, the results of a large randomized controlled trial in *JAMA* in 2008, which involved randomizing 210 subjects with Type 2 diabetes to either a low-glycemic index or high-cereal fiber diet. The HbA1C (which is a marker of glucose control) decreased significantly in the group on the low glycemic-index diet, and good cholesterol (HDL cholesterol) increased, suggesting this diet was a useful intervention for those with Type 2 diabetes. Later, Jenkins adapted these principles to the Portfolio diet, which is a vegetarian diet high in fiber and plant-based cholesterols called sterols.

Specifically for cholesterol, I followed the evidence that foods with soluble fiber reduce cholesterol by binding it. Guided by Jenkins's findings, I ensured I'd have 45g of nuts (almonds) daily, 50g of plant protein (soy, beans, lentils), viscous fiber (okra, oatmeal, strawberries), and plant forms of cholesterol (plant-based yogurt), all of which provide polyunsaturated fats and directly lower LDL. I added almonds, lentils, black beans (soluble fiber), and oats (soluble fiber) most mornings, with foods fortified with sterols and stanols to help with cholesterol absorption.

Jenkins had something to offer both my concerns—my cholesterol, if the dietary changes helped, and my concerns about medical culture. He has become increasingly interested in exploring how medical students lose their ability to think differently and whether the system itself selects for conformists. In 2020, he published a paper looking at the greatest medical innovators, concluding most had, like himself, an unconventional path.

2.

The tale of scurvy might have been one of the first to demonstrate the impact of nutrition on healing. As the story goes, it was the mid-1700s, and France and Spain were at war (the War of Austrian Succession). Scottish-born Dr. James Lind, a junior doctor at the time, was given the title of ship surgeon on the HMS Salisbury, which patrolled the English Channel. By then, it was well known that sailors would suffer from an unusual disease that led to bleeding gums, weakness, and pallor secondary to anemia—it was named "scurvy." It wasn't clear what was causing this: the emerging theory was that it could be prevented by administering substances with a low pH, as in acids.

On May 20, 1747, Lind conducted an experiment—a dozen sailors were ill with scurvy, and he divided them into pairs, with each pair getting either one dose of cider, sulfuric acid, vinegar, seawater, a laxative to induce vomiting, or two oranges and a lemon between them. They were replenished daily. After six days, it was clear that only the last pair improved significantly—they were more energetic, the bleeding had stopped, and their skin color and laxity had been restored.

But this is where Lind's contribution has been overstated: he didn't *actually* draw the association between citrus (or later vitamin C) and the improvement of scurvy. Instead, he presumed the disease was multifactorial, but that diet seemed to have made a difference. Unfortunately, when Lind tried to package the citrus as juice, he unknowingly boiled off all of the vitamin C. This juice was limited in effectiveness when provided to scurvy-affected sailors, and he wasn't able to see the association—because there wasn't one! *

It was also perhaps a case of something lost in translation—citrus as the cure for scurvy was apparently known as far back as 1497 by Vasco da Gama from Portugal, and as recently as 1614 when John Woodall, also from England, wrote in his manual *The Surgeon's Mate* that oranges, lemons, limes, and tamarinds would help symptoms of scurvy. The sad part is because of

---

* Years later, the Bradford Hill Criteria expanded on causality in research studies through nine points. These are strength, consistency, specificity, temporality, biological gradient, plausibility, coherence, experiment, and analogy.

Lind's actual failure to draw the link, citrus was not widely recommended as a treatment until fully a year after Lind died—in 1795. He also died being dubbed one of the first to devise clinical trials, even though that, too, was incorrect. Nothing was logged in the HMS Salisbury logbooks, which were meticulously kept. In fact, the disease scurvy wasn't even documented, so whether Lind even conducted the trial in the first place is debatable. So, Lind's legacy may simply have been that he helped establish that foods impact healing, regardless of whether he was fully aware of the association or not. Criticism aside, in the United Kingdom, the James Lind Alliance (JLA) is a key funder of research studies that aim to address various areas of uncertainty in medicine and science.

Some time has passed since Lind sailed the English Channel, and evidence has emerged that other diseases may benefit from dietary changes, even when medication is needed too. Most prominently, Type 2 diabetes, which is a lifestyle disease, can be reversed through diet, primarily by adding in more complex carbohydrates and fiber. The impact of nutritional changes on heart disease and hypercholesterolemia is also clear —and, of course, it was the latter that got me interested in the link in the first place. For instance, the renowned BROAD Study, based in New Zealand, randomized 65 patients with obesity, heart disease, or diabetes to normal care or to a whole foods-plant-based diet with a vitamin B12 supplement. At the six-month mark, BMI was significantly lower in the intervention group; cholesterol was only slightly so. However, by 12 months, cholesterol was significantly lower.

If I could avoid taking a statin in my early 30s, I'd be much better off, knowing that the potential side effects of muscle breakdown (and pain associated with it) could be challenging. The evidence on nutrition's role in healing is less clear for mental health disorders, chronic pain, cognitive diseases (like Alzheimer's), and inflammatory conditions like rheumatoid arthritis, but this may improve in the coming years.

The research convinced me to at least consider reducing high-glycemic foods that might contribute to high cholesterol, not necessarily eggs or cheese, upon Jenkins advice (which Jenkins suggested to me over a vegan lunch in Toronto afterward; he had been vegan well before it was a trend!). It also meant greatly reducing or avoiding pasta and closely following the Portfolio diet. Within a few weeks, I had more energy and fewer mid-day crashes. I was less anxious, too—but there could have been another reason for that.

*

Chris arrived at Toronto's Pearson International Airport on a Thursday afternoon. Our correspondence over the previous months had turned into a genuine connection, and he shared that he had fallen in love with me. He planned an evening with dinner and a lovely hotel, and there was incredible conversation, which included his sharing things he couldn't on the phone. I was able to share more about my challenges over the previous year. "You must use it as fuel," he said. Chris was unwavering. He didn't seem to care that much of my life was in a state of uncertainty.

While I hadn't been looking for a relationship, the bond between Chris and me grew quickly and deeply. He became my closest confidant, and I, his. I thought I could handle everything life had thrown at me on my own, but I quickly realized that it was much better shouldered with another—and Chris was only too eager to do that.

Two weeks later, he had to return to Geneva as the Syrian refugee crisis in southern Europe was beginning to worsen. He was needed by his U.N. agency to capture data and stories from the field. So, he left for Greece, and we became separate again. "I'm still with you, though — stay strong. I know another opportunity will open up, and this will all be in the rearview mirror. I love you," he said before he left. If only I had known of the roadblocks ahead, but at that point, perhaps ignorance was its own kind of bliss.

3.

Meeting Nira Kehar at her parents' house in St. Adolphe, just outside of Montreal, in the Spring of 2019, I was taken aback by her kindness. Kehar was a chef interested in Ayurvedic medicine, and I had recently picked up her cookbook, *Ojas*. Being South Asian myself, Ayurvedic principles had been a subtle force growing up, especially with my mother making Ayurvedic-based teas when we were fighting off childhood colds, much like how chicken soup serves that role. But with physician parents, it was never front and center. I had read about the doshas, categories of regulatory principles of mind, body, and behavior, and was once labeled a "pitta," meaning "fire" (which might match my "fiery" spirit, perhaps!) by an Ayurvedic practitioner while I was in college.

Food remains a central part of Ayurveda. There are certain foods that are better for different doshas. For instance, as a pitta, cooling foods may be best. But that said, sparse evidence supports eating in an "ayurvedic" way. The one exception is turmeric, which is traditionally used in South Asian and Ayurvedic cuisine. The active ingredient in turmeric, curcumin, has now been studied as a tonic for various ailments, especially rheumatoid arthritis. But any benefit from curcumin would require a much higher dose than typically found in cooking. As Kehar made me an Ayurvedic dish—Kitchuri—I asked why she left a promising career as a James Beard award-winning chef.

"I had breast cancer," she said, almost stone-faced. She was just a few years older than me—how on earth could she have had breast cancer? I thought back to the breast cancer patients I had seen in medical school—none were younger than 45.

Kehar filled me in on more details. She'd run several busy pop-up restaurants in Manhattan. Word got around, and she was invited to cook at the James Beard Foundation in New York. But feeling the pull to India, she gave up New York for New Delhi and opened a restaurant called Chez Nini. "It was what you might call 'nouveau cuisine,' which is essentially French technique combined with my imagination and experience," she said. Chez Nini was one of the most successful restaurants in New Delhi with waiting lists that would number in the 10s to 100s over time. "We'd seat Bollywood actors one evening and a group of expats another," she told me. It was supposed to only be for one year, but she fell in love, got married, and stayed for almost nine years.

One day, just as *Ojas* was published and Kehar was gearing up for her book tour, she began feeling extremely tired and was unsure if it was her erratic sleep schedule or something else. She saw her doctor, who then ordered a scan.

A mammogram identified a mass in her breast, and the pathology results soon determined that it was an aggressive form of breast cancer.

"Suddenly this body that I believed was like totally invincible gave in… And there were so many confusing messages …So of course I had to think of surviving in a way. I knew that I had to take care of my mind. I knew I had to just stay calm." She told me she started to listen to what was happening in her body. "Even when my facilities were weakening and everything, it was just like, 'What is happening here at a deeper level?' I got a chance to really put on the brakes and slow down."

Within months of her March 2018 diagnosis, she began chemotherapy in New Delhi. Sadly, her marriage dissolved, and she returned to Montreal, where her treatment continued. She was familiar with cooking in an Ayurvedic way, and sensing the need to feed her besieged body in a way that was more "pure," she began adhering more strictly to that way of eating.

Kehar incorporated Ayurvedic practices into her cooking, using "cooling" foods for some constitutions and "warming" foods for others. The Ayurvedic way remains a common approach in India and increasingly in the West as a way to balance doshas. Though evidence for the value of Ayurvedic medicine is sparse, there are findings relating curcumin in turmeric, a key spice in Ayurvedic cooking, to improvements in inflammatory conditions such as arthritis. "But then one day, my friend told me about some work her friend, a researcher, was doing on intermittent fasting and that this friend had just written a book," Kehar shared.

The researcher friend turned out to be Dr. Valter Longo, an Italian scientist. Kehar bought his book, called *The Longevity Diet*, and began reading about how fasting could help cancer patients and, specifically, how Longo's trials seemed to show that a specific regimen of fasting just before and after chemotherapy helped improve the effectiveness of the treatment.

"So that's effectively what I did—I would fast 48 hours before, go to chemo, fast another 24 hours, and slowly introduce food again," Kehar said.

Many cancer patients understand the unique cohort they become part of during therapy: often the regimen of chemotherapy is so strict that they see the same people at every visit. At one Montreal hospital where Kehar received most of her care, she began noticing that the others in her cohort seemed more exhausted, had lost more of their hair, and just appeared more ill than she was feeling herself.

"I was convinced that maybe this diet was helping. Even my doctor was impressed," Kehar told me. By the time we met in 2019, her cancer was in remission. And like a storybook ending, she met a Danish musician and got re-married. Her eyes lit up, sharing that last piece of good news as we walked along to the dock in front of her parents' house in rural Quebec to look out onto the lake—Lac Gemont. She currently resides in Copenhagen, Denmark and is working on a jewelry line that combines unique metals with Ayurvedic principles. Creative pursuits, whether designing or creating recipes, were a core part of her healing, not unlike the role narrative medicine plays for doctors.

"I use the creativity of my restaurant to heal my heart and…when you get so practical and you go about the business of healing yourself with something very external like [chemotherapy], your internal world still needs you. … to heal everything now," Kehar said.

Viewing nutrition as part of healing is not without controversy. So-called nutritionists and self-proclaimed wellness gurus with no background in science plug everything from juice detoxes to highly restrictive "raw foods" diets that omit many macronutrients and micronutrients. It's an incredibly touchy area of healthcare—and a booming industry.

One extreme example of the damage that can be done by a highly restrictive diet involves a case in Ontario, Canada, where an 11-year-old cancer patient, "J.J.," with acute lymphoblastic leukemia (ALL), was offered an extreme diet regimen from a group based in Florida. Her parents refused the recommended chemotherapy at a children's hospital, and it emerged that the Indigenous community from which she hailed had received a visit from the Florida diet group, which charged thousands of dollars for their proprietary raw food and juice treatments. The patient died, and the hospital took the parents to court over negligence.

There have been countless other cases, many making the news. An angry op-ed in STAT News entitled "No Food Isn't Medicine" attempted to course-correct the influence of these harmful diet approaches. It was overly simplistic and reductionist, as it didn't address that food does indeed impact how we prevent disease and also, in some cases, how we *heal* from it—whether it's correcting a nutritional deficiency or working in tandem with conventional approaches to help amplify the impact of the medicine. We only need to look back at the story of scurvy as early evidence for the role of nutrition in healing, even if Lind didn't quite know it yet.

Kehar had me thinking as we got up from the dock. "You know, I wrote an entire article two years ago that explained that special diets for cancer patients are bad news. You've now prompted me to re-examine this," I told her sheepishly.

The article was in the *Toronto Star* in 2017, but my focus was more on the harms of extreme diets and those who capitalize on the vulnerability of cancer patients and their families. I concluded that great caution was needed before we made any grand claims about the role of diet and cancer. "You need to speak to Valter then," she advised, as we made our way back to her parents' house. "He might change your mind."

4.

Milan is known for many things, primarily fashion. Perhaps that's why Dr. Valter Longo looked more stylish than the average scientist during our lunch meeting. Outfitted in a black dress shirt with a neatly tailored lab coat bearing his name, Longo's accent was markedly Italian with some Texan inflections. His lush chocolate-colored hair, which was mildly streaked with grey, was coiffed like a model in an Italian shampoo commercial.

Longo has a lab in Los Angeles, based at the University of Southern California (USC), and one in Milan, at the Instituto FIRC di Oncologia Molecolare (IFOM) Cancer Institute in Milan, one of the most prestigious cancer institutes in Europe. Longo was born in Liguria, a small coastal town in northwestern Italy, and he grew up with the classic seafood-rich Mediterranean diet. He would spend summers with his grandparents in Calabria, his days filled with play and exploring. Later, as a teenage Jimmy Hendrix fan, he convinced his parents to send him to Chicago to live with relatives so that he could take guitar lessons with the renowned Steve Piers in Maywood, Illinois. Longo completed high school in the U.S. and was drawn to the University of North Texas (UNT) performing arts school with the goal of becoming a musician. Then, as now, he had the coiffed hair for it—but not the patience. When a professor told Longo that, instead of playing guitar, he needed to lead the school's marching band, he switched his major.

In his third year of biochemistry, and already working in the lab of a professor who studied aging, Longo met Robert Grasey, one of the leading researchers in the field. So, Longo would drive 60 miles roundtrip between UNT and Fort Worth just to work in his lab, studying protein modifications in aging cells. In 1994, at the age of 26, he found an error with a paper published in the 1950s, which was still influencing the work of many researchers. It described the lifespan of yeast but measured aging by counting the number of daughter cells generated by the mother cell, assuming that if the mother produced 25 daughter cells, it would mean it reached a lifespan of 25. This didn't make sense to him, so he came up with a different term called the "chronological lifespan" of yeast, which later allowed him to discover the genes regulating aging and, later, the effect of fasting on aging and cellular protection.

By 2006, years after completing his Ph.D. and starting a lab of his own, Longo submitted a paper looking at intermittent fasting as part of a cancer protocol. The editors were welcoming, but one reviewer, an oncologist who remained anonymous, took issue with the potential paradigm-shifting results. "I still have that reviewer's comments," Longo said with a smile. The paper was ultimately rejected and submitted to another journal, but not before *Science* magazine quoted an oncologist from Memorial Sloan Kettering Cancer Center in New York poking fun at Longo's work.

The paper was eventually published but in a lower-tier journal. "I still think about what might have happened had the paper been accepted. *Nature* as a journal is top tier, so we might have been that much further ahead than we are now," he said. By the time I spoke to Longo in 2020, the benefits to cancer patients of intermittent fasting were no longer news—institutions like

UCSF and Mayo Clinic and, yes, even Sloan Kettering were all reaching out to collaborate with Longo on clinical trials.

Fasting is thought to induce and activate pathways in the cells that help ward off stress, but it can also improve immune system regulation and increase the production of stem cells. The way Longo described it to me was that we must imagine that when fasting, we stop providing nutrients to our cells, and so they must change how they function. Some cells stop growing, others become smaller, and still others die. The cells in the liver, for instance, begin making more sugar to ensure the brain has enough fuel, but the brain's cells (neurons) also adapt to need less sugar and rely on a different sort of fuel, specifically ketone bodies, which are made from fat.

"In general, there is an evolution of the function of many cells, including stem cells, which are active but stand by waiting for food to return to begin the regeneration and replacement of many cells lost during fasting," Longo told me.

But it was an analogy he provided about gladiators that cemented it for me, remembering that a hallmark of cancer, as per a famous 1980 paper authored by Douglas Hanahan and Robert Weinberg published in *Cell* (but updated in 2011), includes cells unresponsive to anti-growth signals. Usually, when we think of cancer therapy, we imagine something like precision bombing used in war to selectively target cancer cells. The problem is that it's rarely as precise as we like. Healthy cells are often affected, which leads to side effects such as fatigue and hair loss. In intermittent fasting, it's more like imagining cancer cells and healthy cells as part of two armies that speak two languages—one Latin and one Greek. Imagine telling the healthy army that understands and speaks Latin to put their shields up and kneel. The cancer army will not do that, so automatically, it's easy to identify them and target the therapy. The fasting protocol effectively sends this signal to the healthy cells to get into protection mode, whereas the cancer cells don't get this signal, so they're affected and starved of nutrients, meaning that the chemotherapy works that much better.

Yet Longo shares that it is difficult to shift the thinking among oncologists: "It's a little like if you imagine putting 100 people in a desert with no water or shade. Sun is the targeted therapy, and water is the sustenance. The people most likely to survive without water or shade are the ones who stay still and conserve their energy. Cancer can't stop running because of unrestricted growth signals, so they don't last as long; the other healthy cells last longer," Longo told me. "What most oncologists do is feel pressure to feed their patients. What this does is fuel the cancer, so it persists. A fasting protocol gets the healthy cells to protect their energy and lets the cancer exhaust itself so that it becomes more responsive to chemotherapy."

In a study included in *Nature Communications* in 2020, Longo, with the Dutch Breast Cancer Research Group, published results from the DIRECT trial, which involved randomizing 131 patients with HER-2 negative stage 2/3 breast cancer (they excluded those who had diagnosed diabetes) to receive a fasting-mimicking-diet (FMD) or regular diet for three days before and during neoadjuvant chemotherapy. The results were remarkable. It appeared the FMD group had a partial response and that the 99-100% tumor cell loss (a system called the "Miller & Payne" response*) was more likely to occur in patients on FMD. It was also found to curtail the DNA damage that is seen in T-lymphocyte cells (see Chapter 2 on DNA damage and repair), and notably the side effects between the two groups were not significant.

Physician-writer Siddhartha Mukherjee has explored other ways diet might benefit cancer patients. His lab looked at low-carbohydrate ketogenic diets in combination with a cancer drug, effectively to decrease the amount of insulin released. For some cancers they tested, tumor growth seemed to be hindered by diet alone, but for other cancers, like leukemia, the cancer grew faster on the diet but was kept at bay with the combination of diet and drug. A review published in the December 2019 issue of the *New England Journal of Medicine* suggested that researchers like Longo and Mukherjee could be on to something: "Evidence is accumulating that eating in a 6-hour period and fasting for 18 hours can trigger a metabolic switch from glucose-based to ketone-based energy, with increased stress resistance, increased longevity, and a decreased incidence of diseases, including cancer and obesity."

---

* The Miller-Payne response is a histopathological grading system used to assess the effectiveness of neoadjuvant chemotherapy in breast cancer by comparing pre-treatment and post-treatment tumor cellularity. It grades the response from 1 (no change) to 5 (complete response with no residual invasive cancer).

There are qualifiers on the good news about fasting, however. Most of the more robust research on Intermittent Fasting (IF) has been completed in mouse or rat models, with only a few small trials in humans. There is also no standard protocol for IF. It could mean restricting the eating window between 4 hours and 12 hours a day. There is some evidence for IF in weight loss, cholesterol and sugar modulation, and blood pressure improvement.

These advances were only possible because Longo wasn't easily discouraged. "I'm not a follower. And that's probably what inspired me about Hendrix. He believed in his music, even when the U.S. wasn't ready. He was okay with moving to Europe where they understood his style, instead of waiting for the U.S. to catch up, which they did eventually," Longo said. "I guess I'm more drawn to what isn't so accepted yet. They say that some of us write chapters in history, so maybe that's the drive."

Longo is now shifting to apply his IF protocol for multiple sclerosis and Type 1 diabetes. But he is most excited about the application to Alzheimer's disease—the idea that fasting kickstarts the body's natural repair process and that this can also apply to our brains. This reminded me of the first time I began wondering about the connection between nutrition and the brain.

5.

Bobby's brown hair skirted across his forehead as he played with the Lego. His fringe was cut unevenly, which I would later learn was because he had trouble sitting still for a haircut. I was in a clinic with Dr. Sandy Newmark, a pediatrician who runs the Osher Center for Integrative Medicine, based at the University of California San Francisco. Newmark is an expert in autism and attention deficit hyperactivity disorder (ADHD), and many of his patients are children of bigwig Silicon Valley types. I was there to work with him for two weeks and learn about integrative methods to manage child development-related concerns. My developmental pediatrics experience, led by several excellent attendings, had taught me a lot. Yet, I was curious to learn about the effects of elements like nutrition and sleep on developing minds, as well as the benefits of (and evidence behind) emerging therapies.

Bobby was nine years old and enrolled in a Montessori school in the Bay area. His ADHD was diagnosed by his general pediatrician a year earlier, and he had tried methylphenidate (commonly in the form of the brand name Ritalin or the longer-acting Concerta or Biphentin) with some improvement, but he still struggled to sit still in school and would often blurt things out without waiting his turn. Now, some of this would not be unusual if he were younger, but at nine, most children understand social norms, especially at school. At home, things weren't much better. He'd often interrupt at the dinner table and would have to eat his meals in two or three bites at a time and then do something else and return to the table. His brain was having trouble paying attention, and he was here because his parents wanted to ask Newmark about increasing his medication dosage.

After watching Bobby play, then interviewing his parents and Bobby himself, Newmark made some suggestions. The boy's typical breakfast was cereal or a bagel with jam, and lunch was a sandwich with ham, which he would barely eat. Since his attention issues were affecting his schooling, Newmark recommended that his mornings start with things that were good for his blood sugar—things that wouldn't cause him to crash, such as eggs, steel-cut oatmeal, and avocado, for instance. Lunch could include a sandwich, but made on whole wheat bread and balanced with healthier unsaturated fats such as almond butter or another form of protein like tuna, which was less processed than ham. Newmark's advice was, by the way, aligned with Jenkins' work on the glycemic index. Newmark wanted Bobby to try a lower glycemic index, higher fat, and higher protein diet. Of course, Bobby would have to enjoy these foods, or he simply wouldn't eat. A week later, during a follow-up visit, Bobby was already showing improvements in his attention, which was heartening. He still required medication, but the previously suggested increase to his medication dose wasn't ultimately needed.

*

Evidence affirms a connection between high glycemic foods and our mental focus. A 2020 meta-analysis and systematic review of seven studies found a positive correlation between sugar ingestion (via added sugar and sugar-sweetened beverages) and ADHD symptoms, but as with most systematic reviews, there were limitations related to the studies not being easily comparable: the term is called "heterogeneity."

The SMILES (Supporting the Modification of Lifestyle in Lowered Emotional States) Trial, led by Felice Jacka of Deakin University in Australia, is probably one of the most compelling studies linking nutrition with our mental well-being. This trial was a 12-week investigation of dietary intervention in the treatment of moderate to severe depression. The intervention consisted of seven individual nutritional consulting sessions delivered by a clinical dietician. Depression symptoms were the primary endpoint diagnosis being studied, assessed using the Montgomery-Åsberg Depression Rating Scale (MADRS) at 12 weeks. Secondary outcomes included remission and change of symptoms, mood, and anxiety. The study, published in 2017, found that participants who received the dietary intervention showed significantly greater improvements in depression symptoms compared to the control group. Additionally, the dietary intervention group had higher rates of remission and reported overall improvements in mood and anxiety levels. These findings suggest that dietary changes can be an effective adjunct treatment for depression.

What exactly is the *mechanism* between food and mood? It may, in part, be due to the impact on our blood sugar, but it also may be related to neurotransmitters and how they relate to our microbiome. Well over 95% of the neurotransmitter serotonin, which is responsible for regulating appetite, mood, pain experience, and sleep, is made in the gastrointestinal tract. Until recently, we didn't know that the tract is lined with neurons and produces neurotransmitters. This is where the microbiome of the gut comes in: good bacteria protect the intestinal lining and prevent inflammation while also allowing for optimal nutrient absorption from food.

More generally, the field of "nutritional psychiatry" is gaining ground as it recognizes that our mood responds to the fuel we feed our brains. Low-grade fuel, like junk food, is calorie-rich but nutrient-poor compared with whole foods that include vitamins, minerals, and antioxidants. Refined sugars can impair brain function and result in inflammation, insulin regulation issues, and oxidative stress while also affecting mood.

A 2017 study found a significant association between an unhealthy diet and mental health issues in children and adolescents. The review included 12 epidemiological studies, revealing that poor dietary patterns, characterized by high intake of junk food and low intake of fruits and vegetables, were linked to increased risk of depression and anxiety among young people. These findings highlight the importance of healthy eating habits in promoting mental well-being in this age group.

Research also shows the gut microbiome interacts with the brain in both directions across neural, inflammatory, and hormonal signaling pathways. The role of these interactions on mental health has been proposed on the basis of the following evidence: emotion-like behavior in rodents responds to changes in the gut microbiome, and it appears that major depressive disorder in humans is associated with alterations of the gut microbiome. Transferring fecal gut microbiota from humans with depression into rodents appears to induce animal behaviors that are hypothesized to indicate depression-like states. A study published in 2024 demonstrated that specific microbiota species have protective effects against anxiety and depression by modulating the gut-brain axis. This study found that probiotics, particularly strains like *Lactiplantibacillus plantarum* D-9, can alleviate anxiety-like and depression-like behaviors through mechanisms involving tryptophan metabolism and the regulation of the gut microbiota composition, highlighting the potential for microbiota-targeted therapies in treating mental health disorders.

The production of neurotransmitters like serotonin—which leads us away from feelings of depression—is influenced by these good bacteria functioning well. Foods rich in probiotics (like yogurt) and fermented foods (miso, fermented olives, kombucha, and kimchi, all of which are rich in probiotics) both promote gut health. Changing one's diet more broadly (the Mediterranean Diet, for example) can also help make the gut more conducive to the flourishing of good bacteria and lead to a two- to three-times reduction in depression.

6.

The importance of access to healthful foods is crucial to underscore—food is ultimately political and linked to equity. Bryant Terry, the resident chef at the Museum of the African Diaspora in San Francisco, was just the person to teach me about this link. Immaculately dressed with a silk spotted shirt under a cardigan and wearing his signature fedora, he shared that his journey from Tennessee to becoming, like Nira Kehar, a renowned James Beard award-winning chef, speaker, and cookbook author, was unique. He recounts the day in high school that set him on a trajectory. "I first heard this rap song called 'Beef' which was by a group called Boogie Down Productions, and the rappers wrote lyrics about how meat can harm human health and the environment. . . so I started eating less meat," Terry told me. A few years later, after he learned about Black vegetarians and vegans in America, such as Coretta Scott King and Malcolm X, he became interested in veganism. But it wasn't until his doctoral work—in American history at NYU—that he learned how an initiative by the Black Panther Party in the 1960s had addressed the intersection of poverty, malnutrition, and institutional racism in a way from which he could learn.

In 2001, Terry founded a non-profit called "B-Healthy" in New York City to teach young people the politics of food, cooking, and how nutrition affected their energy and outlook. It also helped them become more aware of the role food plays in the community. His 2015 TedMED talk about veganism and political change cites the 1969 "free breakfast for children program" run by the Black Panthers and primarily serving poor Black children. (The FBI director at the time portrayed it as a threat to national security.) As such, this was an example of food healing through community and the awareness about food the program built.

Today, after having written his second cookbook called *Vegetable Kingdom*, Terry is focused on creating healthy and socially just communities that gather around healthful eating, making access to healthful foods a priority. In his talk and with me, he shared a mantra that guides him: "Start with the visceral to ignite the cerebral and end with the political."

What all these stories suggest is echoed in a poignant editorial titled "Food Is Medicine—The Promise and Challenges of Integrating Food and Nutrition into Health Care," published in JAMA in 2019: food is a form of medicine, but in more ways than we realize. On balance, the guide put out by UCSF on "Healthy and Happy Eating" in 2019 made the most sense, as it avoids fads and incorporates evidence and common sense. And while supplements are a divisive topic (an overview from the *Annals of Internal Medicine*, published in July 2019, that examined the impact of nutritional supplements and dietary interventions on cardiovascular outcomes, concluded that most supplements do not significantly improve heart health or longevity), we do know that many supplements are helpful. Most of us cannot obtain necessary micronutrients from food, due to the requirement to stick to a standardized high-micronutrient diet, in combination with changes in soil quality and farming techniques that impact how nutritious some food sources are today, compared with even two decades ago. There's good evidence for the use of Vitamin D, iron for those who are iron-deficient, fish-oil, and so forth.* The main concern is around *quality* of the supplement, given that the FDA does not regulate supplements in the same way as medications. In summary, there is evidence for some supplements, not for others, and a balance of assessing quality, evidence, and cost is necessary.

*

Willing to try intermittent fasting to bring down my cholesterol—it would be easy enough to restrict eating to a short window while working—I began skipping breakfast, keeping to only coffee or tea in the morning, and having two meals a day, the first usually between noon and 1 pm, the last around 8 pm. For those two meals, I drew from the Mediterranean diet and the Portfolio diet, increasing viscous fiber, plant-based sources, and almonds daily. I also cooked fatty fish twice a week to take advantage of the omega-3 fats. As in

---

* A helpful overview can be found on the National Center for Complementary and Integrative Health (NCCIH) website: https://www.nccih.nih.gov/health/using-dietary-supplements-wisely

Bobby's case, I opted for fiber over simple carbohydrates due to the impact of such processed foods on my focus and attention—as well as mood, through the microbiome.

Within weeks, I was better able to focus in the mornings with just coffee or tea, though this was just an "N=1" self-experiment that may not be generalized to others rather than a clinical study. By now, I realized that the people I was meeting on my journey to learn about healing—people like Nira Kehar—were also teaching me something I hadn't anticipated: the strength to engage in the healing process and the power of courage.

Researchers like Dr. Longo and Dr. Jenkins showed that it was possible to think outside the box and thrive in medicine and that the courage to challenge dogma was crucial in forming new avenues of learning about healing. And Bryant Terry cemented the key role food plays in how we connect and also the importance of using our passions to fuel social change. My wise self would tell me strongly, during my meditations, that I needed to pay attention to each of these people and channel any residual frustration about this one specific academic hospital environment into inspiration from them to fuel broader change. From where did that wise self originate? Faith.

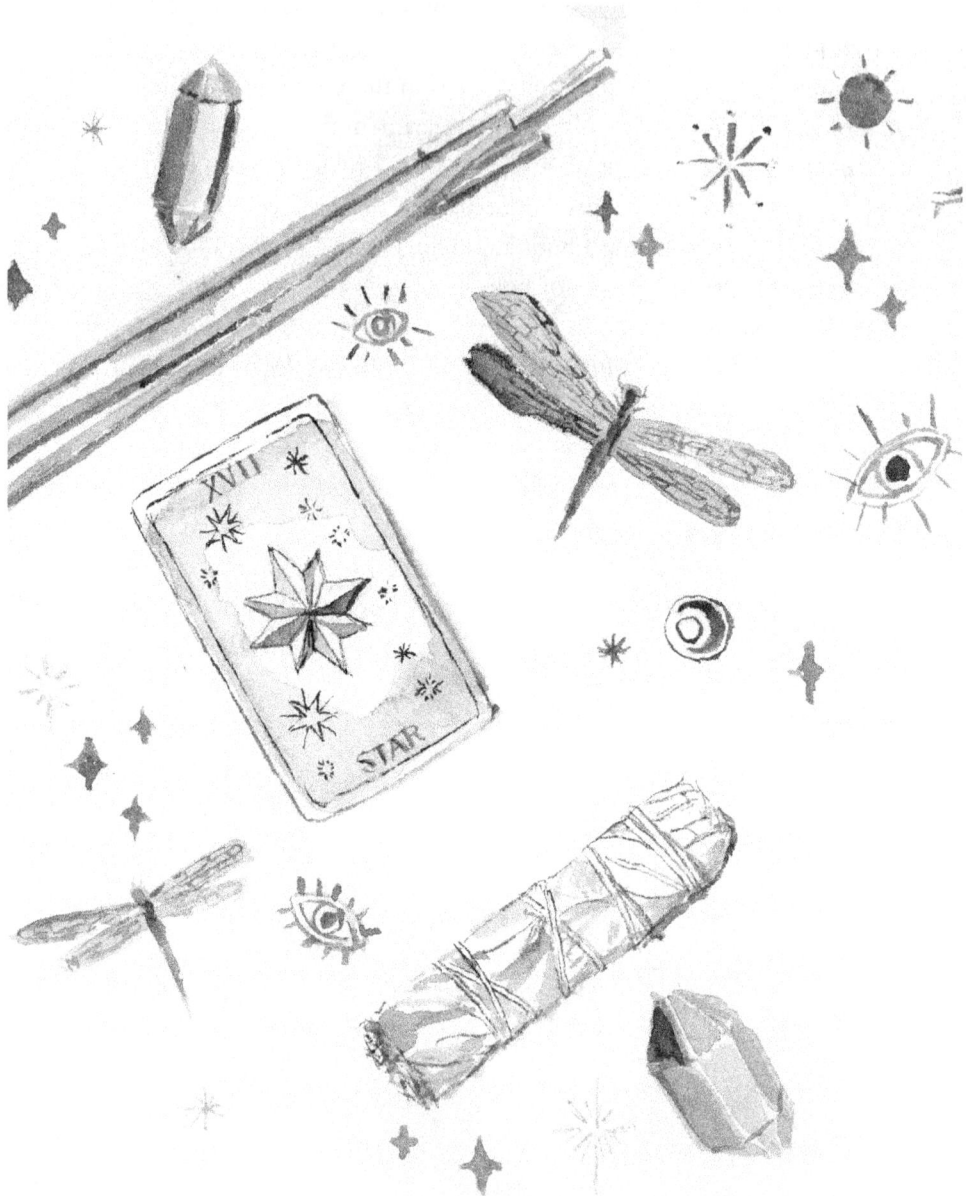

CHAPTER SEVEN

Faith, Spirit, Magic...Woo?

"There is no place so awake and alive at the edge of becoming but birthing the kind of woman who can authentically say my soul is my own...embody it...it's worth the risk and hardship."

—Sue Monk Kidd, *The Dance of the Dissident Daughter*

1.

One frigid January evening, my Twitter (now known as "X") feed lit up with a curious and heartfelt call: "Please. Please. Please. Everyone PRAY for my daughter Molly. She has been in an accident and suffered severe brain trauma. She's unconscious in the ICU. Please RT and PRAY." The tweet came from a woman in Los Angeles named Kaye Steinsapir, a 43-year-old lawyer and mother of three. Hours earlier, her 12-year-old daughter, Molly, had been injured while riding her bike. She was wearing a helmet but had been knocked unconscious. Molly's friend had yelled for help, and an ambulance swiftly took Molly to the nearby UCLA Medical Center pediatric intensive care unit. She was in a coma and suffered from a severe brain injury.

Seeing Kaye's tweet, I, along with thousands around the world, shared our prayers. This started a movement of sorts where Kaye would update us on Molly's status in the ICU. Kaye's Twitter following soon ballooned upwards of 100,000 from a few thousand in just a few days. Molly seemed to be improving but then quickly showed brain swelling, needing surgery. It was a rollercoaster to observe on social media. Much as the Beishes had found comfort online, Kaye did as well. But unlike the Beishes, Kaye specifically requested prayers as part of her daughter's healing—why?

*

On February 11, 1858, 162 years before Kaye's request, a teenager named Bernadette Soubirous was visiting near the mountain valley town of Lourdes, France, with her sister and friend when she had visions of a woman in a nearby cave telling her to "drink from the spring and wash there." Soubirous continued to see apparitions and assumed the woman was the Virgin Mary, and soon many would visit that same Lourdes water, seeking miracles of their own. The Lourdes Medical Bureau became involved to determine whether Soubirous' visions could be deemed a real miracle or if she was fabricating the visions. It was decided that they were real miracles. Soubirous was canonized as a saint in 1933.

Other seemingly miraculous experiences in Lourdes followed. On May 10, 1948, Jeanne Fretel arrived there in a comatose state because of tuberculosis peritonitis. After being given the Eucharist (the disc-shaped wafer used in Christian Mass), Jeanne woke from her coma and declared herself cured. The Catholic church recognized her recovery in 1950 to be a genuine miracle. The area in Lourdes is now a shrine, and when I visited, there were countless devotees praying in front of the statue of the Virgin Mary, each later taking home a flask of holy water. Since Jeanne, the church has documented almost 80 miracles in Lourdes as of 2017. In 2014, a group of scientists and doctors from Lyon and Maryland reviewed many of these cases and concluded that some simply defy scientific explanation. In 2024, Pope Francis deemed a young man named Carlos Acutis the first millennial saint, as several miracles were documented.

C.S. Lewis, who is perhaps most known for writing *The Chronicles of Narnia*, also wrote a treatise on faith-based miracles called simply *Miracles: A Preliminary Study*, in which he interrogates the possibility of miracles, a key part of Christian faith (crucially referenced in the Corinthians Book 1 15:13-14). Lewis defined "miracles" as "an interference with Nature by a supernatural power," which presupposes there's something or someone beyond nature or science, as we know them, that influences events *within* nature. Lewis took skeptics to task for privileging scientific explanations, writing: "Many people think one can decide whether a miracle occurred in the past by examining the evidence 'according to the ordinary rules of historical inquiry.' But the ordinary rules cannot be worked until we have decided whether miracles are possible, and if so, how probable they are." Lewis went on to posit how the supernatural might subtly act on the natural world, which has its own laws: "Each miracle writes for us in small letters something that God has already written, or will write, in letters almost too large to be noticed, across the whole canvas of Nature."

A 2012 *New York Times* article titled "Where Heaven and Earth Come Together" describes a concept called "Thin Places," which refers to "locales where the distance between heaven and earth collapses and we're able to catch glimpses of the divine, or the transcendent or, as I like to think of it, the 'Infinite Whatever.'" And in her book titled *Thin Places,* Jordan Kisner writes: "'thin places' comes from Celtic folklore: that 'the barrier between the physical world and the spiritual world wears thin and becomes porous.'"

I would often experience things that felt like thin places. One night, while out for a run in Toronto, a few months after I received the welcome recommendation to transfer to work in a hospital with a healthier culture, I asked for a sign that everything would be okay. Out popped a white rabbit from the bushes—knowing it was probably my eyes playing a trick, I stopped and snapped a photo (which can be found in the Notes section of this book). It then hopped along for a few minutes toward my house. Logically, it's likely someone had let their pet rabbit loose at that moment, as a wild white rabbit is rare. Or it may just be that there is much more to this world than we recognize, and we get glimpses of it in fleeting moments of serendipity that nudge us along or give us comfort. Or perhaps we look for those things because we so desperately want to believe that someone or something is watching over us. Could it just be this *belief* that provides healing, above all else?

*

The role of prayer in healing is complex. Intercessory prayer, which is the formal name for praying to a higher being for the benefit of oneself or others, may be helpful as an adjunct for pain management among those who identify as religious. It can also help patients create meaning from their experiences. Some, like Christian Science practitioners, believe the soul is key to healing the body. In 2020, a published case report caught my eye: the resolution of blindness after the patient was prayed for, that is, after they received intercessory prayer. But the case happened in 1972. The same group of doctors reported on other cases, too, like prayer for gastroparesis (when the stomach becomes unable to function) in a 16-year-old, but with a heavy reliance on decades-long anecdotal evidence.

In 2006, a group from the Mind-Body Medical Institute at Harvard Medical School reported on the STEP (Study of the Therapeutic Effects of Intercessory Prayer) trial among cardiac bypass patients. The trial involved six hospitals in the U.S. Each participant was in one of three groups: one-third received prayer after not being told if they would or not, and another third didn't receive prayer after being told they may or may not receive it. The remaining third were told they would receive prayer. There was no significant difference among the groups in terms of mortality after one month, nor were there any other major events in their health. The groups were not subdivided according to whether the recipients themselves believed in the power of prayer.

More prominently, a Cochrane review from 2009 examined the question of intercessory prayer and found no beneficial effect compared with no prayer. The study, however, also caught a wave of criticism for failing to "live up to the high standards required of Cochrane reviews." What this suggests is even the mere attempt to scientifically examine the spiritual elements of healing can be met with resistance. But if we cannot lean in close to this inexplicable and otherworldly phenomenon and at least lend a scientific eye, how can we meaningfully say whether or not there is something to the experiences reported by so many?

2.

Christina Puchalski is not your average doctor. She holds an M.D., but for the past 30 years, she has focused primarily on bringing spirituality into hospitals. Puchalski has cropped brown hair, deep blue eyes, and a knowing smile. She has a lightness to her—but balances it with the intensity and grit of an academic. Having grown up in southern California and been raised Catholic, she'd been taught by her parents, who had immigrated from Poland, to be open to the idea of the sacred in all living things. Her bookshelves were filled with texts from various religions.

In medical school, she rotated through a hospice, and when she was extracting a spiritual history of a patient, Puchalski noticed a shift in her perspective. One particular patient shared that she didn't work and that much of her family had passed away: these were things that had given her life meaning and which were impacting her ability to focus on her interest and ability to heal and "return to normal life." Puchalski began wondering if prayer and, more generally, a spiritual practice, could impact healing.

Yet the shift in Puchalski's thinking wasn't a specific lightbulb that went off, she insisted. It was more of a convergence of years of exposure to spirituality. This was particularly interesting for me to hear, as so often our lives shift dramatically after one encounter or event—indeed, that's what happened with me—something that has enough momentum to wake us up and direct us onto another path professionally or personally. With Puchalski, it was different: a slower steering onto a path unlike that of most conventional physicians.

"There wasn't one specific thing that redirected me towards the spiritual needs of my patients. I suppose it was years of acknowledging my connection to the sacred and realizing that so much suffering we see in our patients is of the spiritual kind," she told me, underscoring the intersection between spirituality and psychology. Over the following years, she built a niche for herself as a physician with an interest in understanding the role of "spiritual distress" and that pain can include "spiritual pain."

In her book *Making Healthcare Whole*, she defines spirituality as "the aspect of humanity that refers to the way individuals seek and express meaning and purpose and the way they experience their connectedness to the moment, to self, to others, to nature, and to the significant or sacred." She identifies triggers for potential spiritual growth, including serious illness, aging, loss of loved ones, stress, life change, social events, and tragedies. She emphasized the importance of spirituality in the human quest to find meaning and purpose, "even in the midst of failed jobs, relationships, accomplishments, and unattained successes, especially at the end of life. Ultimate meaning is meaning that sustains individuals in the emptiness of their external lives or as people face their death. The inability to find meaning and purpose can lead to depression and anxiety."

In 1996, Puchalski developed the FICA (faith/belief/meaning; importance/influence; community; address/action of care) spiritual assessment tool, which helped integrate patients' spiritual history into their medical history. FICA caught the attention of physicians across the country and is now a standard tool used in palliative care. Now, having co-authored several hundred papers on the topic, she is most interested in the role of prayer and spiritual practice as it relates to healing and the barriers against bringing spirituality into hospitals, working with everyone from the Vatican to the World Health Organization (WHO). With the WHO, she has advocated to include "spirit" within the definition of health, specifically with respect to palliative care.

Just before the Twin Towers attack on September 11, 2001, Puchalski was working as an attending physician overseeing the care for a patient we'll call Leah, who was dealing with metastatic breast cancer. She had a husband and two kids in school. Leah wanted nothing more than to live to see her children start college. Then, a few days later, the attacks occurred, and Leah learned that one of her close friends had died in the Pentagon, which caused her to feel sad and hopeless. Using the FICA tool, Puchalski assembled a physical, emotional, spiritual, and social plan for Leah in order to restore spiritual meaning to her life. This became a key part of Leah's ability to heal, according to Puchalski, because identifying spiritual distress and attending to it by being present to the patient's suffering helps to resolve the distress. Sometimes, this may include referring to a spiritual professional such as a chaplain.

Spiritual distress specifically is associated with depression and anxiety, and so ensuring it is addressed may improve the patient's overall health and quality of life. Moreover, learning more about the patient's spiritual practices and strengths (it could be spending time in nature, formal prayer, or an artistic endeavor) may impact their decision-making about treatment.

Lastly, the FICA tool can uncover a specifically spiritual community of support, which can also help relieve patient distress. Today, Puchalski leads the George Washington Institute for Spirituality and Health, dubbed GWish, which was established in 2001. It has the primary role of raising awareness about the spiritual aspect of patient well-being. It's the largest center of its kind in the U.S., and possibly globally. To date, Puchalski has worked with thousands of patients clinically while spending half of her time on research.

Puchalski describes how to be a model of spirituality and compassion as part of the full condition of being human when she writes: "We are transformed spiritually through our encounters with patients as they are with us...in healing relationships we find the transcendent, the holy, and the sacred." Indeed, any healing practice is complete only when it takes into account the spiritual journey—of patient or healer—at which point a doctor's practice becomes something more than medicine.

*

Jonah Geffen had rabbis in his lineage, but he didn't want to be one. The 46-year-old New Yorker "tried to avoid it forever," even attending law school for a period. But the calling proved too strong to resist. Geffen was the son of two Jewish community professionals (his father is an educator and founded a school, while his mother is active in various community centers), and law school wasn't sitting well with him. He couldn't accept the idea of having to argue for the "immoral" side of a situation. He also studied conflict resolution in Israel, earning a master's degree in Conflict Analysis and Resolution at George Mason University. There, he met a mentor, a rabbi who worked almost exclusively in helping communities get through conflict. For Geffen, that hit close to home. Now a rabbi himself, he has found a way to provide for his community that is much more aligned with his nature. This relates to what Puchalski described as how taking a spiritual history from a patient can lead to "engaging with a community of spiritual support." Geffen often finds himself the center of that community.

"There's always an element of care involved in it…of people seeking you out to talk about things that they don't generally seek other people out to talk about. And I'd say very often that's someone looking to heal something," he told me. At a moment's notice, Geffen became prepared to run to someone's side in the hospital or in their community.

Indeed, for many people, spirituality is experienced primarily through organized religion. As such, the leaders of those religions, imams, priests, rabbis, and so forth, end up being more than just religious leaders. They take on the role of a "healer," even if the leaders themselves don't see themselves in that light.

"It's amazing how many people spend their lives in a synagogue, paying their dues, going to things, being a part of that, which is being a part of community, and then forget about the part of community which is 'I can let the community take care of me, I can let the rabbi take care of me,'" he said. "In Judaism, there is a tradition of a specific healing prayer made up of 18 blessings, which underscores God as a healer, and it also allows for healing of other people. And this is available for those who go to synagogue every once in a while, as well as to those who pray three times a day."

In the hospital context, the healing element of religion is being recognized, with hospital chaplains often coming from various faith backgrounds, and with faith leaders becoming more involved in the spiritual needs of patients from different religious groups. Geffen adds this last point: Some religious leaders, asked to pray for someone outside their faith, may feel hesitant—but this is slowly changing.

"It's a challenge with some of the rabbis I know, who might be asked to pray for someone. In our tradition, prayers are quite scripted out of the Torah, so the challenge is for them to step out of that and find another way to connect with that person and to God," he said.

3.

The air in Rishikesh was pungent with a mix of jasmine, turmeric, and sweat. But the ashram, a monastic retreat, offered a cool and welcoming respite. It was the fall of 2019, and while traveling to Bangalore, India, to do some reporting on artificial intelligence in healthcare, I took a few days for a retreat in the holy city, which is in northern India. The program at the ashram was run by a Scandinavian couple who had met there two years earlier. Soon, it became clear that most guests were women from Western Europe or North America, the vast majority inspired by Elizabeth Gilbert's *Eat, Pray, Love,* and looking for their own spiritual moment. For the record, I loved Gilbert's book, but it stands alone; her experience is unique and clearly resonated with millions.

India is significant in the history of healing. It offers a now 2,500-year-old Sanskrit text called the *Sushruta Samhita* ("The Compendium of Sushruta") in which a woman named Sushruta describes both medical and surgical techniques for healing everything from hernias to broken bones. Sushruta was an early practitioner of Indian traditional medicine, called "Ayurveda"— "ayur," or meaning of life, and "veda," knowledge.

The father of Ayurveda, Charaka, had already described the roles of hygiene, diet, and plant-based healing remedies. Remarkably, Ayurveda demonstrates synergy with Greek and Egyptian traditions that combine the five elements (water, fire, earth, air, and ether/space) to yield three doshas (vata, pitta, kapha) that are similar to humors (wind, bile, and phlegm). Imbalances in the doshas cause illness; healing requires their re-balancing. This is exactly the approach Nira Kehar took with her cooking.

While at the ashram, I wanted to experience a ceremony that was more akin to what I grew up with when my family would visit the temple, and to do it in Rishikesh—near the holy Ganges River—felt right. So, organized by Ravi at the front desk of the ashram, an Iyer (priest) named Ram arrived on his motorcycle, no less. In his late 40s and pudgy, Ram was pleasant and soft-spoken and spoke only Hindi. He had instructed me the day before to pick up fruit to offer to the deities, and he would bring the rest. It was like Uber Eats but for prayers (likely not scalable anywhere but India).

After breakfast, I met him in the large hall usually reserved for yoga or kirtan (spiritual chanting and singing), where Ram led the Sanskrit prayers, a familiar melody from what I could recall at home. "Om sham shanicharaya namah..." was all I could pick up, which translates to removing obstacles and is often chanted for Ganesha, the elephant-headed god who assists in getting rid of barriers in our path. He also chanted one for the other gods: Shiva and Lakshmi. And then a more general one. It all took a total of 90 minutes.

Finally, I thanked him and got up, shaking my cramped legs, and bent down to help him clean up the old coconut husks. "No, we leave these here," he said disapprovingly, lightly patting my hands away. Then he wrote some things down in Hindi, which Ravi translated right afterward at the desk: "This will be a troubling time for you over the next year, but it will get better by next year."

"Next year?" I gasped, looking up to see Ram had already sped away on his motorcycle. There would be no elaboration.

4.

The trip through the Moroccan souks three years prior was anxiety-provoking, even for the most patient among us. I was on a trip with my friend Jaime—a small getaway, as I was waiting to determine whether a transfer out of my hospital and into a healthier one, would be arranged. Our tour group was being led through the labyrinth of small stalls in Marrakech. The smells of spices, yelling of "yalla" (let's go), trinkets tinkling, and rugs being shaken—it was all a lot for the senses, especially under the beating hot Arabian sun. My friend Jaime returned to the hotel shaken and anxious, wondering how she could possibly be this stressed while on vacation. I had an idea. During my yoga teacher training at Yandara, which had been a year earlier, instruction in a form of therapeutic touch called "Reiki" was offered. I decided to sign up and completed levels one and two. The best way to describe the training was a form of active meditation and presence for another person, a form of massage without touch.

The history of Reiki originates in Japan, founded by spiritual aspirant, Mikao Usui in the early 1920s. There are multiple schools of thought about its value. One is that it's purely placebo and it couldn't possibly be a form of "channeling." But in many scientific contexts, "therapeutic touch" appears to be more palatable. It removes the florid spiritual element, while accepting that, at the very least, the presence of another person in an active way that hyper-focuses on elements of their physical body could have healing potential for the recipient.

By the time I visited Morocco, I had done Reiki on exactly two people, in large part because I wasn't sure myself if it was effective. The first was for my sister and her injured knee (which she believed felt better after Reiki). The second, for Chris, for a migraine that presented on New Year's Eve (his headache went away, but he became violently ill right after – retching for over an hour). Pundits have suggested the violent reaction was a form of "energy clearing" that some people experience. For what it's worth, Jaime loved the Reiki: "I feel so much more relaxed now," she had exclaimed. She still brings it up from time to time. But that night in Morocco was the last time I've offered it.

More than 60 hospitals in the U.S., including the likes of Johns Hopkins Hospital and Massachusetts General Hospital, now offer Reiki and therapeutic touch. But does it work? Studies show that Reiki may improve pain and discomfort, and one study from Italy suggested Reiki might benefit cancer patients, specifically for symptoms of anxiety and pain. The benefits may be similar to massage. The best review of Reiki was published in the *British Medical Journal* in 2019 and reported that there are potential benefits for pain, mood, and quality of life but that firm conclusions could not be drawn. Could it just be another example of the placebo effect? One review, published in 2001 in *Alternative and Complementary Therapies*, specifically reported that it was *better* than placebo.

One limitation to studies of Reiki is that it is often melded together with therapeutic touch, which is effectively a more sanitized (non-spiritual) version of Reiki. It might be biologically plausible to posit that light touch is relaxing and calming, and the downregulation of stress hormones itself (which could be from anything) has an impact. But one study that looked at "distant" Reiki, which is similar in many ways to intercessory prayer, made me wonder if it was better to consider it as a form of prayer, as it involved presence and a genuine intention to heal another person in a way that didn't require any form of physical manipulation.

Whether through intercessory prayer or something more structured like Reiki, how exactly can we "know" whether spiritual elements help us heal? Doesn't this run against the principle of faith, as in a trust and knowing that can't be tested or proven in the conventional sense?

*

Brené Brown's book *Braving the Wilderness* describes finding our own identity through the sense of belonging. She cites Maya Angelou and her quote on belonging: "You only are free when you realize you belong no place—you belong every place—no place at all. The price is high. The reward is great."

It resonated deeply with me, and my faith was a big part of my healing journey. I was in the wilderness, but maybe I was used to it. I had spent my whole life—from a girl in England moving to Canada to one of the only people of color in small towns as we moved from place to place, as a public-schooled kid switching to a private high school, as one of the only Canadians in an American public health graduate program, and as a researcher and master's student in a medical school in which half of the class was right out of undergraduate school—trying to belong.

But here's the funny thing: when your identity is all about trying to find sameness while being so inherently different, over time, with the years and the wisdom, it's the differences you hang onto. I knew that I saw things differently. I could make connections others could not. Being different became what I most prized. And since being an undergraduate, it was what made me stand out and carve my own path, and I was celebrated for it. That is, until I got to that one specific unhealthy hospital environment, faith in what lay beyond kept me grounded.

5.

Though many might poke fun at shows like "Long Island Medium," Laura Lynne Jackson, a medium from Coal Harbor, Long Island, defies the typical image of a psychic. She is trained as a teacher and values science and the scientific method. A former schoolteacher, Jackson has written two books, *The Light Between Us* (about when loved ones cross over) and *Signs* (about the signs we get from the Universe about loved ones who have passed away). It was a 2018 talk she gave with Manhattan-based psychiatrist Mark Epstein, which was posted on YouTube, that made me wonder if there is value in looking more closely at Jackson's practice.

Epstein, a rational and respected psychiatrist, shared that Jackson was able to tap into things about his life, including his childhood, that no one knew, including specifics related to his relationship with his father, who had since passed on. At the event, Epstein himself acknowledged his surprise and reason why he wanted to do the event in the first place: to offer a space for Jackson to engage with doctors, primarily to discuss these seemingly inexplicable experiences.

In psychiatry, believing in magic or psychics or ghosts is labeled as pathological, with an actual diagnosis: schizotypal personality disorder. People with very deep religious faith can also be labeled this way, so the lines between faith and delusion get blurry. I enjoyed both of Jackson's books, and as someone who has prayed nightly since I was a child, I am open-minded about the spiritual, so I felt we should meet. Calling from her office in Coal Harbor on a brisk autumn afternoon, she greeted me warmly and shared more about her story.

As a high school English teacher, Jackson would notice troubles with some of her students. "There was a boy in my class who was off, energetically. I told him he'd get an A and explained that his issues were not about the poetry class I was teaching. It turns out there were some really traumatic issues happening at home, but I was able to reassure him," she told me. "We have a physical part of us but also a soul spirit, and we have free will that allows us to steer the ship. The future affects our past, which is hard to describe."

Most of Jackson's sessions take place over the phone, which eliminates whether a reading is cold or not (i.e., looking at body language or items like a wedding ring). She also works as a medium, without charge, with the Forever Family Foundation, which primarily assists families who have lost a child, and connects them to those "behind the veil," a term Jackson uses to describe the presence of those who have passed on, i.e., that they are closer than we think, even if we can't see them with our eyes. I told her about the teenage patient, Alex, from Chapter 5 who presented with what looked like encephalitis but ended up being anxiety secondary to their sexuality. She had an interesting response: "You healed them in a powerful way and perceived their energy wound. Your soul had a conversation with theirs. Know that."

Jackson is also clear that there should be rigorous objective testing of those who claim to have psychic or mediumship abilities. "You know, with people who want to be hairdressers, they have to get tested, and people that want to be doctors, they have to go through the training and get tested. So how can people who are allowed to go out there and say, 'Yes I can communicate with those who have crossed' not have any training or at least certification of their abilities?" she said.

It made me think back to an essay I had read by Barrett Swanson, called "Lost in Summerland," about Swanson's visit to a psychic fair called Lily Dale in upstate New York with his brother Andy, who had intuitive abilities that couldn't be explained. In his essay, Barrett describes how Andy was tested on stage and how that was enough to convince Barrett that Andy's abilities were real. I felt compelled to email Swanson, who was kind enough to respond, praising an article I had written for the same magazine a year earlier. "After everything I experienced with Andy at Lily Dale, I've grown far more accepting of the possibility that this stuff happens all the time (and that I, too, might be experiencing it but not necessarily registering or appreciating those instances of insight when they come)," he wrote.

There is no scientific evidence that supports the validity of mediumship, but the evidence doesn't exist largely due to the lack of research interest. I can't imagine researchers lining up to submit for grants and other research funding to "test" mediums. How hard could it be to "test" a group of mediums and report on the findings? The closest we get is the work of child psychiatrist Dr. Jim Tucker from the University of Virginia. His work, which was featured in the 2021 Netflix "Surviving Death" series, assesses whether phenomena of past-life "memories" in young children have a basis in truth. Most of Tucker's time and research is focused on traditional conditions:

ADHD, anxiety, and the like. This particular area, as he admitted to me, is highly unconventional and remains inexplicable, but became the basis of his best-selling book *Return to Life.*

"It's hard to explain how a child can have such detailed memories of someone who died decades ago, to the point where they are able to accurately describe situations, point to scenes, and even have nightmares focused on experiences that they themselves never had," Tucker told me. "I'm left, at the very least, with the acceptance that there's more out there that we simply do not yet understand."

When I asked Jackson if she thought of herself as a healer, she said, "Some people get a lot of gratification, especially those grieving at the Forever Families Foundation, but I actually see myself more as a teacher—to teach us that we all have these gifts if we pay attention and use them." But the most interesting thing she shared with me was very personal: an unexpected reading for me.

"Amitha, you're on a personal journey now that started about a year or 14 months ago and will go on for another two years or so, where your path will detour to include, but still be beyond medicine…and it will be much better than you ever imagined," she told me. To a skeptic, this advice may not be ground-breaking. Jackson knew I was writing a book and, having written a few herself, would know the 14-to-24-month timeline from proposal acceptance to book publication. But to me, it was a small bit of reassurance. Maybe it was my optimism or wanting or grasping at strands of hope, but I couldn't help but feel that maybe she was right.

6.

Now that we had been together for over two years, Chris and I had reached a comfortable rhythm, and he was planning on moving from Geneva to the New York office so he could be closer to me. It was a challenge, though. It was almost impossible to switch. He would have to apply for another job or somehow convince his higher-ups that New York made more sense. Chris also explained that he needed to be there for personal reasons, to be closer to me and his mother, who was showing signs that her breast cancer, which had been in remission six years earlier, was now rearing its head again.

Throughout all of this, my meditation was key, but the umbrella around it all was faith. Yet, the story of Beatrice Soubirous and the visitors to Lourdes only paints a sliver of the picture. Faith and spirituality involve *more* than miracles for healing. From Jonah Geffen and Christine Puchalski, I learned that asking if prayer works isn't the right question. We can't possibly know whether it hastens recovery. Instead, we should be driving towards defining recovery more holistically, as in healing for both the patient and their family, one that transcends merely "curing." Perhaps the word "prayer" is unnecessarily constraining. Instead, reframing it as a "compassionate and caring presence" for another, where we genuinely hold their well-being in our thoughts, relegates prayer to a different function in our lives. This might be why mediums like Laura Lynne Jackson are so popular and highly sought out. There's a comforting element in believing our universe is vaster than we realize and that we can potentially connect to the divine, even to our own loved ones who have transitioned.

Prayer may serve a similar function. So, when Kaye Steinsapir eventually shared an update on Twitter that after Molly's tests for brain function came up as showing no activity and that she passed away, it was heartening to read that the family was grateful for the multifaith prayers and the outpouring of compassion from around the world. All of this brought the Steinsapirs comfort and a sense of being witnessed during their unimaginable reality. It left me wondering whether a deeper sense of compassionate presence, which prayer may help amplify, has the potential to *heal* and assist those suffering from a tragedy and the uncertainty that often follows—even if, in the end, we're met with the limits medicine itself places on the ability to *cure*.

Spirituality and faith soon became a core part of how I could navigate through this time. Laura Lynne Jackson, as a medium, gave me comfort, but ultimately, it was a belief in something bigger than myself that extended from more than just the religion with which I grew up. Since I was a child, I had prayed to the Hindu elephant god, Ganesha, the remover of obstacles, honoring part of my family's beliefs.

Now, I had a *real* obstacle in my way—praying extra hard couldn't hurt, could it? At the very least it provided a bit more strength. The Bible's Philippians 4:13: *"I can do all things through Christ who strengthens me"* reflects this. But to me, the Hindu spiritual text, the Upanishads, paints this idea particularly clearly. A passage of the Mundaka Upanishad reads:

> *The student asks, "Sir, what is that by knowing which everything becomes known?"*
> *The sage replies, "Just as by knowing a clod of clay, all the clay becomes known, so is this teaching. Of this mighty tree, if someone should strike at the root, it would bleed, but still live. If someone should strike at the middle, it would bleed but still live. Being pervaded by the atman it stands firm, drinking in its moisture and rejoicing. Bring to me the fruit of the nyagrodha tree."*
> *The student brings it and says, "Here it is, Sir."*
> *"Break it."*
>   *"It is broken, Sir."*
>   *"What do you see?"*
>   *"Extremely fine seeds, Sir."*
>   *"Break one of those seeds."*
>   *"It is broken, Sir."*
>   *"What do you see?"*
>   *"Nothing, Sir."*
> *"My dear, out of that 'nothing,' this great nyagrodha tree has arisen. The atman is subtle, imperceptible, out of which this whole universe has arisen."*

Ātman is the Sanskrit word for "self," as in the universal self, which is akin to the soul or spirit that "transmigrates" after death. The idea is eerily reminiscent of the Gingko and the internal force and architecture that stayed alive even though the external elements of the tree were destroyed or dead. Perhaps my crisis was a trigger for my own spiritual growth? And my own "Ātman" would be the driver to keep moving forward, even if externally everything seemed as though it was crumbling. At the very least, the idea was comforting.

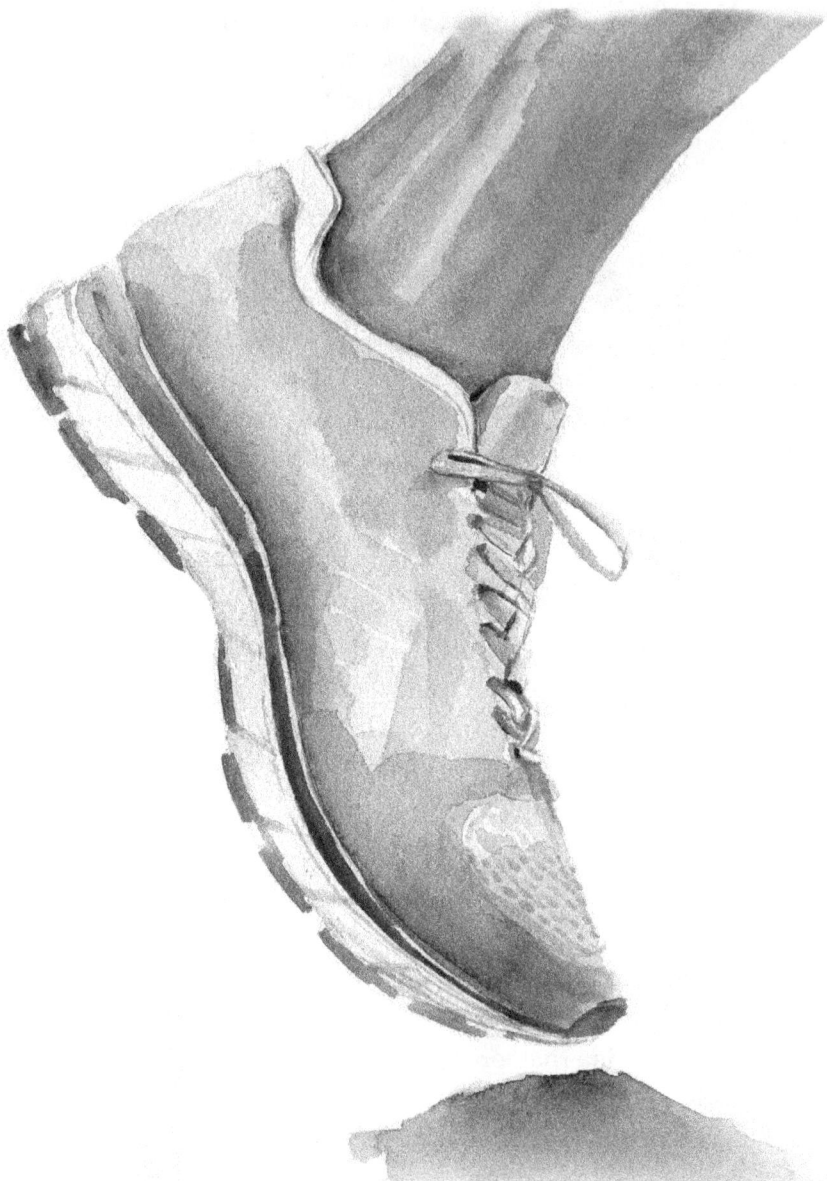

CHAPTER EIGHT

Movement[s]

*"Great spirits have always encountered violent opposition from
mediocre minds."*

— Albert Einstein

1.

In a gym located in an industrial center in Scarborough, part of Toronto,
I found myself meeting with a muscular woman who went by the name
of "Tyra Love." Was Love her real name? No, she told me, cryptically.
Her real name had an Iranian origin, though she was ethnically ambiguous.
Standing at 5'3", with her black curls and caramel skin, she boasted an eight-
pack and bulging biceps. Love could have been Vin Diesel's sister.

"Welcome, Amitha!" she shouted over the soca (Caribbean dancehall) music.
"Don't worry. I used to be a stick like you, but soon you'll get those curves!" She
winked and handed me two five-pound dumbbells. "Start with these, and you'll
be up to twenty pounds in no time."

We started with the battle ropes, my arms aching after no more than 15 seconds.
I tried to take a small break. "Keep going!" Tyra cried out. Love ran a popular
women's fitness "bootcamp," the kind that became all the rage in the mid-2000s,
starting with Barry's Bootcamp™, which spawned other more independent chains.
This workout was effectively a version of Barry's but focused on women who didn't
want to be around all the male grunting and leering.

In the late 1980s, Barry Jay was living in New York as a gay man with
an addiction to drugs and alcohol. "I was this skinny kid that was bullied for

being gay and alcoholism ran in my family, so it was all just a mix of factors," Jay recalled in an essay for the wellness website *Well and Good*. Jay's addiction began first with cigarettes, then a drink with dinner, followed by a drink "to get drunk," then marijuana, until, after he moved to Los Angeles in the hopes of continuing his work in musical theater, "there were drugs all around me—coke, crack, quaaludes…I was numbing and covering up any pain from the past, but really, the damage was done," he told the magazine.

Then, on August 4, 1988, Jay woke up after a night out that ended up in a blur. Shocked he even woke up at all, he realized something needed to change. Several months later, he met a trainer at his local gym and started volunteering with him. He worked his way up to be a trainer himself while also attending addiction recovery meetings. At the suggestion of two of his training clients, John and Rachel Mumford, he started Barry's Bootcamp, which opened its first gym in West Hollywood in 1998, offering a combination of high-intensity interval training built on cardio and weights in a dark room with loud music and red lights. Today, there are 70 studio gyms across the globe, with 100,000 members taking a class every week. Now, the website boasts, "We were first to the party."

For years, medicine has regarded exercise primarily as a tool for weight loss. Diet and exercise are so inextricably linked that they're almost one word: "diet-n'exercise" as the catchall cure for obesity, metabolic syndrome, heart disease, and so forth. But in medical training, we aren't taught exactly what part of exercise actually works. Does walking count? What about all these fitness trends like bootcamps? One of the most misunderstood aspects of exercise is that the name itself implies something vigorous, when it's really movement in general that is at the core of healing. Though, to be sure, specific forms of heavy exercise may be as effective as medicine—at least according to what the science suggests now.

*

The preventative benefits of exercise (for dementia, depression, and chronic diseases like heart disease) are well established, but what about the *healing* aspects? In 2019, a study found that exercise and group sports, specifically in children, could work like an anti-depressant. It's particularly interesting to see this apply to children who have had adverse childhood experiences, which suggests that exercise may decrease the impact of these experiences on adult mental health. A 2013 Cochrane review of 37 trials found exercise as effective as medication for depression, though the low number of trials included was a limitation of the study.

The scientific benefits of high-intensity interval training (HIIT), which refers to exercising in short intervals that increase heart rate above a certain level to burn fat more efficiently, have been explored in several studies. Results show it may reduce overall body mass, improve cardiorespiratory fitness, optimize diabetes markers like fasting insulin, reduce both visceral fat and abdominal fat, and lower LDL cholesterol and triglycerides. There may be mental health impacts as well. A systematic review of 33 studies found improvements in anxiety and depression severity, including among those with dementia.

Part of how HIIT works for chronic metabolic issues may be due to how it impacts body composition and lowers inflammation. In terms of mental health and concentration, it may work primarily via increasing the levels of brain-derived neurotrophic factor (BDNF), a protein that helps neurons (brain cells) grow and survive. That said, HIIT is far from a panacea, and there can be adverse effects, such as rhabdomyolysis when muscle breaks down and impacts how the body is able to function (this can be deadly). As well, hearing issues may arise in HIIT classes where loud music—and, ahem— screaming is common.

Though I was getting screamed at by Tyra Love in the nicest, most motivating way, I was learning how the process of getting physically stronger and more adept could benefit my emotional and mental health. It also had the potential to improve my borderline cholesterol levels while I was at it. Maybe, like David in his battle with Goliath, I needed to optimize my physical strength and endurance for the road ahead. And Tyra Love was helping me do just that.

2.

In medical training, we're often taught about "twin studies." Sometimes, the research involves twins that have been separated at birth, where one might be found later to have a particular disease that the other doesn't. But more often, the twins aren't separated, but one still has a particular condition, whereas the other is spared. The goal, then, is to trace the factors that led to one twin's challenging fate, with the goal of discerning how a given condition can be prevented. It's a bit like the 1998 movie *Sliding Doors* starring Gwyneth Paltrow, in which what seems like a chance event can set one version of the self on a trajectory that is unexpected and more difficult compared to the default trajectory.

In medical research, these studies of twins, with a built-in "control group," help teach us primarily about the role of the environment. As we now know from earlier chapters of this book, environment often plays a crucial role in determining how we are both prone to specific diseases and how well we can heal. Nashville-based Jessica Harthcock, a 38-year-old woman who was born and raised in Indiana, is the living embodiment of one of these studies. We met at a conference in Palm Springs in 2015, and I noticed she was in forearm crutches. Having just met someone who twisted his ankle after a ski trip, I immediately assumed it was a recent accident and expressed my condolences as we spoke over breakfast.

"Oh, I'm a functional T3 paraplegic," Harthcock said, laughing, her perfectly curled chestnut hair flowing gently in the California breeze. I narrowed my eyes, partially because I didn't realize how wrong I had been for relying on a heuristic (or shortcut) problem-solving method to explain her physical condition but also because I found it unbelievable that she was a paraplegic.

"I'm recovering now," she finished quickly, likely sensing my trouble piecing together her words with how she looked, "it's a long story." Long indeed, and it speaks to both her own resolve and how movement—in the context of very specific exercises in a rehabilitation context—can be used to heal from conditions we don't typically expect to improve much at all.

In their childhood home in Indiana, Jessica and her twin sister, Emily, had taken dance lessons since they were toddlers, and both eventually tried out for the swim team. Then, for the first time, they diverged. Jessica started diving, whereas Emily stuck with swimming. Soon, Jessica would be at dive practice for more than 30 hours a week and would be invited to tournaments all over the state. In 2004, at the age of 17, Jessica's path diverged again from her sister's— but this time, very dramatically.

"I was practicing gymnastics in order to improve my springboard diving skills. I went to do a front double tuck with a layout twist. The last move involved going up in the air. When I came down, I landed on my head and broke my neck as well. I heard a crunch and my body went numb. I was in a state of shock and couldn't feel anything or speak. In that moment, on the mat, I thought about Christopher Reeves, that I would be paralyzed like him," Jessica told me.

The next moments were both blurry and rapid. Jessica was immediately sent to the hospital. The scans showed that a cyst had begun to form around the spinal cord, which affected the nerve distribution for everything below the upper back. She needed immediate surgery. Jessica's journey was a long one and involved ten years of rehabilitation with leg braces, and electric stimulation, among other things.

Since she was rapidly placed in a wheelchair, she noticed how uneducated the public was about disability.

"I always grew up conscious of people who had differences in their abilities. One of my cousins has cerebral palsy, so she has been in a wheelchair since she was little. I never thought much of it, and my dad always talked about the ADA (American Disability Act) and how important that was, and how people with different abilities want the same things we all do, so here I was seeing it firsthand," she told me. Jessica didn't let the ignorance get to her. One time, a mother had her child in a stroller, and the child pointed to Jessica, saying, "Look, she's in a stroller too." Jessica would also run into issues with her service dog, Ozzie, as he would get kicked out of public spaces or healthcare facilities, which is effectively against federal law.

So, she had to become her own advocate, and as Puchalski might say, had a spiritual reckoning after her accident, during which she created "meaning and purpose" to help others, especially with the research around spinal cord injury. The first improvement with rehab came after two years and nine months, when she was able to advance her left foot a few inches. "It slowly changed to an actual step, and I remember how shaky my muscles were, just trying to function," she told me.

Jessica combined that with biofeedback linked to gait training, which feeds information to the brain to help signal what to do. It took six years to walk entirely unassisted, and she eventually moved on to having just one forearm crutch. Though being a twin didn't lead to any medical insights here, having her twin sister by her side throughout the healing process undoubtedly helped Jessica stay motivated and optimistic. Love won again: in 2010, Jessica married the man who trained her to walk again. From 2011, she occasionally used forearm crutches when she needed to walk long distances (which is why she had them when I met her). Today, she doesn't need any assistance at all.

The field (of healing spinal injury) has progressed just as rapidly. New stimulators have been invented that can be implanted directly in the spinal cord and brain. This primarily involves trailblazing work out of the Fraizer Rehab Institute in Kentucky, led by Dr. Susan Harkema, who is a leader in this area through her studies with implantable spinal stimulation devices. Other more controversial research areas, such as using stem cells in spinal cord injury, may also show benefits in the coming years.

"We now see patients make incredible strides in recovery, whether it's regaining bowel or bladder control, or whether it's walking or sitting up and balancing again," Jessica told me. "We did believe 30 years ago that spinal cord injury meant someone would never walk again, but the fact that many patients are still told they will never recover and shouldn't even try and are sent home to live the rest of their lives without hope didn't make sense to me."

Though Jessica rejoiced with improvements herself, she knew that her legacy included helping others. During the years she searched for highly specialized rehab treatments, she learned how disconnected and fragmented the healthcare system was for patients like her and how immensely varied the recovery outcomes were. A tremendous opportunity was birthed. In 2013, she created the organization Utilize Health (utilizehealth.com), of which she serves as co-founder and CEO. Utilize Health collects research outcomes for patients with spinal cord injury, looking at various factors: the social determinants, spiritual, emotional, and so forth. It aims to lower care costs for health plans while maximizing overall health for patients with a severe neurological condition such as a stroke, spinal cord injury, or brain injury.

"We get patients from all walks of life, and we're now looking at how we can use big data to tie it together," she told me. The response has been overwhelmingly positive with high engagement results and our health plan partners have experienced lower costs of care."

3.

When most people think of Michael Phelps, they imagine a superhuman-like figure with a wingspan that rivals Michael Jordan, who swam his way to 23 Olympic gold medals. But most people don't know that Phelps struggled with ADHD as a child. In a video for the Child Mind Institute in 2017, he shared how differently he was treated compared to his peers: "I [saw] kids who, we were all in the same class, and the teachers treated them differently than they would treat me. I had a teacher tell me that I would never amount to anything and I would never be successful," he said. "I was someone who was constantly bouncing off the walls—I could never sit still." Phelps has called Ritalin a "crutch" and described how, once he was able to focus his mind, things became better. He also found that swimming, and the discipline involved, helped immensely with his focus—he would practice before and after school, which kept his attention on schoolwork during the day, and he was able to dissipate any excess energy that way.

When I took a course led by Harvard psychiatrist, John Ratey, about integrative approaches to ADHD, one core lesson emerged: physical activity was crucial. Ratey is a tall, bespectacled man with the demeanor of a kind psychiatrist. I soon became friends with his wife, Alicia, a slim blonde who spent years in the television industry, producing shows like "Entertainment Tonight" and several on the HGTV network.

We all kept in touch, and I was most intrigued with Ratey's books, which have a focus on exercise for those with ADHD. In his book *Driven to Distraction*, he describes how ADHD impacts the mind. The book *Spark* details specifically the role of physical activity in curbing ADHD symptoms. More recently, his book *ADHD 2.0* describes advances in treatment over the past 15 years. To be sure, medications such as stimulants *do* help—I've seen good results in patients. But, as with most things, the optimum balance is lifestyle changes combined with pharmaceutical approaches, if needed.

One of the first studies looking at physical activity and ADHD was published by a group of German researchers from the University of Cologne in 2014. They summarized several trials and studies and found that social behavior, motor skills, strength, and neuropsychological parameters all improved with exercise interventions, though the interventions were varied. Other high-quality reviews—from Chile to Denmark to Israel—have reported that short-term aerobic exercise can improve ADHD symptoms. However, a systematic review from Spain of 16 studies didn't draw any firm conclusions for adolescents, and another review found the effect, for both autism and ADHD, was inconsistent across studies.

As such, the relationship between exercise and ADHD is unclear. While Phelps' performance didn't suffer from his ADHD, athletic abilities can, and are, affected by the condition in some children—so much so that in 2011, a set of clinical practice guidelines was published that focused on minimizing its impact.

4.

In 2021, heading up the steps outside of a hospital on North Wolfe Street in East Baltimore, Maryland, I never thought I'd be back. It had been more than ten years since I completed my master's degree in Global Epidemiology and Control at the Johns Hopkins Bloomberg School of Public Health across the street. At Johns Hopkins Hospital, Sapna Kudchadkar pioneered a groundbreaking approach to improve how children in the intensive care unit heal: The PICU-Up! Program.

Kudchadkar still remembers that morning, back in 2010, that shaped the trajectory of her scientific research. She was in the midst of a rigorous medical fellowship in pediatric critical care (also called intensive care) medicine. As she was listening to the hospital's overnight staff summarize how each child did overnight in the unit, and whether the patients had "slept" poorly or not poorly, it hit her. "In that moment, I realized that we weren't really talking about sleep, per se, but sedation," Kudchadkar told me.

As I had learned working in the pediatric intensive care unit (PICU), "sleep" and "sedation" are used interchangeably, but they don't actually mean the same thing. Real sleep is restorative. It's a process that the body uses to get rid of waste and heal. Sedation, on the other hand, is a very surface-level imitator of sleep. The patient looks asleep but is just less awake. Sedation is used primarily to manage pain and prevent the body from using too much of its energy. Kudchadkar suspected that sedation itself could have lasting implications for a person's recovery and long-term health.

Knowing that physical activity enhances sleep, Kudchadkar wondered: would her young patients do better if they were encouraged to move during their stay in intensive care? There was research around this in adults, but it hadn't quite reached pediatrics yet. This lit the match to begin a multi-year study, PICU-Up!, which Kudchadkar would direct in the Children's Hospital at the Johns Hopkins School of Medicine as part of "ICU liberation" in pediatric critical care medicine. The ICU liberation movement more generally seeks to reduce the negative effects of being bedbound and sedated in an ICU, effects which can linger for decades and include everything from lowered muscle strength to depression and anxiety.

One way to do this is to decrease sedation and encourage patients to move far sooner than they have in the past. As with any major culture change, though, there was some pushback initially, so Kudchadkar recognized that she first needed to reassure her colleagues and patients and bring them on board. "There was a collective sigh of relief that we weren't trying to get every kid out of bed walking, regardless of their acuity of illness," Kudchadkar recalls. Still, she adds, "Illness doesn't mean stillness," the program's catchphrase.

Since the 1980s, operating room procedures to keep patients sedated and unalert began being applied in other settings, specifically the intensive care unit. Sedation causes the brain to take on a semi-conscious or unconscious state. Various drugs—such as propofol and benzodiazepines—are used, and they each work differently. As well, other drugs called paralytics render the body immobile (so if a surgeon were cutting, it wouldn't "miss" because a patient moved). Yet the negative long-term effects of prolonged sedation were not recognized.

In 2000, a landmark article in the *New England Journal of Medicine* discussed the benefits of interrupting sedation for a brief period each day. Over the subsequent years, additional research showed that sedation has its own side effects, like cognitive issues, which are often memory deficits. Excessive bed rest can lead to muscle deconditioning. One study found, for instance, that each day of ICU bed rest lowered a person's muscle strength between 3% and 11%, and often, roughly one third left the hospital with significant muscle weakness, which led to years-long impairments.

In the initial phase of Kudchadkar's study, which ended in 2015, the safety of the program was assessed. One patient—Sydney Pearce—was two-and-a-half years old and recovering from open-heart surgery when she was enrolled in the

PICU-Up! Program. Within 24 hours of leaving the operating room, she was up walking and driving a toy car around the ICU. That study, published in 2016 in the journal *Pediatric Critical Care Medicine*, indicated that the mobility program was safe and appropriate.

In a 2021 nationwide U.S. study of 82 pediatric intensive care units (PICUs), Kudchadkar and colleagues found that only 35% of patients received mobility support from a physical or occupational therapist. Additionally, on 19% of patient days, patients remained completely immobile. They also found that mobility was positively associated with having a family member present but that this was only associated in young children under the age of three. In Canada, the prevalence of mobility was much higher at 80%, and family participation in mobility was significant. In Europe, it was around 39%.

Kudchadkar is now leading a multiyear, multicenter randomized controlled trial to look at the protocol's effectiveness. It will measure outcomes such as duration of mechanical ventilation, exposure to sedative medications, and length of hospital stay. Johns Hopkins All Children's Hospital in Florida, Boston Children's Hospital, Advocate Health Care in Illinois, and Our Lady of the Lake Children's Hospital in Louisiana are all participants in the trial. So far, their findings are remarkable, though several results are pending. At the Hopkins PICU, however, they identified that even with supportive staff and families, there were barriers preventing consistent application of the protocol. Such barriers include decisions around sedation, resources, and determining which patients may be suitable for early mobilization.

Kudchadkar and I have a lot in common—we're both first-generation immigrants from the Indian subcontinent, though I was born in the U.K. (and moved to Canada), and she was born in the U.S. after her parents moved here in the early 1970s. Kudchadkar was born in a small city in Georgia called Warner Robins to a father with a background in agricultural sciences, who went on to work for the U.S.D.A., providing loans to low-income farmers and their families. Her mother worked at home and later at Walgreens.

When she was in kindergarten, they moved to Charleston, Illinois, a small town with a population of 19,000. She was the only South Asian person in her entire class, and that would be true for years through high school. Kudchadkar wanted to fit in and even had a paper route, which became part of that desire, as well as helping instill hard work, determination, and grit (she had to get up at 5:30 am every day).

Today, she says it's one of the best things her parents asked her to do when she was growing up. In high school, Kudchadkar joined the 4-H Club, in which kids and teens participate in hands-on projects in areas such as health, science, agriculture, and civic engagement, guided by adult mentors while being encouraged to take leadership roles. She soon got over her shyness and would give talks on breaking stereotypes and the importance of diversity.

"Eventually, I had to make a decision, and I thought, 'why not become a doctor?' Maybe it was because of my Indian immigrant parents and the stereotype, but also because I really felt it bridged my interests and curiosity," she told me.

Kudchadkar then headed to Washington University in St. Louis for undergraduate studies, which "was a rude awakening…it was challenging and I struggled," she recalled.

But she eventually did well in her science prerequisite classes and got into medical school at the University of Chicago, choosing it because it was closer to home.

While college was tough, it was there where she got her first taste of research: "I did pap smears in mice!" she recalled, which made her realize perhaps research wasn't quite for her.

She matched to Johns Hopkins for pediatrics residency, she worked in the pediatric ICU, where she excelled to a point that she decided to do another fellowship in anesthesia. It was there that Kudchadkar began thinking about how sleep and sedation are related in the ICU and whether there was potential to do things differently.

Afterward, she completed a clinical investigator program and earned her Ph.D. at the Johns Hopkins Bloomberg School of Public Health. Sleep research became her main concentration; she felt she had something to bring to the table. She also realized that her interprofessional colleagues did as well. "The nurses were spending more time with the patients, compared with the doctors, for instance, and it was really important to ensure that everyone felt included," she said. But buy-in was tough. For decades, the standard of care for children in the ICU was to rest in order to conserve energy.

"I learned this was a new concept—ICU liberalization in pediatrics—and that we can't just preach to the choir. Sometimes, we have to shout from the rooftop," she said. So began her challenge to transform clinical care in the ICU. Kudchadkar emphasizes that it was crucial to make everybody feel included with the research and, subsequently, the shift in practice.

"You need to celebrate the successes and highlight people's work regardless if they're a nurse or doctor or physiotherapist. Sending out that communication and that newsletter was a big part of sharing the success and sharing the information," she said. "Over time, even those who were very resistant to the idea initially are now very excited about it and will share stories of patients that they've seen that were able to get up earlier and do better."

When I asked her what it is that got her to shift this paradigm and think outside the box, which forward-thinking institutions like Johns Hopkins welcome and support, she pointed to a couple of things. "The biggest was that I needed to go from being a pleaser to being a changer...but that took time. I was initially thought of as bossy, for example, but that transitioned to being 'authoritative' over time," she said. "And the second thing was the importance of mentorship."

5.

My mind was stronger as I prepared to return to the hospital. Taking the time to exercise and strengthen other parts of me was key as well—my mind and my ability to focus, much like Michael Phelps, and my body, through what Tyra Love showed me. Yet the biggest lessons came from Jessica Harthcock and Sapna Kudchadkar. When it comes to changing the broader medical system, there's something about being a bit of an outsider, especially early in life, that forces some of us to adapt. Like Kudchadkar, to many of us, the idea of fitting in was once really important, especially when we were young and trying to find our way and our place. But over time, it's the differences that make us unique and actually drive our identity and purpose. In other words, they become things to welcome as opposed to run from. And so many of us in that position end up doing an about-face in our late twenties to thirties and trying to carve our own niche inside this same nest of difference because that is what our hearts know to be true.

Over time, after leaving her small town, Kudchadkar found her voice and her calling and went on to realize that it was the unique perspective she brought that was of real value in advancing medicine. Indeed, this book is about healing in ways that the traditional medical system doesn't recognize completely. These are the modalities that we know have evidence and are being studied, but it's also important to realize the people behind them. For paradigms to shift and for systems to shift, we don't just need the evidence and research; we need the *people* behind the evidence and the researchers who believe in it and can see it through.

We need people who are not afraid to buck the status quo, those who aren't afraid to be curious and to ask questions. It doesn't mean that we have to be disagreeable or combative. It just means that there is an *art* to understanding how change is made and how to effectively steer the ship in an antiquated system like medicine. With the PICU-Up! program, that's exactly what happened. What started off as a seed of an idea one morning on rounds is now in several hundred countries as a principle guiding practice and will be a formalized guideline in all PICUs in the near future as well. And as a result, thousands of children around the world will be able to mobilize earlier, and then leave the ICU a bit earlier than expected, with healthier bodies and minds. This then will ripple out to impact their lives and that of their loved ones.

And when it came to healing ourselves after a traumatic experience, Jessica Harthcock, who is now a mother of a 3-year-old, underscored healing as physical, emotional, and spiritual. In addition, starting an important movement of a different kind for spinal cord injury patients was a key part of her healing. "I think that people go through adverse times, but you can either let it get the best of you and drown in it or you can tell yourself, 'I can conquer this.' Having that attitude up front is key," she told me. "The adversity I faced led me to the work I do today and the ability to work with amazing people. It led me to my husband, who helped me to walk again. I have an incredible service dog, Ozzie, because of it. It's hard to see the good in a traumatic event when you are in the thick of going through it, but I always knew there was a bigger purpose and bigger plan—I hung on to that."

I let Jessica's words sink in for a few moments. She taught me that even when a situation seems very bleak, where there's no beacon of light, we can be challenged to create our own, and that's exactly what I needed to remember as I continued to heal and face what would come next.

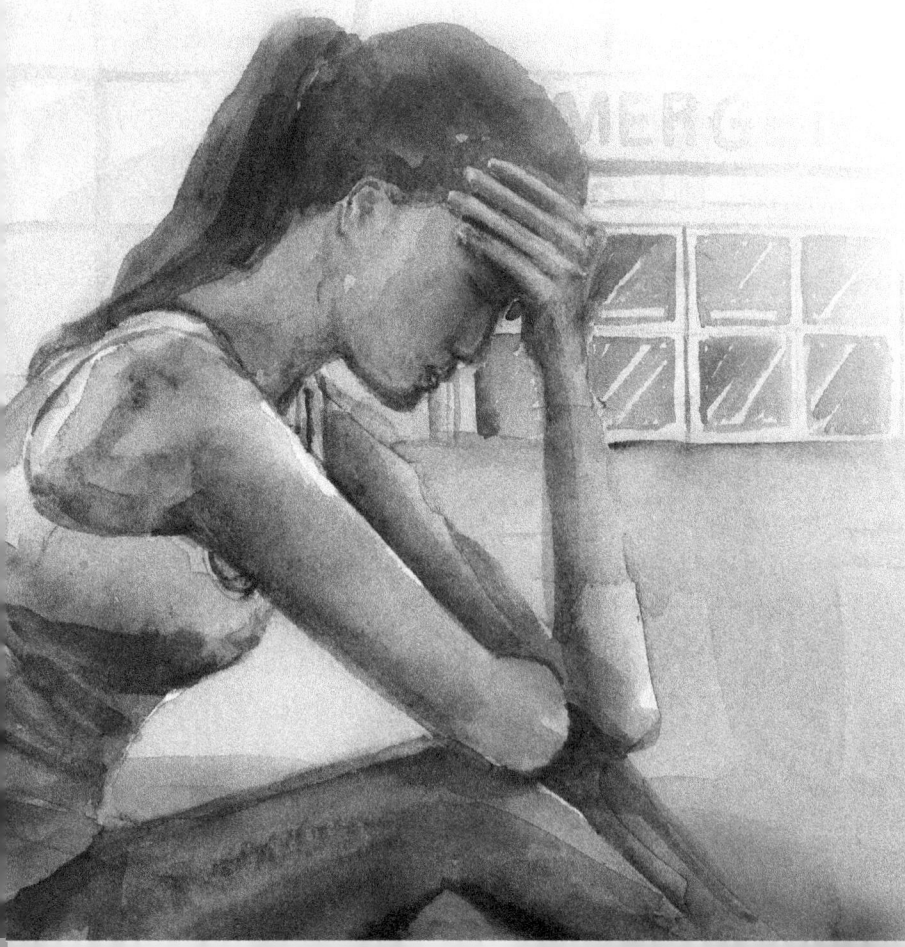

CHAPTER NINE

System Overdrive

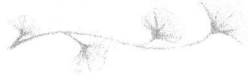

"You never change things by fighting the existing reality. To change something, build a new model that makes the existing model obsolete."
— Buckminster Fuller

1.

A s someone who excelled in school, loved medicine, and always strived to do my best, there was nothing more bewildering and devastating than being singled out for what appeared to be personal reasons. Then I met Kenneth. Over coffee, it became clear that we both left similar academic hospital environments for overlapping reasons. Knowing I wasn't alone helped me start to make sense of what had happened.

Kenneth had experienced nothing but success before entering a challenging residency rotation, where the environment became so hostile that he sought help. The university's wellness officer, who had taken over for a previous staff member, diagnosed him with several unrelated conditions—at one point even suggesting he had an eating disorder. As the situation worsened, a colleague stayed close to Kenneth, worried about his well-being. Thankfully, Kenneth didn't harm himself, but taking a leave of absence helped him realize that the path he was on wasn't sustainable. He went on to pursue a master's degree in public health, where he thrived. Still, whenever we met for coffee or brunch, I could sense a lingering sadness when we talked about the academic hospital. We both knew he would have made an outstanding pediatrician.

I also came to know Kate. Most of her training had taken place in a rural area, but she came to one of the larger hospitals for a rotation that turned into a difficult experience. What began as a minor mix-up on rounds—confusing a patient's name—escalated into unwarranted criticism of her notes and personal attacks on her personality. Kate suspected her direct communication style may have made her more vulnerable to this treatment. As the stress mounted, Kate was formally diagnosed with anxiety—something she had never experienced before. "They failed me on my first probation period," she confided. "Now, I'm just trying to get through." By the time we spoke, she had spent two years seeking alternative training sites, and thanks to her legal team, she managed to complete most of her remaining rotations elsewhere.

Sadly, bullying often leads victims to blame themselves. Perpetrators, too, rationalize their behavior to justify the harm they cause. Research shows that personality accounts for only about 30% of behavior—the rest is shaped by context and environment. As Ross and Nisbett had argued in *The Person and the Situation*, behavior is heavily influenced by the surrounding environment.

Some academic hospitals have troubling patterns—frequent dismissals, transfers, and dropouts—compared to similar programs across the country. It's made more evident when looking at how many trainees may or may not return to work as staff at the hospital where they trained: in part its due to culture. Kenneth's experience as someone who identified as LGBT, and the fact that Kate and I are both women of color, raised important questions about whether certain groups may be particularly vulnerable to toxic environments in medicine.

2.

Although most hospitals are full of good people, the tone at the top shapes the entire culture. When leaders turn adversarial, even well-intentioned individuals tend to distance themselves to avoid getting involved. Others may join in, hoping to avoid becoming targets themselves. Brené Brown refers to this phenomenon as "common enemy intimacy"—a false sense of connection that forms through shared animosity toward someone perceived as a threat. I saw this dynamic play out with an administrative scheduler I worked with early on. After some residents and staff began making disparaging remarks about him, implying he had a mental health disorder, he was quietly dismissed from his role. Common enemy intimacy may not be unusual in a high-stress workplace like a hospital, but residents are not the only victims. In 2019, a study in *JAMA Surgery* reported that surgeons who'd had several reports of "unprofessional behavior" (bullying, aggression, and giving false or misleading information) had patient complication rates about 40% higher than other surgeons. Other research shows that even *witnessing* incivility or bullying can negatively impact performance. I had noticed this among my colleagues.

At one point, in an interview for a major news organization, Dr. Perry, the doctor who oversaw the care of Baby J, came forward and admitted her own experience with depression in this exact environment. "I kept working because that's all I knew how to do," she had shared. Reading that made me realize she'd been empathetic to me in part because she had understood; she may have been affected by the toxicity too.

*

After some time away, I returned to the same environment following a committee assessment that confirmed I had been treated unfairly. I was told that efforts had been made to help me transition to another setting, but nothing materialized. Although I wasn't given specific details, I accepted the situation and focused on continuing my work. Upon my return, I found the atmosphere among my colleagues to be more open and supportive. Some shared their personal challenges with me, and others hinted at exploring ways to shorten their time there or seek other opportunities.

At first, things seemed to be going well. Feedback was overwhelmingly positive, confirming that I was performing at or above expectations, even after my time away. I began to think that perhaps my return would go better than I had feared. However, as time went on and as I worked with those who had previously been hostile, familiar patterns of negativity began to emerge. I was frequently pulled aside during work hours under the pretense of "feedback," leaving me disconnected from my tasks and behind on patient care. Later, I would be criticized for not staying updated—a cycle that felt intentional. Next would be using my research accomplishments or reading as proof that I lacked humility or appeared overconfident.

There were also attempts to undermine my accomplishments. My academic success was reframed as arrogance, and fabricated concerns about safety started to surface. Recognizing the patterns, I began to document everything carefully, though the effort was exhausting and added hours to my day. I had also learned to gather written accounts from colleagues when appropriate. One supportive peer noted in a message: *It made me uncomfortable to witness what happened, especially with someone like Amitha, who is smart and always helpful.* She signed only with her initials, fearing backlash for speaking out.

Even the guidelines I was asked to follow seemed designed to create traps. I was told not to send emails after a certain time, yet senior staff often contacted me late at night. I felt caught between conflicting expectations—either risk being reprimanded for responding too slowly or for not following the rules. These tactics seemed designed to wear me down and justify future criticism.

As I reflected on the situation with trusted mentors outside of the environment, it became clear that the scrutiny I faced was unlikely to stop. No matter how well I performed or how carefully I followed the rules, it seemed inevitable that the goalposts would continue to shift. But this time, I was prepared. I had spent my time away healing and regaining my strength, and I was determined not to lose myself again.

One of my final collaborative experiences was with a senior colleague, Jeff, whose feedback was consistent with my other positive evaluations: *Amitha has a quiet leadership style, excellent clinical judgment, and strong patient management skills. She never hesitates to seek input when needed.* After submitting his feedback, Jeff confided in me that he had faced subtle retaliation, such as being ignored by certain individuals who had previously targeted me.

Despite some optimism from those around me that my strong documentation and performance would shield me from further harm, it quickly became evident that deeper issues remained. Instead of acknowledging progress, new criticisms were manufactured, and efforts to discredit me escalated. This time, vague accusations were replaced with fabricated claims meant to portray me as a risk, regardless of the evidence I presented.

But I refused to back down. I knew that what I was experiencing wasn't just personal—it was reflective of a larger, systemic issue. This fight was no longer just about my experience; it was about standing up for myself and others who had encountered similar challenges in environments that resisted change.

Through a series of conversations with trusted colleagues, I also uncovered troubling patterns. It appeared that many transfer opportunities I was told had been explored on my behalf were quietly obstructed, with informal calls and behind-the-scenes conversations preventing any real progress. Most perturbing to discover was that some of the individuals involved were those the impartial committee had ordered to ensure a transfer. Instead, they seemed more focused on maintaining the status quo than addressing the deeper issues that were harming many physicians.

Despite these setbacks, I held on to the hope that change was possible. Each day was a reminder that the process of healing and growth is not linear, but I knew I was moving forward. The weight of my documentation was heavy, but it was also empowering—it gave me the clarity to see the situation for what it was. And while the road ahead was uncertain, I knew I had the strength to walk it with integrity, determined to ensure that the challenges I faced would not be in vain.

*

Inspired by stories I had heard from colleagues and motivated to address the larger issue of well-being in academic hospitals, I pitched a story to the *Boston Globe* about bullying and mistreatment in medical education and academic hospitals across North America. I believed that grounding my experiences in data and evidence would help me process what I had been through and contribute to positive change. The editors were enthusiastic about the idea, and while preparations were underway for my next steps, I immersed myself in reporting.*

I came across a paper by Lawrence Huntoon in the Journal of American Physicians and Surgeons, stating that "360-degree feedback" in the hospital staffing context is often used as a tool for bullying because it can be rigged so effectively through "sham peer review."** The makers of the 360-degree feedback tool have reiterated it is not to be used as a basis for dismissal (in large part because the tool can be manipulated), but in toxic environments the tool is abused. Finally, I understood why some horrible comments I had received couldn't align with my evaluations.

While searching for answers, I came across the work of David Yamada, a lawyer and expert on workplace dynamics, who described mobbing as a form of coordinated, large-scale bullying often orchestrated by those in leadership. He explained that these situations frequently involve someone at the top pulling the strings—what he referred to as a "puppet master." In my case, it felt as though there a few individuals working in a coordinated fashion against me and others they felt threatened by or envious of, each playing a role. When I spoke with Yamada, he told me, *This is definitely mobbing, but it's rare to see it escalate to this degree—where they block even potential escape routes, like a transfer. It seems as if their goal is to crush you completely, with no intention of stopping until that's achieved.*

As painful as it was to hear, his words gave me clarity. I began to see the situation for what it was—a systemic attempt to undermine me, something that others I knew had also experienced in different parts of the institution. Certain leaders allowed the behavior to continue, either because they condoned it or felt pressured into participating. Reflecting on it, I realized that I should have insisted that any agreement following my initial investigation include a clear, enforceable plan for a transfer—one managed independently, rather than by

---

* This article went viral when it was published on March 15, 2019. It can be retrieved here: https://www.bostonglobe.com/ideas/2019/03/15/america-becoming-doctor-can-prove-fatal/u3x4xfPC9VR2zSCnKArgYM/story.html/. I was humbled that renowned pioneering physician writer, Dr Samuel Shem, author of House of God, penned a supportive and insightful reader letter after publication, which can be found here https://www.bostonglobe.com/opinion/letters/2019/03/18/med-school-bullying-takes-new-form/iRQImyJAeRz9r1x3rPYtvN/story.html

** Dr. Lawrence Huntoon first wrote about this in 2007 (https://www.jpands.org/vol12no1/huntoon.pdf), and published a follow-up editorial in 2022 (https://www.jpands.org/vol27no4/huntoon.pdf). Both are worth the read.

those responsible for the initial actions against me. That had been the approach of others I knew, and it might have made all the difference.

When I shared with my friend Karine what I'd found, she noted the similarity to what she called her ex-husband's "gaslighting"—lying and cheating, but then blaming her for inquiring about her suspicions. "You kept pointing out that something is off because it was," she said. "But they denied it and instead labeled *you* as the problem."

I was slowly learning the interconnections between all forms of abuse. University of Oregon's Jennifer Freyd, in referring to institutional betrayal, coined the term DARVO: deny, attack, reverse victim and offender.* This tactic, often in sexual assault claims, switches the perpetrator and victim to distract from the issue and dehumanize and intimidate the victim. I emailed David Yamada with a question—could DARVO as a principle be applied to mobbing and bullying? His answer was yes—and he went on to write about it on his blog.**

One bright spot during this time was being invited by the Canadian Medical Association (CMA) to contribute to a working group focused on improving policies for both trainees and practicing physicians across the country. As part of the group, we presented several interconnected recommendations. One key suggestion involved ensuring that staff had greater control over their funding, directing it toward their needs rather than through institutions. This change would allow for smoother transitions to safer environments if they encountered unhealthy or unsupportive conditions. We also proposed policies to encourage accountability, suggesting that holding individuals responsible for unprofessional behavior would incentivize better conduct among staff. The idea was to foster a healthier culture where respect, integrity, and professionalism were the norm.

While the CMA's leadership expressed commitment to long-term change, they cautioned that progress would take time and require cooperation from accreditation and licensing bodies. In the meantime, I began hearing from more individuals—both locally and internationally—who shared similar experiences.

---

* Jennifer Freyd's definition can be found here: https://dynamic.uoregon.edu/jjf/defineDARVO.html
** David Yamada's blog about the topic can be found here: https://newworkplace.wordpress.com/2019/03/07/workplace-bullying-darvo-and-aggressors-claiming-victim-status/

Their stories served as a reminder that these issues extended far beyond any single program or institution and underscored the urgent need for systemic reform.

3.

Dr. Uché Blackstock is an impressive Harvard-trained doctor I came into contact with through my work mentoring academics through the nonprofit the Op-Ed Project. Blackstock was hoping to write an article for *STAT News* about why she left academic medicine, which later became part of her autobiography. entitled *Legacy*. I worked closely with her on that opinion article, editing and shaping it with her, as I knew how impactful it would be. The problem was different from mine but had similar themes. The large New York-based medical center that had hired her expected her to take on several "diversity" initiatives, but pushed back on her efforts if they appeared to challenge the status quo.

At first, as one of the few African-American physicians in leadership, Blackstock was happy to do so. She readily identified systemic issues related to diversity and inclusion but was quickly labeled a troublemaker. Any ideas she put forth were quashed. She was alternately given the cold shoulder and treated in a hostile manner. She eventually planned her exit, which is what she writes in much more detail about, including the biases and bullying that I had could relate to.

Blackstock, who now works as an emergency medicine doctor in Brooklyn while also running a successful consulting and speaking company, pointed me to a helpful diagram (next page) that applies to a lot of women of color in non-profits and academia. Intentions might be good initially, but the idea that a woman of color could be in a position of leadership, along with the change that might bring, can make people uncomfortable enough to create a mobbing situation that causes the woman to leave. Clearly, this phenomenon was known enough to have its own framework: it's predictable, in other words, and I wasn't alone.

The 2011 case of United Kingdom-based Dr. Bawa Garba had parallels with Blackstock's experience, as well as mine. Garba, a Black woman, was the on-call medical resident and dealing with a complex case of a child with Down syndrome and sepsis. Her attending staff was unavailable to support her, so she was forced to make decisions and missed a red flag, which resulted in the death of the child. The newspaper coverage was devastating: Garba was presented as an African immigrant with a hijab head covering, in a predominantly white system, and was being blamed by the parents and the system for killing a

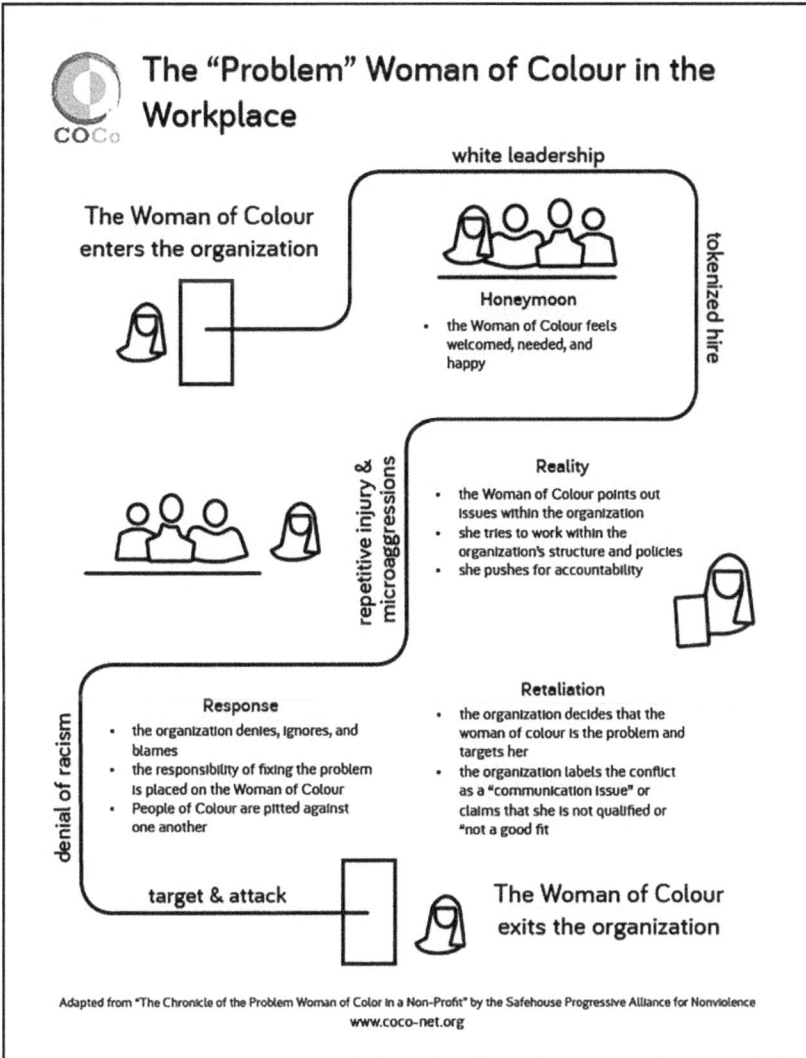

The "Problem" Woman of Colour in the Workplace

COCo

white leadership

The Woman of Colour enters the organization

tokenized hire

Honeymoon
- the Woman of Colour feels welcomed, needed, and happy

repetitive injury & microaggressions

Reality
- the Woman of Colour points out issues within the organization
- she tries to work within the organization's structure and policies
- she pushes for accountability

Retaliation
- the organization decides that the woman of colour is the problem and targets her
- the organization labels the conflict as a "communication issue" or claims that she is not qualified or "not a good fit

denial of racism

Response
- the organization denies, ignores, and blames
- the responsibility of fixing the problem is placed on the Woman of Colour
- People of Colour are pitted against one another

target & attack

The Woman of Colour exits the organization

Adapted from "The Chronicle of the Problem Woman of Color in a Non-Profit" by the Safehouse Progressive Alliance for Nonviolence
www.coco-net.org

Source: Centre for Community Organizations, as adapted from Safehouse Alliance

Developed by the Safehouse Progressive Alliance for Non-Violence, adapted by the Centre for Community Organizations (https://coco-net.org/problem-woman-colour-nonprofit-organizations/)

special-needs child. Though the case dragged on for years, she was eventually cleared. Her attending fled to Ireland and wasn't heard from again. Garba was not supported and then blamed—classic DARVO. Although she is now practicing, at one point, Garba said she "had to hit rock bottom" to remember why she wanted to be a doctor.

Indeed, the ways that female medical trainees are assessed on their performance can be horrifically biased, and the research shows this. Several studies have found that learner assessments during training are biased by gender, even by *female* assessors.* Michigan medical professionals would become among the first to require training in bias. Others would call for structural solutions related to diversity in academic medicine positions.

Two landmark cases from the mid-2000s, playing out in academic medical centers on opposite coasts of Canada, illustrate the broader problem of bias and mobbing within medicine.

4.

Dr. Gabrielle Horne loved all the physiological intricacies of the human heart and easily matched into her first-choice cardiology program at Dalhousie University's medical center in Nova Scotia, Canada. Since she had earned a Ph.D. along with her M.D., she was well-suited to start a rigorous cardiology research program, looking at complex cases of heart failure and examining which treatments might best reverse its impact.

Since funding in Canada is scarcer than it is in the U.S., Horne applied for every grant she could. Her efforts paid off: she received a prestigious grant from the Canadian Institute for Health Research. Her colleagues congratulated her. The division chief, on the other hand, took her aside. "You're going to add me to the grant, right?"

---

* Two key citations here are by Babal et al. 2022 (https://www.ncbi.nlm.nih.gov/pmc/articles/PMC6502889/), Champagne-Lagabeer 2021 (https://bmcmededuc.biomedcentral.com/articles/10.1186/s12909-021-02601-2)

She looked at him, dismayed. The collaborators Horne had identified all had research training and had published on similar topics. This man hadn't. "No, I hadn't planned to," she replied. The chief looked shocked, but Horne thought that would be the end of it. But within weeks, several of her colleagues started accusing her of not caring for her patients appropriately. Then, the chief wouldn't allow her to start the research program, asking for unnecessary documents and paperwork. The delays eventually cost her the grant money because she had nothing to show for it. It echoed the same problem I had endured with the inciting incident around the course I attended.

Horne had been mobbed, and as Eve Seguin wrote in *University Affairs* in 2016, "*Mobbing is social murder* and, by definition, people cannot survive their own murder." Seguin illuminates why mobbing is so common in academia:

> First, because mobbers are not sadists or sociopaths, but ordinary people; second, because universities are a type of organization that encourages mobbing; and third, as a result, mobbing is endemic at universities. The term itself, *mobbing*, describes its four essential characteristics: it is a collective, violent and deliberate process in which the individual psychologies of the aggressors and their victim provide no keys to understanding the phenomenon. Workplace mobbing is a *concerted process to get rid of an employee*, who is better referred to as a "target" than a "victim" to emphasize the strategic nature of the process. The dynamic is reminiscent of Stalin's Moscow Trials: the targets are first convicted, and evidence is later fabricated to justify the conviction. As sociologist of science Brian Martin put it, everything they say, or write and do will be systematically used against them. Successful mobbing leads to any of a number of outcomes: the targets commit suicide, are dismissed (or often at universities, denied tenure), resign, retire early, take permanent or recurring sick leave (the last three being the most common cases for university professors), or have all their responsibilities withdrawn (as in the case of sidelined senior public servants).

As Horne explained in her TEDx Talk,* she decided to fight back. She retained a lawyer, but since mobbing isn't legislated in Canada, the case took a decade to play out. Horne eventually won a landmark settlement in 2016, but the award was reduced on appeal to only cover her legal costs. She has since restarted her program. The division chief of cardiology, who orchestrated the mobbing, is now practicing in another province, but many of the mob participants are still in the Nova Scotia health system.

*

As Horne pursued her case in a Halifax courtroom, Carl Kelly, a family medicine resident at University of British Columbia, was doing the same in Vancouver. Kelly's Attention Deficit Hyperactivity Disorder (ADHD) had caused him to struggle with one rotation, specifically with time management and organization. Kelly was failed and eventually dismissed because of it, even though the school didn't accommodate him to the degree they should have. It's unclear if the attendings he worked with were aware of their biases against his disability or of their legal duties to accommodate physical and mental disabilities. A reasonable accommodation would have involved giving him extra time to complete tasks, being more forgiving if he had trouble focusing, and providing him with extra assistance with multi-tasking as needed.

Since my anxiety and depression were *induced* by the mistreatment specific staff at the hospital, the most obvious "accommodation" would have been to allow me to transfer to a safer place, which had been the recommendation of several third-party physicians, assessors, and committee members. But for reasons we could only surmise, given the pattern of my success on the hospital wards that did not involve the bullies, it was likely that allowing for this accommodation would effectively *prove* that the hospital (and namely, those behind the mistreatment) were in the wrong.

It would take a precedent-setting win to allow for it.

---

* Gabrielle Horne's TEDx talk, entitled "Using medical research tools to survive workplace bullying," can be found here: https://www.ted.com/talks/gabrielle_horne_how_a_doctor_used_medical_research_tools_to_survive_workplace_bullying?subtitle=en

That ruling had come years earlier, in 2013, when the court ruled in Kelly's favor. At that time, he received the highest settlement in the history of Canada's Human Rights Tribunal, which was subsequently reduced by half on appeal by the university. But he was able to finish the remaining year of his training, and he went on to launch a successful practice in Northern British Columbia, where he practices to this day.

In each of these cases, workplace toxicity had damaged people who'd invested heavily in their medical training. It's even worse when that toxicity trickles down to impact those the doctors have sworn to help. Bullying then becomes a matter of life and death, rendering vulnerable the entire system of patient care.

Two stories, which couldn't be more different, confirm this tragic reality.

5.

In 2018, on Twitter, a woman named Ruth tagged me in a story for CBC radio on bullying in medicine and hospitals, in which she detailed a horrific experience with her daughter, Minimosa (Mini), at a children's hospital. She DM'd me and then we spoke.

Mini was a 2-year-old who lived with her parents and younger brother in Eastern Ontario. She loved spelling out words and playing in the garden. One day in October 2016, Mini began experiencing a fever and weakness. Mini ended up in the emergency department and underwent rigorous testing. She was diagnosed with PH+ (PH positive) Acute Lymphoblastic Leukemia (ALL), a severe form of blood cancer. Her white blood cells were mutating and crowding out other healthier cells to the point that her organs stopped working. A chemotherapy standard for ALL was prescribed.

In late November, Ruth, her husband, and Mini were called to have a meeting with her doctors, where it was disclosed that the diagnosis was being revised and Mini was being placed on a more intense form of chemotherapy to target the causative gene. Ruth asked for more information but was told that the physicians' workload didn't allow for more time to explain it. Ruth pressed, and Ruth recalled that the doctors rolled their eyes. Seven months later, in June of 2017, Mini presented with weakness in part of her face. As she grew ever weaker, Ruth became desperate as the doctors kept dismissing her concerns, calling her a "difficult patient" and saying that their family treated the hospital like a "hotel."

More than a year after the initial diagnosis, Ruth headed to the emergency department with Mini and begged that she be retested, since the chemotherapy didn't seem to be working. The testing was halted after confirming a relapse. Fed up, Ruth grabbed Mini and headed home. The family decided to pack up and move to a large metropolitan to seek care at its children's hospital. At that hospital, at the end of 2017, she heard news no parent wants to hear: Mini's treatment was targeting the wrong gene.

"The first relapse [they] hid from us...wasn't discovered until we sifted through all of Mini's files, emails. etc., through RFI [request for information] requests. It was a fulltime job. I didn't work for years," Ruth told me.

For two years, the cancer had been spreading in her body as the chemotherapy killed off healthy cells in scores. Mini was immediately started on the correct therapy and appeared to improve, but soon relapsed again. When nothing further could be done, the family left the hospital. Mini died at home in November 2018.

"I remember sitting there in the clinic in [the larger city] just stunned," Ruth told me. "Completely betrayed [by those other doctors]. Part of me wondered if it was on purpose because maybe I was a 'difficult parent,' but another part just wondered how this could happen."

I told Ruth that mistakes happen—medical errors, devastating as they are, are *human* errors. I frankly surprised myself by jumping to the hospital's defense. Why, when they were exhibiting behavior similar to that which had so hurt me? To this day, I really don't know. It just felt like the right thing to do, especially because I knew that the toxicity tended to localize among only a small handful of doctors in such hospitals, and certainly did not include everyone.

But then Ruth said, "Oh, *that* wasn't the issue. I understand mistakes happen. It was the coverup after." I was taken aback.

Ruth shared that when Mini passed away, it was just the beginning of the nightmare for Ruth and her husband. The records they requested confirmed their worst fears: several mistakes were made, and the "investigation" into the mistake was done by the very people who were involved in the initial decision-making. This was a strategy similar to the one used against me. It's akin to asking an individual suspected of murder to be in charge of their own criminal investigation: it was deplorable. The documents left her horrified but validated: she had a right to have been concerned when she was. Her gut feeling was correct, her fears legitimate. Eventually, an "objective" pediatric oncologist from another hospital was brought in, and as of this writing, the investigation outcome was sealed.

"It just makes me wonder," Ruth said. "Do they even care about children? Why be a doctor for kids if they just don't care?"

Ruth's story left me in tears. I had wanted to believe that at least the patients treated at my hospital were protected from any malicious behavior from the very doctors tasked to heal them. Hearing about Mini's case showed me I was wrong.

Not only was I far from alone, but I was also part of a trend: something sinister was happening within the culture of academic pediatric medicine and medical education.

*

In May 2019, a landmark investigation by Ellen Gabler and detailed in the article "Doctors Were Alarmed: Would I Have My Children Have Surgery Here?"* in *The New York Times* exposed a troubling situation at North Carolina Children's Hospital. In 2016 and 2017, several pediatric cardiologists raised the alarm with members of the hospital leadership about what they suspected to be a higher-than-expected death or complication rate in children after cardiac surgery. Nothing was done. All nine cardiologists expressed grave concerns about being able to refer children with heart issues for surgery within their own hospital for fear they were placing the child at risk.

When pressed by the *Times*, the hospital finally released the data, which placed them among the lowest-performing pediatric cardiac surgery units

___
* Gabler's excellent investigative piece can be found here: https://www.nytimes.com/interactive/2019/05/30/us/children-heart-surgery-cardiac.html

in the U.S., as measured by death rate. In one of Gabler's interviews, a staff member noted "a dysfunctional group...[and] team culture issues." When apprised of this, a critical care physician argued, "There is nothing here that is systematic or systemic that would lead us to be concerned about the performance of operations on children that are high-risk, low-risk, or no-risk." This was an odd declaration, considering that systematic issues in culture are incredibly hard to discern without a formal assessment process.

In secretly recorded staff meetings provided to the *Times*, one cardiologist said, "As a mother of three children, oh my God...it's inexcusable. As a physician, I mean, we all took an oath. We are supposed to do what's right for our patients...that's what you signed up for. And who is he [the surgeon in question] to play God with some kid's life? I can't get past this. This is beyond horrifying." Another physician shared, in terms of referring patients for cardiac surgery within the institution: "I do feel increasingly, morally, ethically uneasy about this."

It turns out the concept had a name: moral distress. Later on, I would know that this is what many of my hospital physician mentors would feel as they tried to advocate and help their mentees who faced harassment and bullying. Any efforts would be futile, leading a sense of failure.

6.

Research shows that moral distress, or the "inability of a moral agent to act according to his or her core values and perceived obligations due to internal and external constraints," can be a major factor in staff turnover. Moral distress occurs when an individual knows the ethically appropriate action to take but feels powerless to take that action due to institutional constraints, legal limitations, or other barriers. It is commonly experienced by healthcare professionals who are unable to act according to their moral or ethical beliefs due to external pressures or policies, leading to feelings of frustration, guilt, and compromised integrity. This phenomenon has significant implications for mental health and job satisfaction among professionals in high-stakes environments. When health professionals feel desperate enough to record private meetings and send them to an investigative journalist, it's clear they're at the end of their rope, torn between their sworn ethics and a culture preventing them from speaking up.

Gabler reported that in 2018, four of the nine pediatric cardiologists left the North Carolina hospital in question, sensing a lack of "psychological safety." Amy Edmondson, the Harvard Business School researcher who popularized the term, describes it in her book, *The Fearless Organization,* this way:

> In psychologically safe workplaces, people know they might fail, they might receive performance feedback that says they're not meeting expectations...[but] they feel comfortable sharing concerns and mistakes without fear of embarrassment or retribution.... They know they can ask questions when they are unsure about something. They tend to trust and respect their colleagues.

Edmondson's Ph.D. research in the mid-1990s looked at the role of team dynamics in medication error at several U.S. hospitals. Edmondson hypothesized that higher-performing teams would make fewer errors. Intuitive, right? Instead, Edmondson found the opposite: high-performing teams made more errors – as many as ten times more. Why? Because rather than cover up mistakes, they felt safe to self-report errors without fear of reprisal. In a paper she published in *Quality & Safety in Health Care* in 2004, she argued that healthcare organizations can learn from their failures only if leadership bolsters psychological safety by supporting reporting, questioning, sharing of insights and concerns, and by actively studying the barriers that affect patient safety.

All hospitals brush shoulders with issues of psychological safety and moral distress at some point, given the traditional medical hierarchy and the fact that lives and careers are at risk. Restoring psychological safety then becomes a crucial aspect of improving hospital culture, and hospital culture is directly linked to patient outcomes. A major study led by Yale School of Public Health scientist Leslie Curry found that risk-standardized mortality rates after a heart attack were significantly higher in hospitals where the culture was deemed less collaborative and open—specifically, concerns about learning environment, senior management support, psychological safety, commitment to the organization, and time allocated for improvement. After the researchers' intervention, every aspect improved in six of the 10 hospitals, and these six also had significant reductions in the risk-standardized mortality rates of patients with heart attacks. With these results in hand, Curry's team created a program called Leadership Saves Lives to improve hospital culture by enhancing elements of psychological safety.

Curry's colleague, Marcela Nunez-Smith, a physician at Yale, has looked specifically at the role of racial dynamics as it relates to the differential treatment of Black healthcare team members. Persons of underrepresented groups fear speaking up. Microaggressions are common. And, as reported by the *BMJ* (*British Medical Journal*), this results in differential attainment—the gap in achievement levels between different groups—among minority physicians during training. The pressures of systemic discrimination cause a leaky pipeline of achievement as it relates to those being 'held back' unfairly. It's the most vulnerable groups that are harassed, even though a 2020 McKinsey report outlined the ways diversity and inclusion make good business sense.

And where bias is a concern with medical staff, it's a concern with patients as well. A story emerged about an Indigenous woman named Joyce Echaquan who hit "record" on her phone as white female health professionals at a Quebec hospital were delivering racial slurs to her. She asked for help; a white female nurse questioned her life choices and suggested she was only "good for sex" and would be "better off dead." She later did, in fact, die, and as of this writing, Quebec—the only province where French is the official language—continues to grapple with longstanding systemic discrimination of other non-white Francophone groups. That particular nurse was charged and dismissed.*

So why can shifting these norms, and ensuring accountability, help both healthcare providers and their patients? A systematic review of 62 studies found

---

* More about this story, published in CBC News, can be found here: https://www.cbc.ca/news/canada/montreal/joyce-echaquan-systemic-racism-quebec-government-1.6196038

fewer deaths, fewer falls, and fewer hospital-acquired infections in healthcare settings exhibiting healthier internal cultures. And physician retention, job satisfaction, and teamwork, all benefit from a strong organizational culture in hospitals. Indeed, the evidence is clear: healthier hospital cultures are good for the doctors (including those in training) as well as patients.

That all sounded great. But what I wanted to know was what could be done to improve a toxic culture like what was seen in too many hospitals – such as the one I was familiar with or the North Carolina hospital. So, I turned to Dr. Jenny Rudolph, Executive Director of Harvard University's Center for Medical Simulation. Rudolph's team is using simulation to build psychological safety.

"Our group works on creating a culture where it's normal to help each other reach 'collective competence' and psychological safety is an important part of encouraging everybody to speak up and contribute. If attending staff invite their colleagues' and their trainees' fresh perspectives and consistently thank them when they do, this helps build a culture friendly to learning and excellence," Rudolph told me. "In simulation, we create an alternative narrative—it's not about perfection. We approach shortcomings as puzzles which invite curiosity. At its best, simulation is a powerful intervention to shift into a growth mindset so we can get better at what we do and keep standards high, while also holding team members in high regard."

In the North Carolina hospital case, due to Gabler's reporting for the *Times*, changes have included creating a dedicated cardiac intensive care unit to watch for and manage post-operative complications and more transparent reporting of mistakes. But results aren't yet in; new data on mortality hasn't been released, and real change will take time and, ideally, an external assessment.

All of this thinking about hospital workplace culture had worked up an appetite and led to an unexpected case study on how one restaurant used the same principles to completely transform their culture to stand above the rest.

7.

On the corner of Ross Street and Wellington Street West, in Ottawa, sits a restaurant called Supply and Demand. With melt-in-your-mouth pasta, fresh seafood from Newfoundland, and inventive cocktails, it has a distinct Brooklyn-meets-Charleston vibe, except the Canadian version.

One frigid winter morning, I made my way to its basement prep kitchen to learn how owner and head chef Steve Wall was able to meet, and most often exceed, the expectations of the hundreds of customers that pass through each week, all while not overburdening the five full-time cooks and bartender that can be found there on any given night. A stereotypical "angry head chef," made popular by countless reality cooking shows, was nowhere to be found. I'd learn that Wall had *intentionally* designed a culture of inspiration and kindness.

The stakes were high when Wall started the business. He'd put his heart and soul and lots of money into it, so he decided to toss in his personal experience with leadership as well. I asked about those influences.

Raised by an ex-military father, Wall grew up with strict but clear expectations, evident today in Supply and Demand's sense of order: even apprenticing chefs note that everything is always in its place. He also told me a story from his chef training job in Nova Scotia—a story he often shares with his new chefs.

"One day I made a mistake where I put a hot pan with a steel ladle on the stovetop, and the chef touched it and burned himself. I apologized profusely but he turned to glare at me, grabbed the ladle, and threw it across the room so it landed up against the wall on another side. Then he asked me to pick it up. 'I got burned, so now you will too,' he said. I had no choice but to do it. I remember getting home that day and crying, which wasn't that rare during that time," Wall recalled. He promised himself he was *never* going to treat any of his cooks like that.

As Wall shared this story, I sensed a fascinating number of parallels between the culinary and medical worlds. Medicine's hierarchy is often compared to the military in terms of blind obedience and the need to "earn" respect;

then there's the battle scars and sleep deprivation. The culinary world was quite literally based on the military, with roles clearly delineated from *sous chef* to *chef de partie*. In medicine we still use terms like "house officer" and "attending," which parallel a junior officer and a sergeant.

It also struck me that "supply and demand" is also the perfect analogy for well-being. When demand exceeds supply in the body, we run into pathology. Demands on the cardiac system during serious infection, for example, can lead to multi-organ failure. When workload demands or undue scrutiny or mistreatment exceed our personal resources, we must meet those challenges; a very real crash—burnout—is the likely result.

When I asked Wall about burnout, he told me about his favorite book, *Setting the Table*, by Danny Meyer, owner of several famed New York restaurants, from Gramercy Tavern to the Shake Shack. When you set the right tone from the start, Meyer argues, staff retention stays high, people enjoy coming to work and serving, and the customer experience is positive. This ultimately results in profits and restaurant expansion.

Wall's wife, Jennifer, who runs the backend at Supply and Demand, said, "New cooks are often suspicious. We counter that by making our transparency a priority. If they have a question, for instance, about their paycheck, we review their hours and how the payments and bonuses and vacation are calculated. We prioritize their rest days to avoid burnout. In the end, many want to stay or come back to us."

The Walls figured out how to cultivate change in an antiquated industry by using very simple, readily available tools— trust and safety. They knew they couldn't tackle the entire culinary world but could start small: with their own restaurant.

The healthcare industry is ripe for that same change, and perhaps it needs to start small, too.

8.

In North America, the toxic medical culture has been called out as primarily responsible for mental health issues among physicians. Data shows that up to two-thirds of trainees experience symptoms of depression, which can manifest in low mood, irritability, forgetfulness, or lack of interest. Surveys put burnout rates at around 45% to 51%.*

And sadly, the endpoint for many manifests as the leading cause of death among medical residents: suicide.

Bullying, mobbing, moral distress, burnout, and a distinct lack of psychological safety create a perverse proving ground for those who are motivated to pursue this rigorous profession.

Reading Steve Hassan's book *Combating Cult Mind Control* made me realize how much toxic medical cultures function similarly to cults. Hassan says cults often have a charismatic leader who controls communication within the environment while applying psychological pressure that makes it difficult to leave ("milieu control") and making it feel wrong to question anything ("doctrine over person"). The culture of silence this creates, which I was all too familiar with, is why the *Harvard Business Review* underscored the importance of obtaining unfiltered feedback to the top.

What might a healthier hospital look like for patients, trainees, and staff? In the *BMJ*, as part of using advocacy writing as a way to make meaning of my experience and help heal the system, I co-wrote an article with a colleague discussing three methods that could work to improve culture for both physicians and patients.** The first was to ensure that culture is measured through staff surveys and objective observations, ideally by a third party. This needs to be coupled with accreditation and regulatory oversight to build in accountability. This worked in Sydney, Australia, where three residency programs lost their accreditation due to bullying of junior doctors, resulting in a heavier workload for the very staff who bullied their trainees. For the journal *Healthcare*, I co-wrote, with another colleague, two case studies that helped illustrate how hospital quality improvement efforts, which include patient care, must be directly linked to creating healthier hospital cultures.***

---

* This is a short article about this topic: https://harvardmacy.org/blog/burnout-addressing-the-epidemic-in-medical-trainees

** This article can be found here: https://blogs.bmj.com/bmj/2019/07/12/for-the-sake-of-doctors-and-patients-we-must-fix-hospital-culture/

*** This article can be found here: https://pubmed.ncbi.nlm.nih.gov/31653584/

Secondly, we must be intentional about hiring talented leaders. In medicine, this means looking at more than just clinical abilities, but also competencies as they relate to empathy, integrity, ability to inspire, and encouraging diversity—not just ethnic diversity, but diversity of thought and work (and learning) styles.

Lastly, organizations should build ways to improve collaboration and amplify voices of marginalized groups such as those with physical and invisible disabilities (e.g. neurodiversity), women, and people of color.

Today, I'd add a few more solutions. Encourage feedback that is productive, not punitive, and limit work hours to allow for rest and recovery. Yet I'm well aware that training well-adjusted future doctors requires more than applying a few Band-Aids to the devastating tsunami of factors that leads to burnout. It will require a massive systems overhaul of the hierarchy that has been riveted in place for too long.

A good starting point is to encourage and reward qualities like kindness, integrity, and civility—traits exemplified by those colleagues I admired most. Creating an environment that nurtures these values could help trainees thrive, ultimately becoming the best doctors they can be. This kind of supportive culture might even prevent the outcomes I feared most.

9.

While visiting a friend in Brooklyn one December day in 2019, a ding on my phone signaled a text from a colleague: there was a suicide. Ryan Seguin, a medical student undergoing hospital rotations, was found dead by his girlfriend. In response, in a Facebook post, one of Ryan's former classmates shared her experience on the pediatrics rotation, which she called the most dehumanizing experience of her life. Her post read:

Please don't feel like you're alone. The road to becoming a doctor is tough. The tragic loss of this 3rd year med student on this pediatric CTU rotation brings back dark memories for me as well. I remember wanting to drop out of med school during this unforgiving rotation and give up. Change has to start from the top, as more senior figures are on the hospital ward, and we have to make sure that our more junior trainees don't feel overwhelmed, underappreciated, and unsupported. This rotation continues to give me a bad taste for pediatric medicine.

I burst into tears and sat on the floor, reading all I could about his young life. He was in his third year of medical school. He served as a wellness ambassador, for crying out loud. He wanted to do internal medicine, pediatrics, or possibly family medicine. He would never have that chance. A few weeks later, I received a call from his girlfriend, the young woman who found him. She had been a fellow medical student and was in shock. She shared more details that I promised I wouldn't share in these pages—those are for her and Seguin's family to share at the right time.

I thought back to a medical student I'll call Marco, someone I worked with closely who had faced unfair treatment from a supervising physician. Marco had expressed interest in pursuing a specialty in pediatrics and had even completed research at a major children's hospital the previous summer. Despite my efforts to advocate for them, the supervisor insisted on labeling Marco as "over-confident" and "unprofessional," leading to a failing assessment. While I had tried to offer support, I realized in hindsight that my own struggle to survive in a toxic environment had left little room to provide the mentorship Marco needed. It was a sobering reminder that others—often younger and more vulnerable—were also trying to navigate the challenges of bullying and harassment in silence. Ryan Seguin was resilient—one had to be, to make it through all the hoops to get into and through med school. It was the culture that broke him to a point where he felt death was the only option.

What if some of the policies I had worked on, such as those with the CMA, had been instituted earlier? Could they have prevented Ryan's death? I would never know for sure. But what I did know was that I could no longer view this as an unwinnable fight—the stakes were far too high. What had started as a mission to save myself needed to evolve into a broader effort to heal the system. For Ryan, Kenneth, Bawa, Kate, all those whose careers had been derailed by unhealthy environments, and for every patient, like Ruth and her daughter Mini, whose care had been compromised by toxic workplaces, more needed to be done. The goal was not just survival—it was about creating a system where future doctors could thrive, and where the people they served would no longer be collateral damage in a broken system.

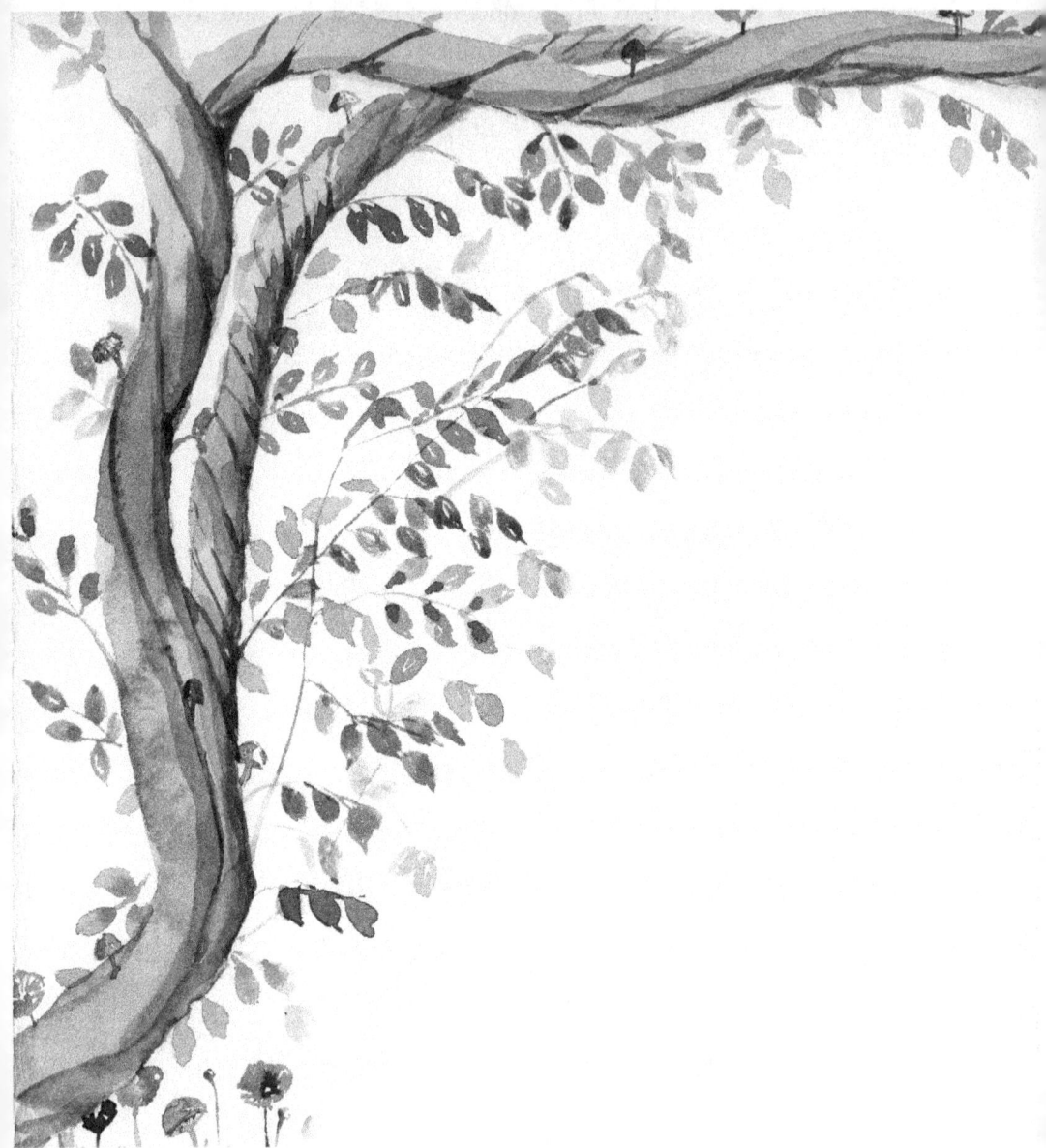

Chapter Ten

Plant Medicine

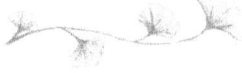

"You drown not by falling into a river, but by staying submerged in it."

—Paulo Coelho, The Pilgrimage

1.

J acob almost convinced me. As part of my book research, I had asked him about his personal experience with plant hallucinogens, a topic I had previously reported on. He had convinced me to refer to Ayahuasca and psilocybin not as hallucinogens but as "plant medicines." That seemed reasonable. We had planned to have me sit in on a ceremony, which would take place at a secret location in upstate New York. That, too, felt reasonable. I'd be a detached and objective observer, taking notes as everyone else "tripped." But the organizers said I'd only be allowed to attend if I participated myself. I was undecided.

Most people who meet Jacob might describe him as one of the most "at peace" individuals they've met. Imagine a Zen monk (he's half Japanese and shaves his head) crossed with a character from the Matrix (primarily as he dresses in navy or black and likes small oval sunglasses). When we met in New York, he was wearing all black with black leather boots. He worked as a massage therapist, but initially he wanted to be a biochemist and began a program in biochemistry for a year at the University of Washington School of Medicinal Chemistry. He quit to brew craft beer in Seattle.

"I would start my day with 2,000 lbs. of grain. There were 55 lbs. of grain in each bag and, one at a time, we would chuck them into a mill and rack off gallons of beer at a time—a lot of physical movements that were really repetitive," he said.

But instead of hellish, Jacob found that these repetitive motions were similar to being in "flow state," in which mind and body seem as one, when so intensely focused on a task, for six hours a day.

"One day, I got into such flow that it was like an all-day meditation, and I fell asleep when I got home. It was like my form of yoga in action," he recalled.

In 2012, Jacob moved to New York City and managed a trendy cocktail bar, which caused him to confront a difficult relationship with alcohol. He drank a lot since it was all around him, and then even more when he was recruited to run a hotel group events team. A few years later, searching for answers, he came across a Tibetan Buddhist monk who was running guided meditation sessions in Bushwick. Soon after, Jacob moved in with a life coach and a guy who ran a travel company. After hearing about an interest in "plant medicines," he then traveled to Peru to learn first-hand about how Ayahuasca was used, participating in his first ceremony in 2019.

"It was a reminder of why I was interested in biochemistry in the first place, which was to understand the human body and the intersection with consciousness," he said.

Through word of mouth, he found a group leading Ayahuasca sessions, first in Brooklyn and then in upstate New York. He now goes to the upstate center several times a year to participate in the ceremonies, takes Ayahuasca at least four times a year, and facilitates sessions at the retreat center over 10 times a year.

"I would attribute my calmness that people remark on to the medicine of Ayahuasca...it took a lot of work to embody this and flow out of a constant anxiety state," Jacob told me.

*

The history of healing is filled with the general theme of imbalances in the mind, body, and spirit as central to healing, and specifically how plant medicine may play a role. Indigenous cultures around the world would use bones, charms, nature, and shamans, as well as herbs, for healing purposes.

Tobacco, for instance, is considered a sacred plant offered to spirits and is used by many tribes today. The bark and leaves of the willow tree, which offer a naturally-occurring precursor to acetylsalicylic acid (aspirin), have been used for centuries for pain and fever relief. One of the biggest contributions to modern medicine may have come from the Mayans of the Yucatan Peninsula, who popularized healers, known as ah'men, who utilized healing remedies like emetics, sauna sessions, mushrooms, or hallucinogens based on a detailed history gathered from each patient.

Across Africa, ill health was often seen to have originated from spiritual causes. Healing thus involved spiritual re-connection by ceremony, and those spirits would advise anything from diet changes to fasting, massage, and chanting. Rituals and animal sacrifices were common. As with many other cultures, African herbalists used plants and mushrooms, as well as the roots and bark of medicinal trees that could be boiled, ingested, or added to joints or the skin. Frankincense was used as well as an inhalant for respiratory issues.

Ayahuasca is a psychoactive plant combination of *Banisteriopsis caapi* and *Psychotria viridis*, usually served as a drink. The chemical constituents are β-carboniles and N,N-dimethyltryptamine (DMT). The latter is an agonist (i.e., it "helps") for serotonin (5-HT) receptors, which causes us to feel "happy" and "relaxed" as the receptors get stickier and can allow more serotonin to pass through the neuronal synapses. There are indications that it may help reduce depression symptoms, but the research is still inconclusive and far from supporting medicinal use. As well, the most common side-effect, excessive vomiting, has its own drawbacks. When we vomit, we release acid out of our stomach, which throws off our blood gases, i.e., the acidity or basicity of our blood, which then affects how our body is able to conduct normal functions. This can be deadly. As well, there's always a risk of aspirating vomit—i.e., when the vomit goes into the lungs. This can also be deadly.

And this gets to why, in the end, I never joined Jacob in an Ayahuasca ceremony in upstate New York. The plant didn't seem to have anything specific to offer me, as I didn't have a health concern that was worth the risks posed by ingesting the plant. Whether there was evidence for its therapeutic benefit was secondary to the potential harm—it wasn't a bet I was willing to make, in other words, at least at that point in time.

But I also realized that the questions I had posed to Jacob, which were around his "trip" experience, weren't the right ones. I should have, instead, asked more about his motivations for seeking ongoing healing from Ayahuasca. So, I texted him: "You use it at least every month, which translates to up to twelve times a year. What is it that you're searching for from that plant that can't be found elsewhere?"

I could see the little text dots pop up on my screen, then disappear, and I wondered if it was a question he hadn't really pondered. A few moments later he responded, but not with the answer I expected: "I know it seems like a lot from the outside, but I'm quite clear and comfortable with my relationship to, and path with the medicine." I suppose I was as well.

2.

Thomas Chan was in a Peterborough, Ontario, basement, as many 19-year-olds may have been, on the late evening of December 29, 2015. It was a Tuesday during a winter holiday week. A classic all-Canadian boy—the son of a Chinese father and White mother—Thomas had played rugby at his private school, Lakefield College, for four years. His father was a well-known gastroenterologist, but Thomas lived mostly with his mother after his parents split up years earlier; both of his parents had moved on with new partners. Thomas was popular and kind and had planned to go into policing. But that December evening changed that trajectory.

He and his group of friends decided they'd spend that night with a bag of "magic mushrooms"—mushrooms that contain hallucination-causing psilocybin or psilocin—which Thomas' friend procured from a dealer. They didn't do this all the time, but when they did, it was fun. Thomas took a lot of mushrooms because he wasn't reacting the way he had in the past: with happiness and lightness. Thomas figured he needed to eat more mushrooms. That's when the experience turned: he became agitated and angry. He went home and got into a fight with his mother and his mother's partner. Then, Thomas walked out into the cold Ontario night, barefoot in the snow, and marched into his dad's house. He began yelling all kinds of things and proceeded to grab a kitchen knife and attack his father—killing him and critically injuring his father's partner.

However appalling, this was a highly unusual response. Psilocybin is not known to result in psychotic breaks, but it can, at high doses, trigger auditory and visual hallucinations, which could, potentially, be acted on. That said, it's not like alcohol, where we know the impact of too much drinking on our ability to make consequential decisions, which could potentially harm others—driving while drunk, for instance. Psilocybin, by most accounts, tends to lead to *improved* insight. But in rare instances, the hallucinations may smother this potential benefit, as in Thomas' case—and indeed, it could be different in someone with a history of brain trauma, which Thomas may have endured while playing several seasons of high school rugby.

When it comes to rare events and criminal justice, we tend to punish the rare behavior, let's call it "Version 2," when the person is in an unusual situation, ignoring the fact that, situational factors aside, "Version 1" (or the "real you") would never behave that way. For *The Washington Post*, I wrote about a prominent case of a young father who, while stressed and sleep-deprived, accidentally left his two infants in the backseat of his car, thinking he had dropped them off for daycare as he started his work in a hospital.* The infants died in the car on a hot summer day of heatstroke. A key point of the article was that the father's actions were unintentional and a result of a variety of situational factors, which any one of us could easily imagine ourselves in. We are accustomed to driving on auto-pilot, especially if we have a high cognitive load to bear, and this worsens when fatigued (the following chapter, "Rest to Recover," dives further into this). So how does that translate to Thomas' case?

The judge in the Peterborough courtroom seemed to understand when he ruled that it was highly unlikely this would happen again and that Thomas didn't pose a threat to society. Dr. Chan's partner, who witnessed the attack, received a sizeable settlement, and Thomas was sentenced to five years behind bars. In 2022, his legal team was able to secure a new trial (as of this writing, a trial date has not been confirmed). As such, his case could be overturned by

---

* The *Washington Post* Op-ed, which helped assist a key piece of legislation getting passed by Sen Tim Ryan, can be found here: https://www.washingtonpost.com/opinions/how-we-can-help-prevent-children-from-dying-in-hot-cars/2019/08/13/b49a016c-be0d-11e9-a5c6-1e74f7ec4a93_story.html

Canada's Supreme Court (which is currently Canada's highest ruling body), and if so, it will be precedent-setting.

Why is all of this important? Psilocybin and other psychedelics have the potential to heal and may lead to insight. But by virtue of how it changes the brain, in very rare and tragic cases it can fuel unusual reactions that would not occur in a person while not on the substance. We can see the same trend with marijuana: many states now decriminalize marijuana, which is seeing its own emergence, especially with cannabidiol (CBD), an active ingredient in cannabis plants, in mainstream medicine. I reported, for *ABC News*, on a marijuana derivative called Epidiolex, used for a rare seizure disorder in children, which is backed by robust research trials but remains prescribed only for that purpose.* Cannabis has evidence-based benefits for nausea (in cancer patients), and anecdotally appears to have an anti-anxiety effect, which is likely why many teens gravitate towards the drug.

But marijuana, via the THC component, can also be harmful, and heavy use is a known risk factor for psychotic disorders like schizophrenia. Indeed, even among a given plant, there may be healing components and components that heal while also posing accompanying risks.

3.

With his glasses, kind demeanor, and grey hair, Mark Haden reminded me of a longer-haired version of Apple's Tim Cook, but he may be more similar to Steve Jobs, given his tendency to think outside the box. When I met him, Haden, 66, ran MAPS Canada, the Canadian arm of the Multidisciplinary Association for Psychedelic Studies (MAPS), which is based in the U.S. and founded by Rick Doblin. We were at his kitchen table, and he had just made me lunch—a salad that included mushrooms (not the psychedelic kind). Haden and I had communicated over email through the years about various stories I had pitched that were linked to psychedelic research. But on that day, I wanted to know more about him: what would cause a mild-mannered guy from

---

* This *ABC News* article can be found here: https://abcnews.go.com/Health/explainer-marijuana-based-pharmaceutical-drug-approved-fda

southwestern Ontario to find himself in British Columbia as one of Canada's biggest proponents of psychedelics, and what did the future of psychedelics look like?

As a child in the 1950s, Haden's father, a prominent psychiatrist in Kingston, Ontario, would discuss psychedelic use around the dinner table—his father would try it with his friends and colleagues (not patients). "It was just normal to me," he recalled. Trained as a social worker, Haden left Kingston, Ontario, in 1980 and made his way to Vancouver, pulled towards the idea of learning yoga and meditation. Later, he dove into the West Coast rock-climbing scene. He then began working with Vancouver Coastal Health in the addictions sector, seeing those with everything from alcoholism to opioid addiction to cocaine and crystal meth addiction. He led group therapy and groups that focused on analyzing dreams.

In 2000, a group from Peru made their way to Vancouver to show interested people how to experiment with Ayahuasca and other hallucinogens. Haden heard about it, and at an event they organized, he tried it. He felt immediately different—calmer, and he felt that certain sense of "stuckness" had disappeared. Then it hit him: could plant-based therapies be useful in addictions or mental health issues? At the time, Vancouver Coastal Health, where Haden worked, thought it was too risky, and the evidence bleak. So, ten years later, inspired by MAPS's founder Doblin, Haden founded MAPS Canada, and subsequently retired from social work practice to run full-time.

MAPS Canada would help facilitate the studies needed in Canada, in conjunction with their partners in the U.S. According to Haden, as it relates to psychedelic use, the focus must be on four factors: set (the drug and its quality, and the intention), setting (where it's taken), dosage, and safety. The dependency potential and toxicity potential for most psychedelics are low, which means the risk-benefit ratio should be low among those who are unable to manage certain severe psychiatric issues.

The research on the potential of psychedelics, specifically MDMA (3,4 methylenedioxymethamphetamine) and psilocybin, for mental health conditions, has become more robust over the years, in large part because there was a 20-year hiatus due to legal reasons (in 1994, most research was halted). The most thorough study on the use of psychedelics for psychotherapy was published in 2020 by a working group of the American Psychiatric Association. In it, the authors reviewed MDMA, psilocybin, LSD, and Ayahuasca. Another systematic review of MDMA, ketamine, LSD, ayahuasca, psilocybin, and ibogaine, which involved appraising 15 articles, found that there were reports of everything from increased connectedness, insights, and altered self-perception to an expanded emotional spectrum. Both MDMA and psilocybin could potentially offer a "single dose, rapid effect model" for treatment-resistant mental illness. Other reviews published have emphasized the promise of MDMA, for PTSD specifically, and psilocybin, for depression and end-of-life anxiety.

MDMA is a form of phenethylamine that is structurally similar to mescaline and amphetamine. In the 1980s, it began being synthesized and sold as "ecstasy." It works in a number of ways—both via the serotonin (5-HT) pathway and also through norepinephrine and monoamine oxidase inhibition. One theory is that MDMA-assisted psychotherapy reduces activity in the brain regions involved in fear and anxiety-related behaviors (amygdala and insula especially) but also increases the connections between the amygdala (emotional center) and the hippocampus (memory center) to assist with processing of traumatic memories. A 2020 systematic review and meta-analysis, which included five trials with 106 participants, found a reduction in PTSD symptoms to be statistically significant. Yet, small-scale studies are not yet sufficient, and the assumption that the results are unequivocally positive is harmful. Others are now looking at applications for alcohol use disorder and anxiety in those with autism.

Psilocybin, the hallucinogen Thomas took at very high doses, is the other major psychedelic with incredible potential, especially for depression and end-of-life anxiety. Psilocybin is derived from several mushroom species and is an alkaloid similar to tryptamine. It is metabolized by the body into psilocin, which is a serotonin transporter inhibitor, and 5-HT2Z receptor, which is a partial agonist. At high doses of between 0.3-0.6mg/kg, it can cause hallucinations (auditory and visual)—this may have been what Thomas experienced. A systematic review and meta-analysis of three trials, which looked at 92 patients in total receiving psilocybin of between 0.2-0.4mg/kg, found a positive effect size on depression and anxiety. Psilocybin may also have an additional benefit when used with mindfulness meditation to alleviate depression.

In a landmark study from 2018, the Imperial Psychedelic Research Group (based at Imperial College London) led by Robin Carhart-Harris reported on results of an open-label trial using psilocybin for treatment-resistant depression. The trial involved 14 males and six females with severe depression, all of whom received two oral doses of psilocybin (10 mg on day 1 and 25mg on day 7) in a medical setting. Symptoms were then assessed at 1 week and then at 6 months. By week five, four patients met response and remission criteria, which was consistent at months 3 and 6.

Notably, no patients sought antidepressant treatment within five weeks of starting psilocybin. A year prior, Rosalind Watts, from the same Imperial research group, reported that psilocybin may work by improving a sense of connection and acceptance—these emerged as themes from semi-structured interviews with patients in the larger trial. Watts researched the areas of the brain, based on fMRI scans, which may respond to psilocybin and determined it may involve less cerebral blood flow to the amygdala (the emotional area) and increased "resting site functional connectivity" in the default mode network. In the 2020 documentary *Dosed*, she described it as "ego dissolution."

Then, in 2021, the same group, led again by Carhart-Harris, reported that a small trial (59 participants) of a daily SSRI (escitalopram) with a negligible dose of psilocybin (1mg) spaced three weeks apart was equivalent to two treatment doses of psilocybin (25mg) spaced three weeks apart with daily placebo, in terms of depression symptoms after six weeks. Published in the *New England Journal of Medicine*, the researchers postulate that psilocybin appeared superior but that they did not perform the statistical correction to assess this.

On the North American end, the most prominent psilocybin trial to date was published in *JAMA Psychiatry* in 2020 by the prominent research group from the Center for Psychedelic and Consciousness Research and led by Roland Griffiths* and Alan Davis. This involved a randomized clinical trial

---

* A pioneer in psychedelics research, Roland, passed away in 2023. A beautiful article interview, led by the incomparable David Marchese, can be found here: https://www.nytimes.com/interactive/2023/04/03/magazine/roland-griffiths-interview.html. His obituary can be found here: https://www.nytimes.com/2023/10/17/obituaries/roland-griffiths-dead.html

of 27 participants with diagnosed major depressive disorder, exploring the impact of receiving either immediate treatment of one session with 20mg (per 70kg of body weight) and a second session of 30mg (per 70kg of body weight) each, or the same treatment but after an 8-week delay. Effectively, this is a "waitlist control" study, in which an untreated group receives treatment at a later date for comparison to the group who receives immediate treatment to help account for natural changes in depression over time, and so everyone received 11 hours of psychotherapy. At one month (week 5), comparison of both groups showed a statistically significant improvement, with over a 50% reduction in GRID-Hamilton Depression Rating Scale scores from baseline.

"Research today has shown positive effects of psilocybin therapy, so to some extent, we were not surprised by finding a reduction in depression, but I think what did surprise us was the magnitude: how *much* their depression symptoms decreased," Davis told me.

Emerging research is exploring how psychedelic medicines may have an epigenetic effect, influencing gene function through environmental and behavioral factors. In New York, the head of Mount Sinai Hospital's psychiatry department, Dr. Rachel Yehuda, has studied the role of epigenetics and mental health, focusing on the descendants of Holocaust survivors. In 2008, Yehuda and her colleagues found that maternal PTSD was more strongly associated with PTSD risk in the offspring of Holocaust survivors, and these survivors were more likely to use psychotropic medication. Recently, they discovered methylation proteins associated with trauma. The mechanism is thought to be two-fold: things that occur during development, such as maternal stress in pregnancy and maternal care after birth, as well as epigenetic changes associated with preconception trauma. Yehuda is now focusing on whether psychedelics, specifically MDMA, might have an epigenetic effect, potentially interrupting the intergenerational transmission of trauma.

Some of what I experienced working within the system, particularly with certain individuals in leadership and supervisory roles, could be understood as trauma, as what psychiatrist Paul Conti describes in his book *Trauma: The Invisible Epidemic* as:

anything that causes us emotional or physical pain, that surpasses our coping mechanisms, that overwhelms our body and mind, and leaves a mark on us…and can include ongoing abuse, neglect, or marginalization.

But when I did my own decision tree on whether it was worth experimenting with psilocybin, even as a small dose in a study environment (where it would be legal), I decided against it. The risk-benefit ratio didn't shake out for me, as it didn't with Ayahuasca. In Davis' work, psilocybin for refractory depression was effective, as was MDMA in Yehuda's work with trauma patients. The alternative for those participants was a life of depression or potentially suicide. By contrast, I was depressed and anxious in one specific academic hospital environment, primarily because I was a target for rampant workplace abuse. But once I was out, I was no longer depressed or anxious: I was able to recover by moving out of that toxic environment.

Other tools, like yoga, meditation, and building social connections, on the other hand, had become immensely helpful to my recovery and to regain my sense of wellness. It was all largely situational, as so many experts had by now pointed out, so experimenting with a new substance afforded more of a potential risk than I was willing to take, even if the chances of having an unusual and negative reaction, much like Thomas Chan, would be exceedingly rare.

This calculation, in general, of the risks and benefits of any unconventional treatment or approach is crucial to understand as individuals but also for physicians to understand when they counsel patients. Scientific evidence often isn't enough to sway us one way or another—it depends on what else we've tried, how much we feel we have to lose, how easily we can imagine an adverse (or beneficial) reaction, accessibility, and just how we, as individuals, accept or tolerate uncertainty and risk. And this principle applies to everything I've covered in this book—from mindfulness to intermittent fasting to HIIT to even spirituality and prayer.

Thinking back to what Mark Haden warned: when it comes to psychedelics, the dose, setting, set, and safety all matter. With Thomas Chan, none of those things were optimized. He was with friends, took way too many mushrooms of unknown quality, and had no medical supervision. There was no "set" or "setting" at play here. Most critically, it wasn't clear whether he was more prone to a psychotic break given his history of head injury compared to someone else in the exact same situation. That said, when the opportunity arose years later to have a guided journey with MDMA as part of Internal Family Systems (IFS) therapy to heal my trauma from that specific work environment, I said yes. As I'll soon share, dear reader, it was everything and nothing I could have imagined.*

4.

The Downtown East Side of Vancouver is notorious for having the highest rates of homelessness and injection drug use per square mile in the country, if not North America. So, when I met Bruce, I was a bit surprised. As I was walking in the area, which was smack dab in the middle of downtown Vancouver, he rode up beside me on a bike and mouthed something. His sunken face and missing teeth suggested he might be from the area. I took my headphones out and asked what he was trying to say.

"I just wanted to say you're beautiful," he said as he rode by slowly. My analytical mind wondered how he would know that if he had been behind me for several blocks. But then I just decided to say thank you. "Are you married?" "Yes," I lied, hoping it would halt the conversation. "Well, lucky guy, have a good day." He then rode off down Cordova Street. That's when I noticed he had a bright pink food delivery backpack on.

On that particular morning, I had been emailing with a writer friend, wondering about including a chapter on plant medicine in this book, trying to reconcile how plants are part of how we heal. I realized Bruce might be part of my answer, so I ran—I mean really, actually, *ran*—to chase down that bike and backpack. Thankfully, Bruce was a slow biker and stopped partway to speak to a Vancouver cop. It seemed like they knew him. After the conversation between them ended, I asked him for his name.

---

* I must leave you in suspense for now, so the experience isn't shared in this chapter; it felt more fitting elsewhere for reasons that will become clear.

"Bruce. Bruce Beadle. Like Beetle Juice but Beadle Bruce," he said. I laughed.

Bruce, then 47 years old, taught me why plant medicine has a harmful side. His battle with opioids started early, growing up on Vancouver Island with a tough upbringing that caused him to be shuffled from foster home to foster home. In grade 10, at the age of 14, he dropped out of high school and was forced to find a means to support himself living on his own.

"I didn't want to work at McDonald's. I felt like I was above that, to be honest, and dealing drugs just seemed to be the easiest way to make money quickly," he said. It started with marijuana, then quickly switched to the higher paying drugs: crystal meth, cocaine, and heroin. And Bruce began using those drugs as well.

"It mostly was because it was just around, and everyone was doing it. But then it became more because the dealers I worked under wanted me to test it before selling," he explained. It soon turned into a situation where he became addicted to those drugs, and to support his addiction, he had to continue to sell drugs. The first time he was in jail—juvenile detention—was at age 16 after he was caught breaking into restaurants to steal alcohol, which he would then sell.

Bruce actually *liked* jail as he was able to meet friends. "It wasn't punishment for me, really," he told me. But it was hard to get clean and get hired after having a record. He used heroin for years and experimented with opioids like Percocet but was now on methadone, a program he has relied on since his early 20s.

Of all the things Bruce shared in his story, one thing he shared in particular stuck out: "People see everyone walking around the Downtown East Side and assume they wake up one day and say they want to do drugs, but it's more that they need to escape the reality they found themselves in, and I think that's why I do it."

*

Opioids originate from the humble poppy, which is often a symbol of past wars fought. The poem, "In Flanders Fields," by John McCrae, is one we would recite every year in grade school on Remembrance Day (November

11th) in Canada, also known as Veterans Day in the U.S. Originally intended for acute pain relief, opioid medications have led to an addiction epidemic, with dependency on drugs like OxyContin and fentanyl peaking in 2018 and surging further during the COVID-19 pandemic.

Purdue Pharmaceuticals has, for the last several years, been front and center with lawsuits related to a potential coverup of the addictive side effects of oxycontin and false advertising of its claims. As of this writing, billions in settlements have been paid out, but many critics believe that the company has not yet been held fully accountable. Fentanyl, and a stronger derivative, carfentanil, have found their way onto the streets and at high school and university parties. It's easily procured from Asia, and even a small dose can induce breathing to stop, followed by death. Reversal requires a drug called Naloxone, which is not always easily available.

Cocaine has a different root, a coca plant that grows in places like Bolivia. Chemically, it is a stimulant and can cause intense happiness. Crack cocaine is the kind that mixes cocaine with water and baking soda. It's cheap and highly addictive, given its highly concentrated nature, fueling the crack cocaine industry that began in the early 1980s, primarily in big cities across the U.S.: New York City, Baltimore, Miami, Los Angeles, and Philadelphia, to name a few.

Drug dependency and addiction used to be differentiated. In medical school, we learned the *Diagnostic and Statistical Manual of Mental Disorders*, fourth edition (DSM-IV) distinction, where dependency requires tolerance and withdrawal symptoms, while addiction requires a change in behavior secondary to brain alterations due to the substance, causing a heavier focus on obtaining the drug. The DSM-V doesn't include that distinction, and the scientific community much prefers the more umbrella term "substance use disorder" to define addiction or dependence on a substance like a drug or alcohol.

Adding to the complexity of substance use disorders, especially in the U.S., is that drug use, specifically cocaine and meth, but also street versions of opioids such as fentanyl, is criminalized. What often happens with plant-based drugs is a vicious cycle such as the one Bruce fell into: a person gets drug addicted, thrown in jail (leading to a criminal record), gets released, and can't find a job because of their record, so making money selling drugs becomes the only option. Fundamentally, it's an issue of a lack of choice.

In 2017, for a Canadian magazine, I reported on an initiative called Police Assisted Addiction and Recovery Initiative (PAARI-USA) that involved policing in Boston with the idea that individuals would be provided with treatment as opposed to jail time. PAARI's elevator pitch is "a no-arrest, direct referral for drug detoxification and rehabilitation treatment." I learned how the program—in partnership with the Gloucester, Massachusetts police department—had helped a man named Steve Lesnikoski, who had developed a heroin addiction. Lesnikoski credited the program, dubbed the "Angel Program," and months of treatment for setting him on the right foot, where he now works as a drug counselor.

The program's costs for participants are covered for Massachusetts residents, but Lesnikoski needed private funding to participate, given that he hailed from Oakland, California. There are well over 160 police departments across the U.S. that are part of PAARI-USA. In 2016, a Boston University Medical Center team presented data on the Angel Program in the *New England Journal of Medicine*, in which it was clear that PAARI-USA helped ensure a 95% referral rate to rehabilitation and detoxification facilities in and around Boston, which was up to four-fold higher than referral rates seen out of emergency rooms. "The fact is, we know the medical care system historically has not been welcoming or effective for people with addiction," said David Rosenbloom, a member of the Boston University Medical Center study team. "Many providers still refuse to see addiction as a disease. Cops wouldn't send them to the street, but emergency room doctors do."

When I spoke to Rod Knecht, who was then a police chief based in Edmonton, Alberta, Canada, he was quick to point out that focusing on the social determinants is key. "I like the model [...] of having the police be facilitators to connect those with addictions to get help," Knecht told me. "But I would want to emphasize the wellness aspect. It's more than just rehab and detox. Housing is also a big part of it." That said, the "detox and rehab approach" to opioid substance use disorder is imperfect.

Unfortunately, there's a downside. A 2017 exposé in *STAT News* found that some referral programs that send participants to expensive rehabilitation centers out-of-state have become lucrative businesses, with potential kickbacks for the referrers.

Other researchers have found that those participating in in-hospital or in-facility programs may lose drug tolerance, which can increase the risk of death during a relapse, so outpatient programs based in a community may be more effective. One researcher had written a letter to the *New England Journal of Medicine*, shortly after Rosenbloom's work was published, pointing out the flaws of a "detox-for-all approach" and their high relapse rates—up to 81% of those surveyed in the dataset apparently had previous detox attempts and a large number were recurrent users of the program.

*

Gabor Maté's book, *In the Realm of Hungry Ghosts*, described addiction in the following way:

> ...addiction is neither a choice, nor primarily a disease. It originates in a human being's desperate attempt to solve the problem. The problem of emotional pain of overwhelming stress, of lost connection, of loss of control, of a deep discomfort with the self. In short, it is a forlorn attempt to solve the problem of human beings: all drugs, and all behaviors of addiction, substance dependent or not, whether to gambling, sex, the internet or cocaine, either soothe pain directly or distract from it, hence my mantra. The first question is not why the addiction. But why the pain?

In a podcast with Tim Ferris, Maté described psychedelic experiences as facilitating a "super-highway for self-awareness"—that it takes "one day for what may typically take 10 years." With respect to the duality between opioids and psychedelics, it appears that opioids numb the pain and cover up its root cause, whereas psychedelics bring the pain to the surface. It's somewhat like comparing simply covering up a weed (addressing the surface level) with digging under the ground or soil to unearth the cause of the weed to address the root cause.

In our conversation, Maté shared: "Broadly speaking, what we call 'drugs' in medicine have a temporary effect…they suit the symptoms, but don't deal with the underlying issue. If I prescribe opiates for you, you're going to be taking it every day, but it's got nothing to resolve your underlying problem. A psychedelic experience with psilocybin, for instance, when properly used, you don't keep taking it. You have a few experiences, and it's what *happens* during these new experiences that promotes the healing. So, we can't compare the two things…they aren't the same at all."

Maté and I spoke as well of my view of normal reactions to abnormal situations, like what I had faced in one specific academic hospital environment. This general topic—how our minds adapt initially to protect us but then may become maladaptive—is a big theme in his newest book, *The Myth of Normal*. Maté also shared a personal experience with this theme: early in his medical career, he was a workaholic and had maladaptive responses in the form of anger which led to a firing from his initial job. After experiencing a moment of contemplation and awareness, he then embarked on a brand-new path, working with those with addictions on the Downtown East Side—people similar to Bruce Beadle.

A proponent for how plant medicines can heal trauma, Maté also spoke of how trauma may play a larger role than we realize in the manifestation of various illnesses, such as multiple sclerosis, and that the mechanism may be related to abnormal inflammatory responses. The pivotal role of trauma was best described in a 2021 book by Bruce Perry and Oprah, called *What Happened to You*, as it underscores how both early childhood events and later life events can radically impact our responses to both abnormal and normal situations.

When I shared with Maté that initially, Dr. Morgan thought I had M.S., even though depression was likely the more common cause, he offered: "Well, but you don't know if that [M.S.] would have developed. Perhaps you just missed it." The experience left a lasting emotional impact that was later identified by a therapist as trauma. One clear sign was my tendency to avoid certain areas altogether, as just being near those places triggered overwhelming anxiety. Reflecting on it, I realized that if I hadn't made the decision to step away and focus on healing, the chronic stress might have taken a serious toll on my health. It's not far-fetched to think that prolonged exposure to such an environment could have contributed to the development of an autoimmune condition, like M.S., or another stress-related illness.

Maté's point made me think back to the axolotl regeneration pathway Dr. Currie discussed in Chapter 2; whereas humans tend to go down the pathway of scarring, axolotls go down the regeneration pathway. Perhaps resilience works the same way, and because I got out of that toxic environment just in time, I was lucky to have gone down the "regeneration" route.

Wanting to know how the medical community might respond to what might be a major paradigm shift when it comes to using what are now classified in the U.S. as Schedule 1 drugs for clinical use, I decided to ask Dr. Andrew Weil. Weil, who had been divisive in the medical community for his contrarian views, though he does promote an evidence-based approach when it comes to complementary approaches, founded the clinical integrative medicine fellowship at the University of Arizona that I would pursue. He has explored (and experimented with) psychedelics beginning in the 1960s. But for decades, his experiences were ignored, so I was curious to know how he felt now that the psychedelic world was experiencing a resurgence in research and clinical applications.

"I still think most doctors are very poorly educated in the proper uses of botanicals and, you know, don't understand them, but that's something we're trying to remedy… I've always known that I was on the right path, and I was able to not let all the ignoring and criticism affect me that much," Weil told me. "And it's been very gratifying to me to watch the change because I think there are many people who are forward thinkers who don't live to see the culture catch up with them. And I feel fortunate, you know, to see that that's all changed in my lifetime. Back then, it definitely felt lonely, not getting much validation, especially from my medical peers, and that obviously gets old. As I say, it's gratifying to see this now."

I was beginning to see a theme—Jon Kabat-Zinn, Max Ortix Catalan, Bryant Terry, Roger Ulrich, Steve Nygren, Christine Puchalski, Uché Blackstock, Amy Edmondson, Jessica Harthcock, Valter Longo, Ruth, Gabor

Maté, Sapna Kudchadkar, Mark Haden, and others—the doctors, pioneers, patients and researchers who stood up against the status quo and dared to think and dream differently about healing, ultimately benefiting thousands of patients as a result.

5.

I had planned to move to New York City with Chris in late 2019, so we began looking for apartments in Manhattan. I was finally ready for this step, as it was the perfect place to be to write this book. But we went back and forth about which area would be best. He preferred the South Street Seaport area, which is far from central, maintaining that it had character. I wouldn't budge—there are a few streets in the West Village that always captured my heart. Perhaps subconsciously, I knew that it used to be a hub for creatives and writers— people like Patti Smith and James Baldwin.

We soon realized it wasn't just about where we wanted to live. We couldn't see eye-to-eye on many other things as well: we had grown apart. So, in December 2019, Chris and I found ourselves on either end of a burgundy couch on the 13th floor of a building on 34th Street and Broadway with a lovely couple therapist who looked like an ethereal mermaid with her silver hair worn in a side braid and blue shell earrings. I really wasn't sure what would happen next. It appeared there was a pattern of dishonesty with himself and others that impacted family members and loved ones. The therapy session provided him with insight, and the remaining details are for his own story of healing, should he ever share it.

The therapist then asked more questions of us. Chris' mother's recent passing, on top of a series of other disconnects over the previous few years, had contributed to his own depression and anxiety, which had worsened when his mother got sick. I shed some tears; it was time for me to support his own healing journey. Chris kept looking out of the window into the distance onto the Hudson River. We left arm in arm and shared a kiss and embrace as he had to go back to work in midtown Manhattan. But I resolved to move to New York City a month later in January anyway. I felt a pull there and that it would be the best place to work on my book. I would realize why soon enough, but for now, it was simply just a feeling.

In Glennon Doyle's beautiful 2020 book, *Untamed,* she describes love this way:

> Love is a river,
>
> and there are times
>
> when impediments stop
>
> the flow of love...
>
> Healing is not the reward
>
> for those who love the most or best.

Chris came into my life at the most perfect point in time, right as I was embarking on my journey of healing. He was with me every single day, as a supporter, champion, and ally. When I look back at Chris and his role in my life, so much of his love, which I experienced so deeply and consistently, was healing. I couldn't have gotten this far without him. Years ago, thinking back to college, it was crazy to imagine that we would reconnect. Love is healing. Even the hormone dubbed the love hormone, oxytocin, is used in childbirth to help facilitate labor. It may also help the heart. Chris helped heal me as much as anything else I did on my own, and that, too, was truth. We loved the most and the best, but it wasn't enough—our relationship had completed.

I had intended to spend the following 10 days— between Christmas and New Year's—at a silent Vipassana meditation retreat. But I left after five days. My heart hurt too much to sit in a room, trying not to feel it at all. The guide, Anna, was disappointed when I explained it. I tried to chalk it up to being anxious, as I didn't want to give her the impression that my personal life had anything to do with my distraction. In hindsight, perhaps I should have just been truthful. Instead, I spent the last five days of the year mourning my relationship and trying to explain to my friends and family why I felt like I needed to listen to the pull to head to New York City soon.

*

Following that intuitive nudge to head to New York City to work on this book, I arrived at my studio apartment on tree-lined Charles Street, close to Greenwich Avenue, on a frigid mid-January evening in 2020. I had planned to stay for only two months. The apartment was quaint, with a huge desk placed in front of a window that overlooked the street. It was truly the most perfect place to write, in other words. I spent the first few days unpacking and decorating so it resembled a peaceful meditation studio: it was my creative healing cocoon.

I began dating casually but didn't have the motivation to continue. I did, however, get into a healthy routine—yoga, Pilates, eating healthful and nourishing foods, daily writing at a women's coworking space, and catching up with New York friends a few times a week: many people I hadn't spent as much time with over the years. It all felt necessary. I still spoke occasionally with Chris, and we caught up when we could. But my focus remained on my writing and my healing.

On my third morning—January 18, 2020—I bumped into a prominent writer on the street whom I had long admired and whose work I had studied. I greeted him formally, and he stopped, a bit jolted. We ended up speaking for several minutes, and I quickly shared my writing work to make it clear that my greeting didn't come with a request for "writing help." He offered it anyway, over coffee. I refused—"I think I'm okay for now actually" (something several friends would be shocked at—who would deny an opportunity to learn from one of the best?), but shared how it was lovely to have met him.

The Writer cocked his head, seeming a bit surprised, and narrowed his eyes. I offered my card as a way to smooth over the awkwardness, and we smiled and said farewell. I immediately texted my siblings and best friends: "You won't believe who I just met." I smiled all the way to the grocery store. It was a sign. The chances of bumping into a successful writer on a cold morning in a city of almost 9 million felt like serendipity, that yes, taking that leap to come to New York City, and specifically the West Village, was the right choice: that strong pull I had felt to this specific area for months was real.

Three days later, the Writer emailed me: "It was nice running into you the other day, Amitha. Let's get lunch!" Over the ensuing weeks, we emailed several times a day and met up for friendly lunches and coffees. Weeks later, after a lovely walk along the tree-lined streets of the West Village, he invited me to his apartment to retrieve a gift, a book he wanted to give me. I chose to sit on the stoop outside, much to his chagrin. "Bye, Amitha," he managed after he handed me the book: one his mother had written, which he had specially bound. A bit conflicted, I returned to my own apartment alone, head spinning, but with the treasured book in hand. Though our emails would continue, in large part due to the world slowly turning upside down, I wouldn't see the Writer in person again for almost two years.

Two months after I first landed in New York—on March 13, 2020—Chris and I, enjoying a newfound close friendship, were at dinner talking, sharing oysters, wine, shrimp pasta, and a Caesar salad at Jeffrey's Grocery down the street from my apartment in Manhattan. We were discussing what appeared to be an evolving and devastating situation affecting our world, which now had a name: the COVID-19 pandemic. By mid-March, New York City was the epicenter of a worldwide pandemic, with millions of lives lost before a vaccine was developed months later. We were about to experience a total lockdown—that meal at Jeffrey's (a Caesar salad and shrimp pasta) would be my last meal inside a New York City restaurant for well over a year, as the world was about to embark on its own challenge of healing.

6.

The experiences of Jacob, Thomas Chan, and Bruce Beadle helped cement the core element of how plants can either heal us or destroy us: it's a duality, a rose with thorns so to speak. In Bruce's case, opioid addiction was primarily a response to his long-standing trauma, beginning as a foster child. It was, as Gabor Maté would suggest of all addictions, a *rational* response to a traumatic problem. The system itself didn't recognize that and criminalized Bruce's addiction, which only retraumatized him and entered him into a cycle of ongoing emotional and personal destruction, a cycle he has still not completely escaped. When our criminal justice systems reframe drug addiction as secondary to trauma and stop criminalizing it, it would allow us as a society to address the upstream factors: poverty, food insecurity, systemic racism, social isolation, abusive and unstable homes, and the lack of meaning, among other things, to prevent the trauma in the first place. This is not unlike our earlier discussion of adverse childhood events—many ACEs do indeed contribute to drug addiction.

With Jacob, something else was brought into full view: the "self-help" and "self-improvement" industry can be an addiction itself.* The quest for "total healing" is elusive, one that cannot be obtained through a magic bullet, whether it's a plant, meditation, a special diet, or a psychic. These are merely *tools* to assist healing. The hard work, which leads to sustainable change, remains within. This is ultimately why trying psilocybin myself, even under controlled study conditions, didn't appeal to me: I had the tools I needed. I just needed to use them to buttress my own ability to heal my body and mind.

My mind led me to regain my academic prowess: I completed a clinical fellowship in integrative medicine, journalism training at the University of Toronto, and lifestyle coaching from York University, on top of mindfulness training through Mindfulness Without Borders. Yet, I still needed to focus on the task at hand—the last and final opportunity for justice, despite inevitable delays occasioned by the pandemic, a pandemic that had suddenly placed the challenge of healing front and center for the entire planet.

---

* I explored this idea in a 2022 essay for the *Globe and Mail*, found here: https://www.theglobeandmail.com/opinion/article-are-we-done-self-improving-yet/

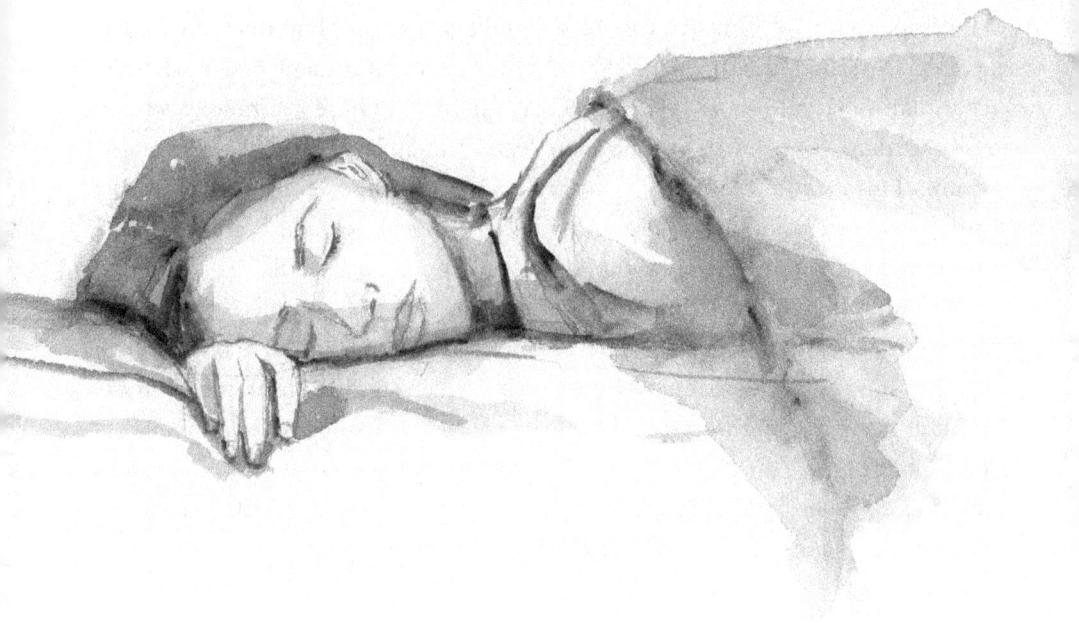

CHAPTER ELEVEN

Rest to Recover

"If your voice held no power, they wouldn't try to silence you."
—unknown

1.

It was 11 pm and 2-year-old Laila was sleeping peacefully in her hospital bed, snuggled up with her mother and several stuffed animals. Laila was admitted to us with a mysterious condition that we hadn't quite figured out. Her breathing was quiet and soft. Her bedside heart rate monitor, which glowed a faint yellow in the dark hospital room, was turned to "silent."

"Sorry, I have to take a listen to her heart," I whispered to her mother, tapping her shoulder lightly. I was on call, and her mother and I had a good relationship. I had served as an advocate for her daughter several times during her seven-week stay in the ward. She had a rare disease that had been a medical mystery for the hospital for many months, but she would be transferred to a more specialized center soon.

While I hated to wake her, I had been scolded by a senior colleague earlier in the day for waiting to examine her until after a nap. "You can't care about that. If you do, you'll never examine them. They have to get used to it—they're in the hospital, after all," he said.

Though this was a colleague who had been fair and wasn't known to bully, I couldn't understand why he didn't seem to see the impact on the patient, and it suggested I simply wasn't aligned with how doctors practiced here. Laila was exhausted. She had been disturbed several times and poked for blood work

209

or taken down to get an MRI or a CT (CAT) scan at different times during the day. Her exam—I was able to check her vital signs (heart rate, breathing) examine her liver and spleen, check her heart, and her perfusion, while also listening to her lungs—was stable. I backed out of the room slowly.

The next morning, Laila's mother seemed bothered. She asked kindly if there was a need to examine Laila while she slept and asked a very good question: "Wouldn't a good night's sleep help with her condition?" At the time, I wasn't sure.

Now we know from research that sleep disruption isn't just inconvenient and doesn't merely just affect our moods or increase the risk of disease. Disrupted sleep can, in fact, drastically affect how well patients heal from the condition that brought them into the hospital in the first place. As I wrote in *The New York Times*: "If sleep were regarded as a continuous infusion of a medication that helped a patient heal faster, provided them with emotional stability and ensured they were in the best mindset to understand the risks and benefits of that care, we would think twice about disrupting it."

*

Considered part of Connecticut's "Gold Coast," New Canaan is one of the wealthiest communities in the U.S., with a median household income of $800,000.

It has one of the best public school systems in the country, named officially the best in the U.S. in 2008, and currently stands as one of the best in the state. The students in New Canaan excel in school as well as various sports, including football and soccer.

I was meeting with Katherine Price Snedaker, the founder of an organization called "PINK Concussions," a non-profit founded in 2013 that focuses on brain injury among women and girls. It wasn't until her 10-year-old son suffered a concussion in 2008—which forced him out of school for an entire year—that Katherine, a licensed clinical social worker by training, reflected back on her own experience as a 16-year-old with several concussions from car accidents.

As a fraternal twin, her son offered another 'natural' twin experiment (not unlike Jessica's experience in Chapter 8)—the effects on the concussed twin were obvious. Her son had a total of six concussions over 12 months and then had two years with no concussions. He missed school for most of the 6th grade (he had a tutor at home) and was found to have a significantly slowed processing speed compared to other boys his age.

Katherine is a pearl-necklace-wearing blonde, with a spring in her step, and an optimism that is contagious. But when she thinks back to where it all started, it's clear that her path was anything but typical.

"It really began with my son. I began looking at alternatives to just the 'rest until symptoms went away' idea. I quickly gathered a long list of medical experts and researchers working on concussions, and everything else followed," she told me.

Over time, she founded several concussion-specific websites and support organizations like "SportsCap" and the "Concussion Aware and Prepare Program" to integrate the CDC information into the sports world in New Canaan. And she testified at the national level for children with concussions while also making presentations to schools and youth sports teams, including the National Football League (NFL), an invite which she believes was in large part because she was plugging a message they resonated with—that only a quarter of concussions were sports-related.

However, it wasn't until she became aware of gender differences in concussion recovery that she found her niche. In 2009, Katherine began working for two different concussion clinics, and over time, as people found out about her personal interest in concussion, given her son's experience, they would call her at home, and she would advise them free of charge. But soon, she began noticing something. The parents of girls with concussions were coming in late for care, often a full week or two after a concussion, and they weren't resting at all, so they would be doing their normal activities and arrive in very bad shape up to 10 days later.

"They'd say things like 'I'm three months out,' and I didn't really know girl moms since I only had sons—they were the ones we would see from across the playground, and I'd wonder, 'Why are these girls so far out and just finding services now?' A girl missing a month and a half at school because they just didn't' know what to do didn't make sense to me. At first, I thought the parents were irresponsible," Katherine said.

Years later, Christina Master from the Children's Hospital of Philadelphia found girls are systematically taken in for care much later compared to boys, and this might be a reason girls take longer to heal after a concussion. To understand why, Master and her colleagues completed a retrospective cohort study, published in 2019, of pediatric patients admitted to a subspecialty service for pediatric concussion secondary to sports. They found that, on average, girls presented later for evaluation after a sports-related concussion compared to males, and took longer to recover—this included how long it took for them to return to school without needing accommodations, time to return to exercise or full sport, time it took to heal from neurocognitive issues (measured on computerized testing) and clinical recovery of vision and balance. However, when the time to presentation for care was controlled, the differences disappeared, which suggested that early identification of concussion made a major difference.

So, Katherine ended up running a girls' group for athletes and worked with an athletic trainer who tried different movements, but it became too much. Katherine then suggested yoga, as this allowed for "restful positions" such as propping themselves up with blankets and pillows to open up the neck and shoulders. She also invited speakers in twice a week for two hours per session.

That's when she came across Tracy Covassin, now Director of the Sports Concussion Laboratory at Michigan State University. Covassin's research on girls with concussions found that female collegiate athletes were at a higher risk of concussion in sports such as soccer, basketball, and softball compared to males playing that same sport. Further, as compared to men, women are concussed more often and at a higher *rate* than men, even though overall, in sports, men have more concussions. Women report both more symptoms and higher symptom severity (which includes how long they experience symptoms). Women also take longer to recover—though this is controversial. The thought may be that male axons (the tail end of the neuron or brain cell) are larger and more complex in structure, so more able to withstand force, whereas women's finer axons may be more prone to breakage and ion influx during damage, leading to degeneration and dysfunction.

Inspired, Katherine started a website in 2012 dedicated to sharing this information on concussions in women. She called it PINK Concussions. It became a non-profit in 2015 and expanded to focus on sports, but also concussions created during domestic violence, military service and accidents. The first summit was held in 2016 at Georgetown University Medical School with 65 experts and 220 participants attending. It has grown exponentially since then.

"I was also interested in how researchers were connecting at this conference —before, it seemed that the brain injury experts focused on domestic violence weren't really speaking to the sports folks. But here it was like speed dating for researchers who were working on the same organ but looking at different things. Many walked away with potential new collaborators," she recalled.

The summary statement from the 2001 consensus conference on concussion in sport, held in Vienna, recommended strict rest followed by a graduated return to play. Though rest has been prescribed for several decades for concussion, despite minimal evidence, this has been called into question. One randomized controlled trial (RCT) study of adolescents from the emergency department showed that participants prescribed five days of strict rest reported more symptoms and had slower symptom resolution when compared with those prescribed light activity.

Dr. John Leddy, an orthopedic surgeon at the University of Buffalo, created the Buffalo Concussion Treadmill Test, which involves assessing the degree of exercise tolerance in someone with a concussion by looking at heart rate thresholds with the idea of recommending a safe level of activity without worsening of symptoms. His subsequent work was pivotal to shifting the dogma around rest. In one study, he found that the group allocated to absolute rest after concussion had a statistically significantly longer recovery time (16 days) compared to those advised to exercise (13 days). Another study, this time of adolescents, found that 30% of those with concussion had delayed recovery when advised total rest, compared with those who were advised to do some exercise. Then, Leddy's work in 2018 on how aerobic exercise can increase the speed of recovery from sports-generated concussions echoed some of the principles that are similar to Sapna Kudchadkar's work on PICU patients.

"Before, it was all about rest. We'd put dark coverings on windows, decrease brain stimulation to allow for rest, and so on. John Leddy's work became a major factor in why I shifted my thinking," Katherine told me. But why did Katherine begin questioning the role of rest and what it meant? And what made her take note of the potential gender differences in recovery? It might be Katherine's early life challenges that caused her to question the status quo: growing up with dyslexia, ADHD, and an auditory learning disability since grade school almost forced a rebellious streak.

"I would always go left when someone went right," she told me. She would memorize words instead of reading them, and in short, adapted to whatever challenges presented to her. By college, she told me she suffered from more than 20 concussions (but these were usually not from sports but from things like hitting her head against a cement wall accidentally, getting hit by a lacrosse ball, and later from two severe car accidents). Career-wise, despite her limitations, Katherine excelled—first in an advertising job, then with accounting and basic programming using Excel spreadsheets. As a developer, she ended up using a software product to help residents in her community communicate with one another and built a website for her children's school. "I was ahead of the curve because at that time I was told schools don't need websites," she said.

Like so many others in this book, Katherine was changed by lessons learned earlier in life that force a questioning of the status quo and help to shift paradigms. For Katherine, it was to advocate for concussion sufferers that rest combined with some activity is the best treatment, while also raising awareness of gender differences in concussion recovery.

2.

Michael Grandner and Meeta Singh couldn't be more different, though they are both powerhouse researchers in the world of sleep and medicine. Grandner, a pleasantly round-faced man with dark brown hair, began studying the link between sleep and disease in athletes as part of his work directing the Sleep and Health Research Program at the University of Arizona and the behavioral sleep medicine clinic at Banner-University Medical Center in Tucson. With almost 9,000 research citations, his focus more recently has been on sleep and healing.

"The main job of the immune system is to regenerate every cell of the body, and that happens most often during sleep," Grandner told me. "Our blood pressure lowers at night to allow for this, as well as for the genes to upregulate. Think of it this way: if we want to construct a road, it's better to fix it when no one's on the road. The brain works the same way."

This is true. For example, growth hormones are regulated during stage 3 non-REM sleep, and this is involved in repairing tissues and muscles. The G-lymphatic system turns on during sleep, and our brain, as researcher Amy Bender told me, is like a dishwasher with our glial cells shrinking so fluid flushes out amyloid and tau proteins.

Singh, a slender Indian woman, embarked on sleep research as a medical doctor, trained in psychiatry, but she is also board-certified in neurology and completed her sleep medicine fellowship at the Henry Ford Hospital in Detroit, Michigan. She has advised several professional sports teams, such as the National Basketball Association (NBA) and National Football League (NFL), and these teams tend to be more focused on the link between sleep and performance. For instance, a UCSF study in 2011 found that male Division I college basketball players who stayed in bed for 10 hours per day for 5-7 weeks were able to increase their sleep duration to between 6.6 and 8.5 hours, which translated to a 9% increase in free-throw accuracy and reduced sprint times of 16.2 to 15.5 seconds. Also, when it comes to performance, knowing sleep schedules could help predict which NBA teams would win based on how much sleep the players would get, predicting that East Coast teams would typically lose when playing on the West Coast. These were dubbed "Red Alert" games.

But sleep is also key to recovery and healing. Singh shares, "In addition to the recovery process and healing process that occur during sleep, sleep also functions in our pain response. If you don't get enough sleep, you're more likely to feel pain, and the requirement for pain medication actually increases, so recovery and healing can be affected by this, for instance, because the higher need for medications can interrupt the healing process." She also underscored that the hospital environment itself, with light and noise, is also not conducive to sleep.

Grandner wants to change the idea that sleep is just rest—it's more than rest; active things happen. But his most compelling paper may be one published in 2020 that looks at sleep and elements of recovery. While he underscored that sleep is important as an element for injury prevention, there is plenty of other research to back this up: for instance, the impact of sleep loss on sports injuries in teens.

Yet, the mechanism of sleep impact on healing isn't clear. It is believed sleep affects the release of growth hormone and how much cortisol is secreted, as well as increasing inflammatory markers like C-reactive protein and interleukin-6, which affect the immune system and how well muscles can recover and repair damage from training and athletic performance. This builds on what researchers have found about the role of sleep in upregulating genes and rebuilding cellular components.

*

It's clear now that for concussions, rest must be distinguished from sleep, and that sleep deprivation, specifically, appears to hinder recovery— this has also been established in research from the University of Kansas Medical School. Grandner's work has also found that National Collegiate Athletic Association (NCAA) Division-1 athletes with clinically moderate to severe insomnia severity, because of their nighttime sleep deprivation, were at a higher concussion risk. He has also reported on the role of sleep and performance among athletes.

Among children, poor sleep quality was strongly associated with worse symptoms and a longer time to recover after a concussion. David Kalmbach, while at Johns Hopkins Hospital, looked at 238 patients who presented with a head injury and found that those with mild traumatic brain injury (TBI) had higher insomnia rates and shorter sleep, which in turn impacted TBI recovery, thus showing a bidirectional relationship. Sleep deprivation may be responsible for a 3- to 4-fold longer recovery time among athletes in a study of 13- to 18-year-olds. Females may also have more sleep disturbances.

The link between sleep and concussion is tough to tease out, though, as we know that concussed individuals have sleep disturbance as a result and that this sleep disturbance can worsen outcomes. For instance, research involving 13- to 33-year-olds found that a history of repeated concussions results in worse sleep disturbance and longer concussion duration and that sleep deprivation itself, after repeated concussions, is linked to severe headaches and mood and cognitive issues.

Today, a big gap remains regarding the optimal amount of rest for concussion recovery among youth. In Canada, the idea is to move towards less rest and earlier activity, as we learned from Leddy's work. In recent years, the research and recommendations around childhood concussions have changed significantly. The recommendation used to be "rest for long periods," but now the recommendation involves lots of sleep (usually 10 hours for children) but with very light activity. In a 2019 Canadian guideline led by McMaster University's CanChild Centre, Carol DeMatteo suggests five minutes or less of activity during the first 24 hours after a concussion, with little screen time or reading time. Children need to be able to concentrate for 30 minutes without worse symptoms before they return to school. In terms of supplements, melatonin does not directly reduce post-concussive symptoms. However, it appears that melatonin may improve sleep among children with concussion, which can help alleviate symptoms of depression.

This is why a group of researchers led by Dr. Ginger Yang at Nationwide Children's Hospital began the Rest Evaluation for Active Concussion Treatment (ReAct) project. The study looks at athletes aged 11-17 and follows them over time to monitor physical and cognitive rest, and concussion outcomes. These results changed concussion policy in 2024 by balancing rest for concussion recovery needs with preventing deconditioning and slow return to activity: sticking to "sleep" as opposed to just "rest" is key.

*

Singh underscores the element of the circadian clock and how sleep allows the injury to be repaired more *efficiently*, though the exact process is unclear. A 2018 study published in the journal *Sleep* reported that among patients presenting to the emergency department with traumatic brain injury, the mild sleep-onset insomnia and shortened sleep experienced may, in turn, prevent recovery. A 2020 study reported poor processing speed among those soccer players who regularly headed the ball, which then also impacts attention when sleep is disturbed. Interestingly, if sleep duration was increased, neuropsychological attention was preserved, which suggests that sleep (or lack thereof) can be a risk factor *or* a protective factor.

One of Singh's most interesting papers, published in early 2021, looked at the role of sleep among players in the NBA and was followed up by a commentary on sleep in professional sports in general. She and her collaborators underscored the impact of the number of flights, flight times, number of games per season, and what is often insufficient recovery time, and the impact on players.

The consequences of poor-quality sleep and insufficient (less than 7 hours) sleep are clear: it negatively affects athletes' mental and physical health, increases injuries, and decreases performance. Interestingly, it links to medical training too: rookies often have the biggest learning curve in terms of adjusting to the grueling schedule, similar to first-year medical residents.

In her paper, Singh cites Sacramento Kings assistant coach Jason March in an interview where he shared: "I think the biggest challenge for the rookies is fatigue; it does take a toll on them." Sleep is also an issue for coaches, who spend hours into the night reviewing game film. Damningly, March says, "You ask anybody in the room, the thing I talk about is sleep…I think in a couple of years [sleep deprivation] will be an issue that's talked about, like the NFL with concussions."

Uniquely, with the COVID-19 pandemic forcing players to play in a "bubble" in the same time zone, sleep actually improved. ESPN's Baxter Holmes quoted a Western Conference General Manager noting the players felt better, and an Athletic Trainer was quoted as saying, "This is the advantage that we have not had. We're always tired...[now] our guys have been rested. They've been fresh. We've been able to get them recovered again and again." Post-pandemic, the focus may have shifted away from the old guard style of coaching through sleep deprivation and poor recovery. In 2023, Boston Celtics head coach, Joe Mazzulla, shared that he prioritizes rest and recovery for himself and his players, using wearables to help track their recovery and practices such as breathing techniques to assist stress management and sleep. As I submitted the final draft of this book, the Boston Celtics had just won the 2024 NBA playoffs.

3.

With the global pandemic now in front of me, death front and center, I thought back to when things felt normal before the pandemic. Two moments stood out. The first, on January 30, 2020, I was emailing the Writer about an article I came across in *The New York Times* that included a graph about a mysterious coronavirus. Even though there were no known cases in the U.S., something seemed amiss: it didn't strike me as a virus in Asia that could die out very soon. He wrote back a short line: "Jesus, this isn't good." The second date was March 13, 2020, the night to dinner with Chris in New York City—we were indoors, and physical distancing was a new concept. No one wore masks. The city still had some semblance of normalcy. The following day, most restaurants in the city shut down, as did many other businesses except for the most essential.

Over the following weeks, ambulance sirens spaced five minutes apart had become normal. There would be thousands of cases and thousands of deaths. Huge freezer trucks would be parked on street corners to store dead bodies piled one on top of another—a far cry from the dignity we afforded cadavers like Joe in our anatomy labs. New Yorkers would be locked in their apartments, afraid. It would be months before anyone had a clear sense of what the symptoms were— there was so much misinformation and fear, as well as flip-flopping of advice, like whether to wear masks (as the public health messaging was contingent on science, and the science hadn't yet evolved).

Indeed, by that summer, the COVID-19 pandemic showed no signs of slowing, and I had to move back to Canada at the end of July as my visa in the U.S. was only valid for six months. Two weeks before I was scheduled to drive back to Canada, I climbed onto a chair in my apartment to reach something, slipped on the chair's mesh covering and fell backward.

My left hand broke my fall, and miraculously, I didn't hit my head or neck. I lay there on the floor, feeling my face flush. The adrenaline kept the pain at bay. I felt a sharp pain in my left wrist, and I couldn't move it. I stayed calm as different possibilities ran through my head—I had seen this with patients in the emergency room. It could just be a sprain. Or it could be worse: a break.

And here I was, in a country with a healthcare system so unfamiliar to me that I avoided using it when I was in graduate school in Baltimore a decade earlier. I needed to figure out a plan just as I would for my patients. So, I mentally went through the steps. Step one: get up and take a look at the injury. Step two: ice it. Step three: call my friend Daniel, an emergency medicine doctor in the city. He'd know where to go. And then I'd go from there. I looked at my wrist. It had deformed. And it was tender in the places that are tender only where there might be a break. It was more than a sprain.

When I called Daniel, he thankfully had the presence of mind to think ahead: "You can't go to any emergency room. It's best to go where they have orthopedics on call." He offered to arrange it. He called me back, saying that his friend and colleague was working at a Mount Sinai emergency room that morning and would add me to her list. I just needed to get there. I was grateful, which made me realize how much harder it is for someone who didn't have an advocate or an "in" with the system.

I thought back to patients like Roger and Baby J and how part of my role was advocating. Finally, I was at a point where I needed someone to do that for me. I got it casted and, trusting second opinions from Daniel, my brother, and friends in Canada who were emergency doctors or orthopedists, all who looked at my X-ray, relieved I wouldn't need surgery (even though it was the recommendation from the NYC orthopedic surgeon). The U.S. just tends to be more aggressive with interventions, they said, and I agreed. Many physicians in the U.S. are incentivized to do more invasive procedures, as payment is up to 20 times more, and conservative management is not the first choice. It's why, as I described in the Introduction, healthcare spending is such a high fraction of the country's GDP. But now I was stuck—I could fly out of New York, but I couldn't drive my stuff back home with my wrist in this state.

One thing I had come to learn was that there was so much we couldn't control about our situations. COVID-19 was a big example: We still had no idea when it would let up, and while a vaccine was in sight, it would take months, possibly well into 2021, to acquire herd immunity.

After all these years, I had focused on healing my mind and soul. I had just healed my heart, and had made changes so that my cholesterol was better. Now the universe was throwing in something extra: a physical injury to see how well I could heal from that while also getting a glimpse into the U.S. healthcare system that was as broken as my wrist. It was a lot. But I knew this pattern as well—I could observe it, acknowledge it, but stay forward-focused.

So, I flew back to Toronto with my broken wrist, knowing that things would make sense very soon. The one thing I *could* change, which I couldn't change in my hospital, was my environment. It was now August, and I was back in Canada. The fall would quickly turn to winter, which was around the corner in Toronto. A second wave of the virus was lurking. The tenant who stayed in my Toronto apartment told me she was stuck and asked if she could remain there. I took that as a nudge to relocate: Vancouver, with its temperate climate and proximity to both forests and the Pacific Ocean, seemed fitting. The virus was less prevalent there, so yoga studios and Pilates studios were safely kept open. I could get back into my routine now that my wrist was on its way to healing. My physiotherapist and orthopedic surgeon remarked on how quickly I healed, wondering if I had some inherited factor that predisposed me (nope, I smiled; resilience was just literally in my bones, perhaps).

I eventually responded to a series of emails from the Writer. "Sorry, I've been busy. I'm giving a talk on grief for a hospice organization, and I have a piece for *The New York Times* that I'm sending in." He wanted to take a look at the talk, so I sent it over, and he replied right away. It was a talk on attachments, our mutual obsession for the year. "I loved it," he wrote, "but maybe you can omit one section and replace it with more about you and how you felt. You were doing a lot of un-attaching in New York, weren't you?" I wasn't sure what he meant—was he referring to Chris? Or something else?

Chris, knowing I had left my things with my neighbor in New York City and that I was unable to drive back given my injury, performed a grand gesture of bringing it all to me in Toronto. He drove more than 400 miles with his car packed to the brim.

When I realized he had driven almost nine hours with limited visibility, I questioned for a moment if we had made the right decision to end our relationship. There was clearly a lot of love there. When he dropped it all off, we had a sweet chat and it felt clear: Chris would remain one of my closest and most loving friends, but our romance had completed. I packed and took a flight out to Vancouver the following week.

*

I landed in the neighborhood of Kitsilano, a block from the beach. My apartment had a view of the mountains and ocean. I would spend some mornings down by the beach with my coffee. I would keep my windows open to let in the sunshine and a soundscape of seagulls, Canada geese, and ravens. I dove back into my fitness routines, joined a coworking space, and began cooking for myself again now that my wrist was almost healed. And, of course, I was writing—a lot. I stayed in touch with friends virtually, as many of us did, and a few in-person, in our own "bubble."

While I navigated the next steps in my journey, I noticed signs of systemic change beginning to emerge. Regulatory bodies issued public statements acknowledging the need to address systemic discrimination in healthcare. Attention in the media also turned toward concerning practices within certain institutions, where security measures appeared to disproportionately affect certain individuals, raising questions about bias and unequal treatment. Reports of discriminatory language surfaced, prompting further scrutiny. Additionally, legal actions against academic and medical institutions began to shine a spotlight on long-standing issues. Although these changes were gradual, they signaled the beginning of an important shift toward greater accountability and fairness. Other advocates, like Dr. Uché Blackstock, would speak out about race-related bias in academic medicine on a national and international scale calling for change. Still others, like Drs. Peter Attia and Casey Means would, in their own books, speak to the role of hospital culture and their personal experiences as a driving force for entering the world of tech and entrepreneurship instead. Things were shifting; I could sense it.

Anyone who has ever faced the odds in a battle for what's right, while clouded in tremendous uncertainty knows this: this sort of change rarely comes at the flip of a switch or a tipping point. And sometimes, just like an abscess, it takes digging deep first before it can get resolved. It was then that I was reminded of the quote by David Whyte, which applied not just to me but to all of us during what would feel like an immensely challenging year with so much loss: "Courage is the measure of our heartfelt participation with life, with another, with a community, a work; a future. To be courageous is not necessarily to go anywhere or do anything except to make conscious those things we already feel deeply and then to live through the unending vulnerabilities of those consequences."

4.

Sleep deprivation is one of the oldest forms of torture. It was used in Guantanamo Bay, among prisoners, as an interrogation technique along with waterboarding. Why? Because it works. Sleep is the most natural and primitive need we have. So, the fact that doctors are forced to learn but also take care of patients safely while chronically and acutely sleep-deprived makes little sense. But even I thought that there was some rationale for it because why make something so against our intuitive understanding of "wellness" mandatory in so many training programs and hospitals at large? Yet the long days and on-call shifts of more than 26 hours straight have an interesting origin, which I never knew until a friend mentioned it casually over dinner in SoHo one night.

"You know, the whole on call idea came from a guy who pretended he could function but was high on coke all the time, right?" she said as we were picking at our gambas al ajillo (my favorite dish at my favorite tapas bar in New York— Boqueria). We had been sharing academic hospital experiences.

"What?" I almost spit out my sangria.

That started a long discussion about who Dr. William Halsted was, the person who is perhaps most responsible for why thousands of medical residents are consistently bleary-eyed and work 26-36 hour shifts every 2-3 nights as part of their training. The story, as is detailed in the 2017 book *Genius on the Edge* by Gerald Imber, is worth a read—it's a good one.

In 1852, Halsted was born into a life of privilege in New York but was a mediocre student who made it to Yale and picked the profession of medicine for disconcerting reasons: he had a bizarre fascination for cadavers. During his surgical training, anesthesia became standard, and the germ theory was established, leading to more rigorous sanitary standards, which, as we learned in Chapter 2, drastically improved outcomes. Cocaine was used as an anesthetic, and Halsted took a particular curiosity towards the substance for—ahem—personal use, though arguably, it may have begun as an innocent self-experiment. He even published a paper on cocaine as an anesthetic that was so poorly written he became a laughingstock, but he would soon after leave another legacy.

Halsted attempted to get clean of his drug habit and was able to leave New York for Baltimore, taking a job at Johns Hopkins Hospital, where he rose up the ranks, becoming a well-respected surgeon, even rising to chief of surgery. And he was a skilled surgeon who took his time, rarely having to deal with complications.

But it seemed his addiction loomed large. His behavior was unusual, and he would go missing for long periods, leaving his trainees in the lurch. When he was around, however, he would push them to stay for long shifts, which often included his hours-long surgeries. When they complained it was inhumane, he reminded them that he was older and still able to stay awake. What he didn't disclose was that his "alertness" was due to his heavy cocaine use.

So how did a 19th-century doctor with a clear substance use disorder involving cocaine help influence work hours among trainees today? The history of medicine has been unfairly kind to Dr. Halsted until Imbers' book was released, which finally shares the shadow side of medicine: it is riddled with perfectionists willing to resort to anything that might give them an edge, even at the expense of leaving a cultural legacy on the profession that would be harmful.

*

Several medical cases over the years have ended in tragedy, shining light on the particular issue of sleep deprivation. The case of Libby Zion is probably the most prominent. Zion was a teen who, in the spring of 1984, was admitted to a New York hospital for a high fever, muscle aches, and joint pain. She had a history of psychiatric issues and was treated with phenelzine (a medication that inhibits a substance called monoamine oxidase), but had also been prescribed an opioid called Percodan after a dental procedure, with two other medications: an antibiotic (erythromycin) and chlorpheniramine (an anti-histamine for allergies).

For the fever, she was given Tylenol and evaluated by both a resident and an intern. However, when her chills went unabated, she was prescribed an opioid called meperidine. Apparently, around 4 am, Libby remained upset and hard to console, and she was given an anti-psychotic usually reserved for psychiatric patients, haloperidol or "haldol," and placed in physical restraints to prevent her from leaving her bed. Haldol was exactly what my patient Alex had been given that night before the "Code White" when I was on-call.

By sunrise, Libby's fever remained unabated, and she remained agitated, so she was given a cooling blanket and cold compresses. Shortly after, she stopped breathing, which then led her heart to stop—respiratory arrest just before cardiac arrest. Seven hours after she was admitted, Libby Zion was declared dead.

Zion's father, Sidney Zion, was a prominent Manhattan-based journalist, so wearing both his hat as a journalist and a father, he became concerned after learning that the two trainees on call, tasked with making decisions leading up to his daughter's death, had been up for more than 24 hours. And that was on the lower end of what can be up to a 40-hour shift.

The Zions successfully sued the hospital, basing it on conditions that he felt influenced the poor decision-making that led to Libby Zion's death. This then led to a domino effect in media: stories popped up about unsafe work conditions in hospitals and interns who were too exhausted to function. Changes happened as a result. In 1989, the state of New York limited work hours for trainee doctors to 80 hours per week, and in 2003, all U.S. training programs mandated the same limit, specifying the 24-hour cut-off of continuous duty and mandating at least one day off per week.

Since 2003, there has been a flood of research linking prolonged duty hours to everything from medical errors to car accidents after a shift. For instance, in a study by Harvard's Christopher Landrigan, interns made over one-third more errors on a 30-hour shift. These errors encompass wrong site surgery, missing both obvious and rare diagnoses, omitting a crucial patient-care issue, calculating the wrong dose for a drug to be administered to a patient, and so on. And this doesn't even include communication challenges that happen to all of us when we're overworked and fatigued—empathy can be tough even when we're well-rested if the day is hectic. With no rest, professionalism is at stake.

Then, in 2009, a study by Medicare, which almost undid the work in Landrigan's study and others, found that a fifth of all hospitalized patients suffered harm from medical errors and that decreasing trainee work hours had no measurable effect. The intent of this study was to show that continuity of care may benefit from longer shifts, and the mediating factor was hypothesized to be the errors induced during "transitions," as in handing over one set of patients to a new physician who is taking over for the previous physician on shift. It's a bit like a broken telephone, where messages can get misconstrued, so Landrigan shifted his work to understanding how to better standardize the handoff process.

Beginning in early 2011, nine hospitals across Canada and the U.S. implemented a new initiative, led by Boston Children's Hospital, called I-PASS (which stands for illness severity, patient summary, action list, situation awareness and contingency plans, and synthesis by receiver) with the aim of reducing the percentage of medical errors which could be linked to poor handover. Handover, or "handoff," is the term that describes when a previous medical team (either the on-call team or another daytime team) transitions hospital care for a series of patients over to a new team. It is a vulnerable time: the handover period has been linked to a variety of poor outcomes and, according to the Joint Commission for Transforming Healthcare, is responsible for up to 80% of major adverse events in hospitals, primarily due to issues with communication. The most infamous handover period that remains controversial happens on July 1, known as the "July Effect," when new residents and medical students begin. Patients tend to fare poorly during this period.

The I-PASS study group, led by Harvard's Dr. Amy Starmer, along with Landrigan, decided to ask a simple question: if handover were standardized to more easily identified priorities which reduced the 'noise' involved in miscommunication, that can trickle down to patients, what might be the impact on medical error and preventable adverse events? This was an involved process that required standardized verbal and written handoffs, training in communication for handoffs, as well as ongoing faculty development and frequent observation (and feedback) of handoffs. What they found, published in the *New England Journal of Medicine* in 2014, was remarkable: the medical error rate dipped by 23%, and the rate of preventable adverse events decreased by 30%—both were statistically significant decreases. This has since led to an entire I-PASS curriculum implemented in hospitals across North America.

So now that the handoff problem has been addressed, why does limiting hours on duty remain controversial, even while the premise behind excessive work hours is completely flawed and can be traced back to an unreliable authority figure who was addicted to cocaine? Why is the medical industry unwilling to yield, even when we know how high the stakes are?

5.

A recent study in the journal *Anaesthesia* found that sleep deprivation among healthcare workers was directly linked to DNA damage. Research has found that a lack of sleep among resident doctors is a risk factor for depression in a profession that already struggles with mental health issues. Also, shifts that are near the 24-hour mark increase the risk of a hazardous driving event (40% of attending physicians have reported they've fallen asleep while driving).

Dr. Michael Farquhar, a British-based sleep expert, writes that many hospitals remain unaware of the impact of this issue. Particularly for night shifts, he writes: "We are not evolved to be awake at night. Our circadian rhythm, the powerful drive that helps regulate wake and sleep, means that we are at a physiological low when working at night."

He started a campaign called "HALT: Take a Break" that offers ways to reduce fatigue while also decreasing the stigma associated with simply asking for a break to rest and recuperate once one's limit is reached. The National Health Service (NHS) in Britain has even instituted nap-pods for tired doctors. In the U.S., other initiatives for patients, such as a nursing-led project at Yale New Haven Hospital, try to give patients their medications before they go to sleep to minimize sleep disruptions.

*

Dr. Matthew Walker, a professor of psychology and neuroscience at the University of California, Berkeley, has explored the issue of sleep in his research and in his best-selling book, *Why We Sleep*. In his 2017 paper, "The Sleep Deprived Human Brain," published in *Nature Reviews*, Walker and his colleagues detailed a variety of cognitive effects of sleep deprivation, such as problems with working memory and attention, as well as emotional issues, such as failure to discriminate between others' emotional signals, and to modulate our own (our amygdala is more active when sleep deprived).

Currently, Walker serves as an advisor to companies like Google and the Oura Ring, focusing specifically on how tracking our sleep quality can make a difference in our ability to prioritize sleep. "Sleep is one of the most powerful, freely available healthcare systems you could ever wish for," Dr. Walker told me. "But the irony is that the one place a patient needs sleep the most is the place they're least likely to get it: in a hospital bed on the ward."

Walker's study in *Nature* found that sleep disruption is directly linked to atherosclerosis, a buildup of plaque in blood vessels. It also impacts immune function. More disturbingly, interrupted sleep could actually affect how well we heal in a hospital. One study found that sleep affects wound healing, including wounds from surgery or any type of procedure. Using the Pittsburgh Sleep Quality Index score, the researchers looked at patients with inflammatory bowel disease, such as ulcerative colitis or Crohn's disease. These diseases are characterized by wounds primarily in the bowel and treated most often by medications to suppress the immune system. The wounds took longer to heal among the patients who had lower sleep scores.

Indeed, sleep's impact on healing has been linked to everything from wounds to oral ulcers to atherosclerosis and ß-amyloid (a protein that builds up in the brain of Alzheimer's patients). During the COVID-19 pandemic, it was postulated whether melatonin, a hormone that signals that it is time to sleep, specifically may work to block COVID-19's various effects through being an anti-inflammatory, antioxidant, and antiviral.

As it relates to patients, Walker suggests providing patients with ear plugs and a mask if they are expected to stay overnight in a hospital, and encouraging doctors to be more mindful about when they wake patients for a question or an assessment: things I had tried to do for little Laila.

As to why American doctors must work brutally long hours to be properly trained, Walker counters: "Countries such as France, Switzerland, and New Zealand train physicians in the same amount of time despite limiting resident shifts to less than 16 hours, yet these countries continue to rank in the top 10 for quality of medical care and practice. It's worthwhile remembering that after being awake for 22 hours straight, you are as cognitively impaired as if you were legally drunk. Nobody would accept medical care from an inebriated doctor. Yet we must accept medical care from doctors who are similarly impaired due to the lack of sleep the system imposes on them."

6.

Gregg Popovich, head coach of the San Antonio Spurs, helped pioneer the NBA's Do Not Play (DNP)-Rest strategy, which prevents players from playing back-to-back games to allow for adequate recovery and to decrease the likelihood of fatigue and injury. In 2012, Popovich sat Tim Duncan out for a rest day—this was his first implementation of DNP-Rest. But the policy remains controversial.

Not every team incorporates DNP-Rest—it's dependent on the coach. Most notoriously, Pat Riley, then coach of the Miami Heat, was quoted as saying: "We don't rest. I don't believe in it. I think it's gotten to the point where it's become a travesty, an absolute travesty. Blatantly. I don't care how many players you're resting or who. Who are the ones entitled to get the rest versus who doesn't rest? We don't rest." Notably, the Heat hasn't won a championship since 2013 and lost a star player in Chris Bosh once he was out with blood clots in 2016 (the link between fatigue and risk of blood clots has not been established, but the link between blood clots and immobility due to frequent travel has).

In March 2017, Cleveland Cavaliers' Lebron James, upset that he played almost 40 minutes in a game, took a rest day against the Clippers. He came back rejuvenated, scoring 34 points against the Lakers. Fans of that game were impressed, but the ones who bought tickets to the Clippers game were angry. They had paid to see "The King" play, after all. James ended up taking a total of five rest days that season with his coach's blessing.

In contrast, in European soccer, fans tend to be more concerned about player health, pushing coaches to sit players out if they seem fatigued or suffer an injury. But this difference is less about the type of sport and more about the type of *fan*, which means it really comes down to culture, and the push-pull factors are ultimately about business; professional sports is a billion-dollar global industry that depends on its fans. Anything that could potentially push fans away, even if it means risking a player's health, is avoided.

This all harkens back to the Greek tragedy of Milo of Croton. A celebrated 6th-century wrestler, he found himself in a forest, curious as to why a tree trunk had split in half but remained intact. Attempting to pull the pieces apart, his hand became stuck, resulting in his inability to break free. He was devoured by wild beasts as a signal that testing one's strength can be humbling or, perhaps on occasion, deadly. Known for his strength, Milo of Croton died when he pushed himself to test it.

In North America, the "hero" ideal of pushing beyond one's limits to achieve a goal is prized, and fans pay a premium on sports tickets to watch "their" player play. It's owed to them. However, in parts of Europe, rest and leisure are appreciated, from daytime siestas to more vacation days. Soccer fans prioritize the long-term health of their favorite players so that they can have the pleasure of watching them over the years.

In other words, it's also about immediate versus delayed gratification and temporary versus long-term pleasure. And this gets to why knowledge alone isn't enough—the situation and culture must support a shift to become aligned with knowledge, and that's particularly the case when it comes to aligning with new recommendations that deal with our health.

In 2021, several athletes, from Simone Biles to Steph Curry, either didn't attend the Tokyo Olympics or backed away for several days in part to focus on rest. During the 2024 Paris Olympics, Curry and Biles each won gold in their events.

7.

Decades before DNP-Rest came to be in the NBA and work-hour limitations were placed on medical trainees in parts of North America, there was the work of Christopher Johnstone. As far as doctors go, Johnstone is the U.K.'s answer to Mister Rogers. Now 63 and based in Scotland, he has a soft British accent, a gentle manner, and sparkling eyes. I had stumbled upon his work on resilience entirely by chance, work that he does through his organization called, aptly, the College of Wellbeing. But his sweet demeanor hides something bigger: an incredible strength.

The year was 1988, and Chris Johnstone, working as a junior doctor at the London Maudsley Hospital, had become depressed and a shadow of himself. Just six years earlier, he had moved to London from the south of England at the age of 17. His dad was a family doctor, and Johnstone excelled in math and science, so it seemed natural to follow in his father's footsteps.

However, Johnstone chose medicine for other reasons. "I wanted to do something to improve the world, and I could see that was possible with medicine. I didn't really have enough of a sense of what life was about and to make deeply considered decisions about my life's path. It was more like [medicine] was an easily available pathway to me," he told me.

Johnstone got involved in the peace movement in the early 1980s when there was a threat of nuclear exchange, and, knowing how anxious his peers were about this possibility, he became interested in psychology and the use of biofeedback for stress reduction. He ended up conducting experiments on biofeedback in medical school at the University College London— experiments like placing a subject's hand in a bucket of ice-cold water and measuring reaction times before and after a hypnotherapy exercise. He was interested in looking at what factors might build resilience.

But then he rotated through six months of surgery, then obstetrics and gynecology and another in geriatrics, combined with back-to-back hospital shifts where he was on-call every two or three days without protected time off. As a result, he became a wreck. So, he and his colleagues began a campaign for improved working conditions. Until one day, after driving home after an extended overnight shift, he almost died behind the wheel.

231

"I opened my eyes and realized I was driving on the wrong side of the road, so I swerved to avoid an oncoming car and crashed," he told me. After his car wreck, Johnstone hit a limit. As he was home recovering, it struck him: he needed to do something to affect change for others. So, after he finished his training in family medicine, 26-year-old Johnstone began thinking he should help change the very system that almost killed him before it could harm others.

He recalls that the moment "was about, literally, life and death. It became a threat to my life to continue working the way that I was working, and talk about toxic culture, you know, working as a doctor where you're supposedly acting as an agent for health improvement, but in a way that was so clearly wrecking my own health. It just felt, sort of…kind of like a paradox, really."

Speaking to a well-known expert in stress research, Johnstone was advised to "get measured" as part of his cause. This involved hooking up a portable EEG monitor to his head as he worked overnight shifts.

"It's very compelling evidence, you know, data is. There was a time when the Health Minister had said it was all just a fisherman's tale, or a tall story, this idea that doctors would fall asleep at work, but actually I had evidence of all the microsleeps I was having while I was helping with operations during the nighttime," he said. The pattern was one of extreme exhaustion. And the press responded with a mix of dismay and amazement. A local news article read: "Dr. Chris Johnstone has wired himself up to look like a walking Frankenstein monster to prove to his bosses that a 120-hour work week is not good for humans."

What started as a well-intentioned public relations stunt ended up gaining the attention of a young lawyer who, at a party, suggested Johnstone file a lawsuit against the hospital, believing he had a good chance of winning. She pointed out that employers—even hospitals—have a legal obligation to provide a safe system for work, but the contract Johnstone and other junior doctors had signed, in which they agreed to an average of "88 hours a week," meant there was no real upper limit—it could technically be 168 hours a week which is effectively 24/7. So, Johnstone filed it with the backing of his peers and the local medical association.

It was a long, drawn-out ordeal, and one which a top judge, Lord Denning, in the United Kingdom, at one point described as being "highly unlikely" to be successful for the underdogs. Johnstone and his peers were funded by pro-bono legal work and private donor funding, but it still took almost six years and more than 10 hearings. In the meantime, Johnstone explored other vocations, in part to rehabilitate his soul after the car accident and the additional dehumanizing experience of the justice system. "I learned how to garden," he told me shyly, "and realized I was rather good at it, in fact, and resolved to do that should all else fail." During the years-long ordeal, a good friend of Johnstone's, in his medical school year, sadly collapsed and died after an extended shift on the obstetrics ward as well. This only served to reaffirm the cause.

By then, given he stood up against the status quo, the possibility of working seemed dismal. "I was viewed as a troublemaker, a whistleblower," he said. Johnstone applied for a variety of jobs but was never selected. "One interviewer was honest with me and said I was qualified, but I would be an 'industrial relations nightmare.' And so there was that kind of sense of 'Well, maybe I burned my bridges, maybe I've blown it as far as a medical career is concerned,' but I did find my way back in, and in some ways, it's interesting because when you take a stand for something that's important to you, as it was to me, there will be people who won't approve, and who will block you, but they're not the people I'd wanted to work with anyway," he told me.

Then the most unlikely thing happened: Johnstone *won* the final hearing in 1995. And it set a precedent that changed the way the law in the U.K. was understood. Previously, occupational injuries, i.e., injuries "on the job," only applied to physical injuries—things like breaking a wrist or hurting one's back. Damages could be claimed for those. But now "psychological injury" would count as well. It set one of the very first precedents for injuries secondary to work stress and those related to the mental distress of working in a psychologically unsafe environment. Other claims and large settlements soon followed from a variety of industries, including healthcare.

For Johnstone, then, his healing from depression and suicidal ideation had little to do with therapy or medication. Instead, it had everything to do with being empowered to change the very system that caused his illness in the first place. Today, he has a thriving practice focused on resilience for healthcare professionals and non-healthcare professionals alike. And he still enjoys gardening.

When I asked what made him decide to pursue that case, to stand up against the status quo, and potentially risk it all, he gave me an answer I didn't expect:

"For years, there was a period of time where it was just accepted, that things like the transatlantic slave trade or apartheid were accepted as normal…that it was just one of those things that happened. And there were a lot of powerful vested interests that would block any attempt to change it," Johnstone told me. "But over a period of decades, there was always one particularly committed action. There were people in history who said, 'You must draw a line,' or said, 'This is wrong, it's got to change,' and they took a step, and sometimes they were stomped on, but sometimes…sometimes other people rallied behind them in a way that led to bigger change. And so, I could see that process and thought, 'Well, if I'm really serious about this, what's stopping me from playing this kind of role?' Somebody had to do it."

8.

And now, we return to little Laila, the patient we met at the beginning of this chapter. When I spoke to Laila's mother months later, I learned that Laila ended up being transferred to the Toronto hospital a few days later and eventually discharged. For a long while, she was assessed in a clinic for her medical care and finally got onto a regular sleep schedule at home. Would she have healed faster if her sleep had been less frequently interrupted in the hospital? We will never know. Maybe the sleep interruptions were justifiable for other reasons that could have improved her care. But the opportunity to have stretches of restorative sleep in a more comfortable environment at home were all part of keeping her well.

We know that the broader attention on sleep—everything from Arianna Huffington's advocacy among industry leaders and even the new trend of sleep concerts (think: hundreds of people piling into an auditorium to sleep on individual beds, to the sound of classical music) suggests that the role of sleep in our culture is shifting.

While robust data isn't available on how effective DNP-Rest is, correlation data suggests that games missed due to injury or illness declined dramatically in the 2016-2017 season. Extrapolating data from the COVID player "bubble" might provide a more convincing case for other NBA coaches—this is exactly what Singh explored. So why does it, with all the research we now have about the harms of sleep deprivation on our brain, recovery, and performance, remain so controversial? And why does the controversy extend to other industries—like medicine—where performance can literally mean the difference between life and death? For the lack of a better word, it's probably time to give the controversy a rest and focus on changing how we work and play, to ensure sleep is prioritized and prized, knowing the dividends on performance and well-being will emerge.

This then reminds us of Steve and Jennifer Wall, who we met in Chapter 6 at their restaurant on the corner of Ross and Wellington Streets: it takes committed and skilled leadership to change the culture, and this applies to restaurants, basketball courts, and, of course, hospitals. It's the same problem we saw with how European soccer fans (and coaches) view rest compared with American fans of the NBA—and it all stems from one core issue: a different understanding of how knowledge should translate to change. France, the U.K., New Zealand and Switzerland, by the way, all have top-notch soccer teams and lower prevalence of burnout in the medical profession. It's not a coincidence.

Elizabeth Lesser's book *Broken Open* is instructive, and she talks about this idea called the 'Phoenix Process': the moment when there is a line in the sand that clearly demarcates our lives and identities 'before' a tragic event—a natural disaster, a health crisis, death of a loved one, losing a job, divorce...a pandemic. The moment when we are forever changed as a result. Indeed, we all need to bravely welcome the new dawn after these transitions.

Part of that, for me, was being open to new opportunities, like starting a psychotherapy course offered to physicians; it opened my eyes to what causes people to behave the way they do—often, they are driven by early life experiences. This gave me more compassion for those that bullied others in the academic hospital. It was also a reminder that I had come so far. Then, through an interesting series of events, I was recruited to work with Twitter as a consultant to help improve the health and well-being of their platform, and I would later be recruited to consult for startups as well as other Big Tech companies venturing into healthcare.

I asked Johnstone what he would share with his 26-year-old self, knowing what he knows now or what he'd share with a junior doctor. "Recognize how larger stories of change can happen through you, that you can play a role in a larger story of change that goes beyond what you might think of as possible. So, I think my advice to somebody in their 20s now would be to seek a beautiful life that's good for you and good for the world," he said.

I then shared with him my own challenges. By then, there were legal cases and stories of everyone from gymnasts (who reported on abuse by female coaches)* to postdoctoral researchers to teachers. It was as though this issue was being fought in multiple industries—and women (not men) were emerging as the common perpetrators; indeed this was also true for my own experience. Johnstone's parting words couldn't have come at a better time:

"Culture happens through us. We also have the choice about what kind of culture we express. And it's how we really think about power and what's beyond our power and how we expand our sense of what we can contribute to. But one of the big ways we do that is moving beyond the story that it's just about me, and I," he shared. "It sounds like you're on the path. Writing is a big part of that, and you're finding your voice, and writing your book is part of that too…so really—good luck."

It was exactly what I had gathered from the cases of Horne, Garba, Kelly, and Blackstock. Johnstone was just filling in the gaps I needed to understand it all more completely. I knew exactly what I needed to do.

The poet David Whyte perhaps best encapsulates the role of rest more generally in his poem in his book *Consolations*:

Rest is the conversation between what we love to do and how we love to be. Rest is the essence of giving and receiving; an

---

*   Mary Wright (https://www.nytimes.com/2020/11/06/sports/gymnastics-coach-misconduct-safesport.html) and Maggie Haney (https://www.si.com/more-sports/video/2020/04/30/maggie-haney-suspended-eight-years-emotional-verbal-abuse-athletes), both women, were investigated in 2020 for severe bullying of female gymnasts.

act of remembering, imaginatively, and intellectually but also psychologically and physically. To rest is to give up on the already exhausted will as the prime motivator of endeavor, with its endless outward need to reward itself through established goals. To rest is to give up on worrying and fretting and the sense that there is something wrong with the world unless we are there to put it right; to rest is to fall back literally or figuratively from outer targets and shift the goal not to an inner static bull's eye, an imagined state of perfect stillness, but to an inner state of natural exchange.

Finally, I recognized the importance of harnessing every other tool I had discovered so far: nutrition, movement, mind-body approaches, psychedelic medicine (or, in this case, recognizing that it wasn't the right tool at the time), leaning on my social support, optimizing my environment, and advocating for systems change and placing my experiences in the context of "story" in order to make meaning. So now, it was time for me to rest.

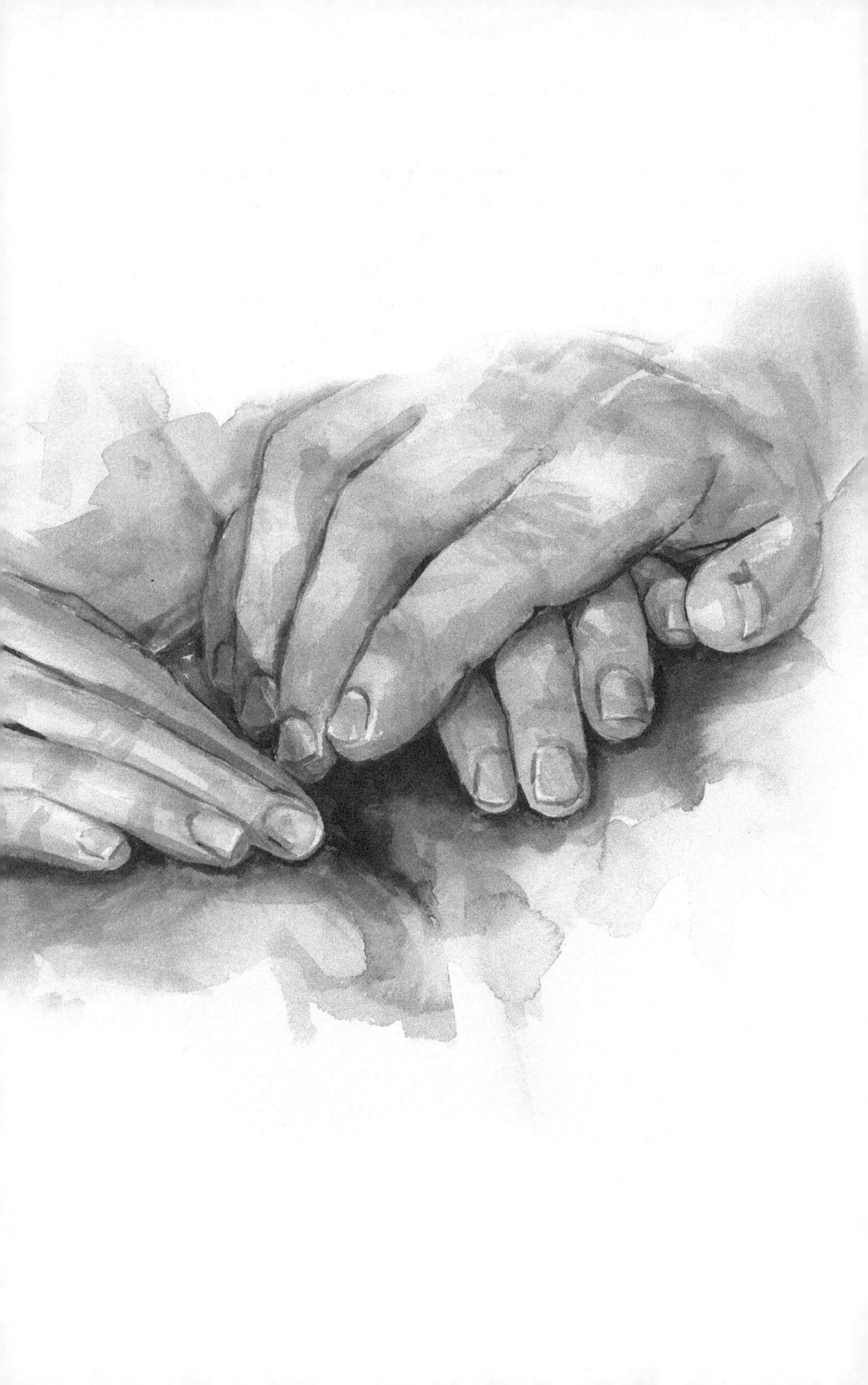

Chapter Twelve

Sweet Surrender

"Hardships often prepare ordinary people for extraordinary destiny."
— C.S. Lewis

1.

Priya lay there, the whites of her eyes jaundiced and her skin resembling a mix of yellow and brown. Her straight black hair, which was greasy from not having been washed for two days, hung in a loose ponytail. The skin on her forehead glistened with beads of sweat from being moved around and fighting what was a losing battle with her own body. Perhaps it was her heritage—her parents were from India, that did it, but I saw myself in her. Except, instead of being a fighter, she lay there meek, almost expressionless, staring at me.

The intensive care unit (ICU) team, which included myself, was wheeling her to the CT (CAT) scanner on the second floor. It was a feat. An aide carried the portable ventilator. The respiratory therapist had to ensure she kept breathing. In that moment, my responsibility was to ensure her lines and tubes stayed untangled while monitoring for any changes in her status that would require intervention on the fly. The CT scan was ordered to see if her lungs had noticeably worsened. A fungus, we had thought. It's interesting how that genera could mean anything from charming toadstools in an enchanted forest to massive clumps of mold that digest an immunocompromised patient from the inside. Priya's cancer had relapsed, and the fungus had caused

239

multi-system organ failure. She seemed to have some understanding that this was the end.

As we entered the elevator, I wondered what we would do if the scan showed that, indeed, her lungs looked worse. Perhaps, we could start an anti-fungal medication. But it was a temporary measure. If there was fluid build-up, maybe we would administer a diuretic medication (a "water pill") to cause her body to urinate the fluid out. Another short-term fix. Surgery was out of the question at this stage—too risky, and she could die on the table. Temporary measures were all we had, and it was *because* her doctors cared, not in spite of any apathy, that those choices were made.

Her mother was frantic—"We must save Priya," she had pleaded. Priya's dad had stood by stoically—seemingly embarrassed at the commotion but also helpless in consoling his wife. The tragic circumstances undoubtedly placed additional strain on their marriage. Grief has a wide spectrum.

After the scan, we found ourselves all together again in her small ICU room, trying to choose between acceptance of the end and a few other quick fixes to buy more time—without buying more "life" per se.

Priya took her last breath in an ICU bed in the early hours of a Monday, or so I heard. I was sleeping at home; my co-resident, Greg, was on call. Her family was around her, he shared, and one other doctor and her nurse.

When I heard about it the following morning, I thought back to the yellows of her eyes and my inability to translate whatever the wishes were behind them. I wondered who the last person she looked at was, if they saw the same expression I had. I wondered what her last glimpse of this world might have been and if the last sound she heard might have been the beeping of the bedside cardiac monitor. I would never know if she understood why all these interventions were taken or if her disease prevented any understanding in the cognitive sense. If she could, would she have protested against all of the short-term fixes?

With Priya, I learned for the first time that *healing* was entirely separate from *curing*. One can be healed without being cured, and perhaps vice versa. Healing was what Priya most likely wanted and perhaps what her family desired as well. Instead, due to the complexity of anticipatory grief and the sense of futility doctors often feel when nothing they proposed had any impact, she received unnecessary procedures and testing. And so, Priya had passed away, as a slow withering out of this world, while her mother fought her own resistance around letting go among the machines and cords and fluorescent lights of a small ICU room.

2.

The term "anticipatory grief" means grief that appears before actual loss or death. That's what Priya's mother likely felt—death was near and she, like many parents, wasn't ready, and so it manifested as anxiety and the need to do everything for her daughter to prolong her physical time on earth. Surrender wasn't just difficult, it likely felt like the harder option, an option that would leave any caregiver feeling guilty about making the more morbid choice. Just like the small boy, Nixon, that Karine had rescued from the rubble in Haiti and subsequently was forced to leave behind, the hardest part of choosing is the letting go part that must often come first.

But what does it really mean to surrender, to really *let go*? Throughout the previous ten years, this was the one area I still couldn't grasp. How long should doctors keep fighting for our patients? And for ourselves? When does letting go make sense? As doctors and as patients, how are we supposed to "know" when to let go? And is that knowing the same for everyone?

I thought back to my grandfather ("Tata") who died in 2016 in Colombo, Sri Lanka. I was fortunately able to see him a year earlier. When I did, it was clear his health was failing. He was still active: able to walk to the market every day, for instance, though it was more challenging with every passing day. His blood pressure and cholesterol had been managed with medications, and he still saw his doctor every month or so, but it didn't take away from his tiredness.

My grandfather had been a fighter, though. Raised in an orphanage in the Dutch-colonized northern village of Delft, he succeeded in school and also social causes: he was a socialist. He would donate to orphanages around the country and sponsor children who needed school uniforms. He would protest against the discriminatory policies affecting the Tamil minority in the country.

In recent decades, epigenetic research, largely from Holocaust survivors (part of Dr. Rachel Yehuda's work described earlier), has suggested that many of our personality traits may be inherited, including those hardened by trauma. I wondered if my fighting spirit came from my grandfather. But, at 91, he was clear with my mother and aunt: his time on earth was drawing to a close. He even said that he would probably be dead by 92, joining his wife who had passed away thirty-five years earlier. When I saw him though, he had a certain calmness about him: he just seemed ready.

*

The field of palliative care was created after World War 2, after a British doctor, Dame Cicely Saunders, founded the first known hospice center in 1948 to serve patients who were terminally ill. In that year she writes that she encountered "a Polish Jew whose few poignant words proved a powerful catalyst of a new worldwide movement. His statement 'I will be a window in your Home' gave a challenge to openness of all kinds; 'I want what is in your mind and in your heart' set scientific enquiry alongside personal encounter; his very personal journey into peace gave the demand for space for freedom of spirit in facing the mystery of death."

This led first to the concept of "hospice care," which emphasized end-of-life wishes. Yet it wouldn't be for another 42 years, in 1990, for the World Health Organization to formally recognize palliative care as a unique area of study and medical specialization focused on relief of suffering and optimizing quality of life for terminally ill or seriously injured patients. It is described as the "prevention, assessment, and multidisciplinary treatment of physical, spiritual and psychological problems," and is now distinct from hospice, as services can be offered through palliative care services without being end of life. According to the Center to Advance Palliative Care, between 2000 and 2011, hospitals in the U.S. increased palliative care beds by up to 157%, which speaks to the recognition of the value it brings.

Uniquely, in her essay, Saunders writes, "The losses of parting cannot be removed, but their devastating effects can be ameliorated. For this we must give attention to the whole person, with all the insights the humanities can give us." In other words, she gets exactly to the definition of healing, which makes the most sense, and echoes again the work of American writer, Wendell Berry: it is a return to *wholeness*. But how do we reconcile wholeness with death and surrender when, at face value, these ideas appear diametrically opposed?

3.

Though the name "PEACH" brings to mind a soft orange fruit that is pleasant and juicy, it also happens to be the name of an initiative that brings palliative care to the homeless in inner-city Toronto. It stands for Palliative Education and Care for the Homeless and is the first of its kind in Canada and possibly the world. PEACH provides mobile medical care and is founded by palliative care specialist Dr. Naheed Dosani at the Inner City Health Associates in downtown Toronto.

Toronto is much like many big cities in North America. Homelessness has increased over the past few decades significantly and now there are more than an estimated 5,000 sleeping on the street on any given night in the city— people much like my patient, Roger, back in Chapter 2. PEACH began in 2014 with Dosani and a street nurse making informal visits to the homeless and has now expanded to a 24-hour service with more than a 100-client caseload at any given time. It integrates housing and homecare with four palliative care staff physicians, a nurse, a psychiatrist, and a healthcare navigator. The U.S., England, and Australia have followed suit, starting smaller pilot programs inspired by PEACH.

During an interview for Canada's CBC news in 2018, Dosani pointed to the mirage that many cities like Toronto have, when it comes to homelessness: "I think about how a city like this can look, like everyone's really well supported, and really, it appears that way," Dosani said. "But there are so many people falling through the in-betweens, falling through the cracks. And it's this invisible sense of vulnerability, it's hidden to the naked eye, which is dangerous."

Dosani is, as far as palliative doctors go, probably the exact opposite of Dame Cecily Saunders. He looks young and approachable: someone who doesn't fit the typical image of an assistant professor at a large academic institution (he is on staff at the University of Toronto medical school). Dosani doesn't meet most of his patients in a fluorescent-lit clinic or hospital ward. Instead, he goes to bridges, alleyways, and public parks—he goes *to them* to address their pain and general healthcare needs, including at the end of their lives. It's a calling towards a population that epitomizes the impacts of the social determinants of housing and income disparities. Research shows that homeless individuals are at a higher risk of almost every chronic and acute disease, from heart disease to cancer to infectious diseases like Hepatitis C.

It's partly linked to exposures, like injection drug use that Bruce Beadle experienced, but also to risks associated with chronic stress, daily uncertainty, and unmet basic social and physical needs. It probably makes more sense to frame homelessness as "choicelessness," which is the stance I took when I wrote one of my first articles for the *Huffington Post*, inspired by news that a homeless man in Toronto had been found dead in a bus shelter, after what appeared to be several days.

Dosani has dedicated his life to this cause. It's likely because what brought him into medicine in the first place was unusual. The son of two refugees from East Africa, he grew up as an Ismaili Muslim. Ismailis keep as a core value community service, which was instilled in him early on. In terms of stature, he was always the smallest among his peers, so he needed to make up for it in other ways. School was always a priority, as his parents prized academic achievement, as many first-generation immigrants (my parents included) did. He particularly excelled in the sciences.

Dosani sought to stand out in Scarborough, a particularly rough section of Toronto with a lot of gang violence and crime, especially in the mid-1990s. "I got caught up in the wrong crowd at one point, but I was also part of my high school student council, and I played recreational basketball and football," he told me. He was fast too—able to run past the bigger guys, many of them from the West Indies and easily a good six inches taller than him. Dosani also dived into music and saw the potential of radio, creating a radio station called the "Bethune Blaze," a play on the name of his school—Dr. Norman Bethune

Secondary School.* Yet what interested Dosani most was the potential of the radio station to act as a youth program at his school.

"There were youth—from disadvantaged backgrounds...one-parent households, where maybe there was gang involvement or maybe they just skipped a lot of school or got into drugs—that were in a stream the school called 'high risk' and this was really stigmatized. We all knew who those kids were. So, I thought it would be cool to create a before-school program for any student—regardless of the stream they were in—to be part of this radio thing...to choose music or start conversations on the air that no one was having, and lots of these things related to the factors that made life challenging for all of us," he told me.

The radio station was a way to allow these students, who had an entirely different trajectory in life and were branded for it, to feel like they *belonged* and, more importantly, to *give* something unique of themselves. It was meaningful and facilitated a sense of shared purpose and community. For Dosani, the first taste of social impact at a school named for Dr. Bethune was how medicine came to appeal to him: it was a vocation that allowed the blend of advocacy and science.

Medicine attracts some of the brightest among us—but it has traditionally looked for one thing in its candidates: the ability to memorize facts and understand challenging science, and effectively regurgitate it. Caring for the ill requires much more than that. Today, almost anything can be looked up on the internet or in a textbook. The speed at which medicine progresses is mind-numbing for those tasked to keep "up to date," so much so that most doctors rely on a database called "UpToDate" when consulting with patients to ensure they're aligned with the most recent and accepted way of approaching and managing a given condition. Now, artificial intelligence (A.I.) takes this idea further, with its ability to comb recent guidelines, synthesize research, and provide clinical reasoning to guide doctors.

---

* Norman Bethune was a Canadian physician and medical innovator known for his pioneering work in mobile blood transfusion during the Spanish Civil War and his contributions to battlefield medicine in China during the Second Sino-Japanese War. He is celebrated for his humanitarian efforts and his dedication to providing medical care in war-torn regions.

The good news is that over the past two decades or so, most medical schools began to prioritize well-rounded candidates: those who demonstrate an understanding of humanity and empathy and who come from diverse upbringings and experiences. That said, the system is set up so that the most ruthless can effectively "hack" the process by sprinkling in a few volunteer activities and superficial research to *appear* well-rounded. But that's getting harder to do, thankfully. The payoff for well-roundedness and inclusiveness of experience is clear in Dosani's case: without his upbringing as a son of refugees and familiarity with navigating the many worlds of urban Toronto, as well as his own deep understanding of how it feels to be on the fringes of society and empathy for "the other" (the overlooked, ignored and the stigmatized), Dosani may never have founded PEACH in the first place. And without it, Toronto and other cities would be much worse off.

*

In 1915, Dr. John Scott Haldane, a Scottish physician, became one of the first proponents of "sentinel animals," those that provide us with warnings of impending danger. He was one of the first public health physicians in the U.K., and investigated the effects of toxic gases—the "Haldane Effect" is named after his work. Haldane was credited with using canaries and white mice dropped into a coalmine to signal the presence of carbon monoxide. Their fast metabolism would lead them to present with symptoms of carbon monoxide poisoning much earlier—indicating when miners should exit to prevent death by asphyxia. The idiom "canary in the coalmine" comes from Dr. Haldane's observations.

When I was at Johns Hopkins for public health graduate school, we learned about this story, but it wasn't until I became a physician that I realized that among us are human canaries, the most vulnerable who live at the extremes of the human experience: the homeless, refugees, impoverished children, and so forth. To get an accurate idea of how our society—a specific city, country, or neighborhood—is doing, we need only look to these communities first for patterns. The moment we see a worsening, we know that something is fundamentally wrong and must be changed before it has a ripple effect outward.

And this gets at another meaning of surrender, the more traditional conception of it: the willful *giving up* and dismissing of these canaries in our midst. In other words, being a bystander, or turning a blind eye because it hurts too much and feels too hard, to confront the challenge head-on. Because, at some level, we feel our futility more than our strength. That's likely what we had all felt with Roger that day when I was a medical student on 14 Cardinal Carter West at St. Michael's Hospital in Toronto, knowing we were discharging him back to the street, to exactly the same situation that brought him to the hospital in the first place. We couldn't see an alternative or chance to make another reality possible for him.

But doctors like Dosani refuse to surrender in this way, possibly because their own lives were, in part, catalyzed by a degree of optimism or perhaps an ounce of necessary self-delusion, making that alternative more visible and more visceral. And by helping lead the charge in his small corner of the world, in Toronto's alleyways and bridges, parks, and shelters, Naheed Dosani gave permission for others to see those same possibilities and willingly follow suit.

4.

When I met Darren Sudman in 2014 at the TedMED event in Palm Springs, I didn't expect that his story would be one I would return to time and again as I began examining what makes us thrive and heal after difficult times. Sudman introduced himself as a former lawyer and a founder of a non-profit, but I was most inspired by how the non-profit came to be. In 2004, Sudman and his wife, Phyllis, experienced every parent's worst nightmare: their three-month-old son, Simon, was found motionless in his crib. He had passed away from sudden infant death syndrome (SIDS), later deemed to be secondary to a heart rhythm disturbance called Long QT Syndrome.

Sudman's non-profit, Simon's Heart, was created with the purpose of screening children early in life. But it was what Sudman shared about how he *emerged* from this unspeakable tragedy and his ability to move forward that has continued to stay with me, particularly as I thought of the collective re-emergence after the pandemic.

"My daughter was two, and she needed me to get out of bed every day. She was really young and didn't have a grasp of what was going on, and I had to take care of her. That forced me to wake up and live every day as best I could—she was my motivation," Sudman told me. "I [also] got some unique advice from a co-worker who really had no education or expertise in the field of grief. His advice to me was, 'When you feel grief, let it pull you under and don't resist it—it's temporary, and when you're ready, you'll come back up.' This idea continues to work for me."

Though I didn't appreciate it then, this was perhaps the biggest lesson I learned from Darren Sudman, which I hope we can all put into practice as we re-emerge stronger and more whole from the situations that ail us. Sudman's intentional efforts to steer his family's crisis into an initiative that could help other parents helped offset his personal horror of re-emerging as a grieving parent.

"We had just suffered one of the worst tragedies, but through it, we [created] new narratives that involved helping prevent this from happening to other children and meeting families with similar experiences," Sudman said. "When Jaden, our third child, came home, he brought another ray of sunshine to our house and reinforced the fact that life goes on, and there's still goodness in life."

*

For Alua Arthur, working in grief counseling or end-of-life work was not the plan. The daughter of two professionals who migrated from Ghana in the 1970s, she pursued a career in law, heading to the University of Colorado for law school, and became a full-fledged lawyer by 24 years old. Arthur grew up with a strong sense of justice and agency. Her sister, Bozoma Saint John, rose up in Silicon Valley's tech sector, with leadership positions at companies like PepsiCo, Netflix, and Uber. Her father took her to the family farm when she was a child. Upset after she witnessed the killing of one of the farm animals, Alua became a vegetarian.

In the Fall of 2012, Arthur hit a wall. She had been working in Los Angeles as a lawyer for the Legal Aid Foundation of Los Angeles, representing the most marginalized, much like Dosani. It took a toll.

"I had to separate myself. I'd be hearing about this heartbreaking domestic violence case, and I'd sort of just be thinking, 'I don't have the time for the sob story, we need to get the affidavit in, I'm looking for evidence.' But over time, it was constantly a fight, and I'm a lover, not a fighter," Arthur told me.

Over time, Arthur became depressed. Her hair was thinning. She'd spend most of the day crying. She was a shadow of herself. During that time, she was supporting her sister, Bozoma, whose husband was dying. Then she felt a nudge pulling her elsewhere.

"I went on a leave of absence and one thing after another happened where I kept getting these signs to go to Cuba," Arthur told me. She ended up visiting Cuba and met several people in succession who spoke with her about a terminal diagnosis of cancer. Then, while in Cuba, she came face to face with her own death—after stepping off the bus, she almost got run over by a car. The woman in that car was later on the same bus and disclosed her battle with uterine cancer.

"That was just the final straw: it just felt like I needed to be with people at the end of life, like how I was with my brother-in-law. It was a crash course, in Cuba especially, with my life's work," Arthur shared. "So, I got trained to be a death doula."

Arthur herself had to mourn many things. As a first-generation immigrant, prestige and the law profession were huge. "My student loans are still speaking to me," she said. She also had to grieve her old life as a lawyer. But what opened up for her was immense: now she wakes up every day with a sense of purpose. Arthur's story is also a lesson in surrender.

Indeed, only when Arthur let go of that old life could she sense the draw to another place, where she would birth her new life and enter her life's work. But she had to surrender and choose discomfort and courage over what was comfortable and safe.

More people are seeking the assistance of death doulas like Alua Arthur. And there are even journals like "Exit Planners" that assist in preparations for the end of life. Events like Death Over Dinner bring up to ten strangers together over a meal to talk about end-of-life to help reduce the stigma of these conversations. When I attended one in San Francisco, I learned more about a set of seven strangers and their end-of-life wishes and experiences with grieving loved ones than I knew about my closest friends.

And we're seeing a burgeoning industry and interest in grief community work as well. When I interviewed Claire Bidwell-Smith for an article in *The Atlantic* and asked her about how her work relates more generally to surrender, she shared this:

> My work helps people navigate transitions more generally. Loss is always about change and transition, so it becomes part of understanding a narrative of loss...and asking how the relationship continues. We never get to keep anything, and life is about letting go all the time, so even for me personally I've learned to grieve deeply.

The medical profession has tried, with some success, to allow physicians and patients to have formal processes around processing grief. There are Schwartz Rounds, which focus more on physicians having permission to share their vulnerability, whether it's the death of a patient or another cause, in a formal way. Balint Groups are similar but focused on the doctor-patient relationship, where challenges are shared around everything from grief to boundaries to challenging interpersonal situations with patient families.

5.

During my last week in Vancouver, I took the time to get outside as much as possible. The draft of the book you're now holding was almost complete. I had extended my time for a month, knowing how dreary Toronto is in the winter. I ran along Kitsilano beach almost every day and hiked in the nearby forest, aptly named Pacific Spirit, as much as I could. While there were no Gingko trees in that forest, I was reminded of what botanists call "marcescence." The marcescent leaves are the ones that refuse to let go. They're the shrivelled brown ones that stay stubbornly stuck on the branches throughout winter, failing to join the rest on the dusty ground. Eventually, they molt off and sort of disintegrate right on the branch, often months after the new buds have emerged in the spring. Such leaves provide a nice contrast to the idea of 'atman' or the individual soul—the essence of the tree that is deep underneath, even as its leaves shed each season. The marcescent leaves may be akin to impossible attachments, while the trunk represents true, consistent Being. When we let go, in other words, it doesn't mean we give up.

In late April 2021, I boarded a flight back to Toronto, feeling at peace with leaving Vancouver behind. That chapter felt complete, much like other transitions I had made along the way. New opportunities were on the horizon, and I was ready to embrace them. I had several exciting offers to consider— one in the Bay Area for a research fellowship, another in New York in medical journalism, and the possibility of diving further into the tech world. Each path presented its own opportunities for growth, and I felt empowered by the choices in front of me, knowing that whichever direction I chose, it would align with the next phase of my journey.

The Writer and I stayed in touch, sharing laughs and reflecting on how the past year had shaped us since we first met on that frigid January morning in New York. We became a bookend in each other's lives, marking the clear shift from "before" the pandemic to what came after, tethered by this shared memory and the ways it defined who we were before and after COVID-19.

When I returned to Toronto, I saw my family doctor, Dr. Bacci, for my updated cholesterol results. My mind was feeling at ease now, but was my risk of a heart attack what it was several years earlier? I had tried to be strict with what I ate but slipped from time to time, especially when stressed. The good news: my levels were lower, hovering in the normal range, suggesting that the changes I made had worked.

I also had a chance to catch up with Kate. She shared a brief update, explaining that things had improved after she won her case. Following a firm legal warning to the program's leadership, the mistreatment she had faced subsided.

"I think they were just being careful after that," Kate said during our conversation. "But I've learned my lesson. It's best to keep some distance from that environment."

Kate had managed to complete her remaining rotations at a smaller, community-oriented hospital, where the physicians supported each other and prioritized well-being. By the time we spoke, she had passed her board exams that spring, and it was clear that her "happy ending" was within reach. I was genuinely happy for her and asked if she had any advice for me as I approached the final stretch of my journey.

"I had to get to the point of just letting go and being okay with whatever happens. I thought about going to pharmacy school. Or maybe research. But I sort of just *let go*," she told me. "So that's all I can really advise."

6.

In 2016, when I met Sacramento-based graphic designer, Liz Salmi, I misjudged her. I had presumed she was another eager young woman in tech. Maybe a co-founder of a start-up. Maybe an investor. She was funky and cool—with dark, spiky hair, sparkly, thick-rimmed black and white eyeglasses, and deep dimples. But then I realized that my assessment of her might have been accurate if I met her 10 years earlier. You see, Salmi, like so many in this book, took a devastating problem she was presented with and, instead of being intimidated, turned it around and used it as fuel to create something entirely different.

Around April 2008, Liz, then 29, began experiencing severe dizziness, headaches, and what were later known as partial seizures. "I would be on my computer working on a design and feel dizzy and like I wasn't in my body," she told me. Finally, after a few weeks, she dragged herself to her family doctor, who thought the likelihood of something serious was slim. In July, during her first week of work at a large architecture firm, just after her new boyfriend took her out for a birthday lunch, she began feeling dizzy while her team had gathered for a "standing meeting."

Liz's dizziness got worse, and she noticed her boss's voice becoming faint. She felt that "out of body" sensation again and sat herself on a nearby chair until she couldn't sit anymore. "I felt myself sliding out of the chair and slowly onto the ground," she recalled, "then I felt one side of my body begin to jerk, which was painful, and the jerking made its way into the middle of my body, which I now know meant the seizure was traversing throughout the brain, and then I was out."

After her boss called 911, she was rushed to the hospital in an ambulance. In the emergency room, the doctors reviewed her previous records and concluded she was too young for the seizure to be secondary to a series of medical issues. "I remember one of the docs saying that maybe I had stayed up too late or drank too much," she said. But then, in front of the doctors, another seizure happened. She was wheeled in for a CT (CAT) scan, followed by an MRI, which showed a mass. The medical team presumed that it was likely a first presentation of multiple sclerosis, which can present as areas of inflammation that can look like a mass on some general MRIs. So, Liz was sent home with anti-seizure medications and instructions on when to return.

At home, she had more seizures, forcing her to return to the emergency room. She was then transferred to a higher acuity specialized center where she had more tests done, including a spinal tap and another higher-resolution MRI of her brain. There, the neurologist concluded it was a tumor of some kind and that she was likely stable enough to go home but would need to be followed up. After another follow-up MRI three weeks later, she got another call: the tumor had grown. "They decided they needed to operate. It was definitely not MS, which is what I had been hoping for since it was better than, you know, *cancer*," she recalled.

Liz noticed some red flags. In medicine, we term "red flags" as those signs that should shock a physician out of their cognitive biases—the things that should make us think of the zebras, not horses, when we hear hooves galloping, so to speak. According to the American College of Radiology, for headaches these include seizures, nausea, vomiting, and unexplained vertigo. Liz had almost all of them, but her age and apparent health led to a diagnostic bias that is all too common. Like Liz, when I had my MRI years earlier, I recall vividly the moments in the machine. For me, it was the uncomfortable—almost anxious—knowing that someone, in that case, the technician running the scan, had for a period of time, more information on my own body than I did, the *owner* of my body.

For Liz, she recalls the banging and clicking of the MRI, but that wasn't what panicked her. "The only thing I remember thinking was that this big crazy thing in my life means things will never be what they once were, and my life could end soon. But I also knew I felt less afraid than my family did," she told me. "And while I know many people mourn their old 'healthy' selves, I was more mourning my independence, I guess."

Having grown up in an unstable family situation, Liz had lived on her own since the age of 17. For years, she handled her own bills while juggling school and part-time jobs. She was very "self-sufficient." That was her identity and all she knew for the previous decade: that she could do it all on her own. "Now, suddenly, this boyfriend I had just started dating had to take care of me. My best friend's dad would get angry at the doctors because of the lack of information and uncertainty," she recalled. "I just remember feeling embarrassed and ashamed at the help I was getting…because I didn't ever need anything close to that before…and didn't dare ask for it. I suppose I had to surrender to that. So that's probably what I grieved more than my tumor-free brain."

*

There's a moment between the unknowing and the knowing that is as comforting as it is frightening. It's sort of a grey zone. I remember first feeling it vividly one winter during my surgery rotation in medical school while eating dinner in the cafeteria at St. Michael's Hospital in Toronto. The TVs suddenly blasted "breaking news" to report on a massive car accident where two young people were being airlifted to the nearest trauma center—which was our hospital. As I was on call, I was paged immediately into the operating room to join my attending, a popular and skilled female trauma surgeon, whom I'll call Dr. Mohamed, and the surgical residents.

The patient was a girl, around 18. Mediterranean, possibly Greek. She was in the passenger seat of her boyfriend's sedan and they had skidded on the ice and rammed into a pickup truck—uncannily like what Chris Johnstone had barely missed earlier. The boy had minor injuries and was admitted for observation. The girl, however, was stabilized in the emergency room trauma bay, but it was all hands on deck to try to save her life.

Her face had swollen up—it was hard to make out any features except for heavy black eyes that were from makeup combined with severe bruising. The neurosurgeons had to shave her curly hair and drill bore holes through her skull to release the pressure from her swelling brain before it herniated, though one of her pupils looked "blown" (entirely black), which suggested things were progressing quickly. After the surgeons stopped the bleeding, which was primarily coming from her abdomen, she was wheeled into the intensive care unit. There, she was hooked up to a ventilator, and it appeared she may be brain-dead.

By then, around six hours had passed. It was well past midnight. One of the other medical students on-call, a visitor from another school, had Googled the girl's name and pulled up her profile photo on Facebook—I couldn't look. "You can't look people up like that," I pressed. In hindsight, I realize this was his way of compartmentalizing the horror — to recall she was once just like us. Eventually, I turned my head to look. She was beautiful. In the photo, she was dressed up; her tight dark brown curls, which had been bloody in the operating room, were flat-ironed straight. It was a photo that looked like it could be from a school dance. Maybe even prom. I wanted my mind to replace the earlier image with this one. I tried to force it to.

I pulled myself away to grab a coffee. It was going to be a long night, and I needed a moment to get away and process it all and something to keep me alert. As well, the family was set to arrive any minute. They were driving from their home hours up North. I took the elevator down to the first floor and could see the statue of Saint Michael in the distance—nine-foot-tall, with large wings and a sword held up high to attack what looked like a dragon below him. Dr. Serge would smile and refer to him as "the urban angel," which was the hospital's slogan, especially when our team would find ourselves advocating for the most marginalized patients, to remind us in a way that those who chose to work at that hospital had a duty to protect the most disenfranchised, something for which St. Michael is known. It was a sense I would viscerally experience mere moments later.

As I passed through the lobby, the glass sliding doors of the hospital's front entrance opened, and a family walked in, stopping for a moment in front of the statue. They looked Mediterranean. They appeared worried. One of the women looked a bit like the girl. Something just told me it was the girl's family. We made eye contact briefly as they rushed by. It's a feeling I'll never forget: the knowing that we, as physicians, hold information, even for a few moments, before those who are most immediately affected. It felt unfair. In that moment, the family was fearful but likely still hopeful. They had no status on their daughter's condition: she could be dead, but it could very much have been a close call. Or maybe a devastating situation with a miracle just ahead. I could imagine the series of possibilities that would have run through my own head if I were in their shoes. But I wasn't in their shoes. They didn't know what lay ahead. I did.

The information desk by the front entrance was closed after hours, so when patients or visitors walk in later in the evening, they often have to ask a passerby for directions. After we made eye contact, I had quickly glanced towards the floor—partly out of cowardice, but mostly out of fear. I couldn't trust myself not to break down or have my face give away anything that could suggest I knew how her daughter was faring. In hindsight, I think a big part was my attempt to allow them to hear the news from someone else: someone more experienced, and while at their daughter's bedside, not in a cold hospital lobby. And certainly not from a lowly medical student who just happened to be on-call, but from someone experienced and knowledgeable like Dr. Mohamed. The family would forever remember where they were the night they were told that their young daughter was brain dead. I suppose as well, knowing I had nothing to offer, I wanted to give them a few more minutes of hope, to offer a small sense of protection. I saw a nurse in the distance—someone I recognized from another floor who could instruct them objectively. So, I headed for the coffee shop. This was the grey zone just before we get certainty that punctuates so many moments in medicine; it would punctuate my own life in that MRI scanner a few years later, and I was hearing it again from Liz.

*

Liz received her results from the follow-up MRI, and it was the worst possible scenario: astrocytoma, a severe and incurable form of brain cancer. And it was advanced. Terminal. It was immediately operated on that fall and again the following January. Liz began chemotherapy in early 2009 but was told that she could still work if she wanted to, if she had the strength.

"And, unlike a lot of other patients, I didn't look sick on the outside. I had my hair. I wasn't that pale. I felt horrible inside, though, but I felt I could handle that," she told me. And what emerged after the shedding of her old identity was something new: she found a job working in communications for a labor union that worked closely with the Obama campaign.

"I began learning about what it meant to be part of a community and to fight for what your community needed," she recalls. Then Liz started a blog called The LizArmy, where she detailed her experience with a newly diagnosed brain tumor. Over time she posted her scans online and amassed followers. Soon she began asking for her patient notes, and posting those as well, along with other reflections. Others quickly signed up to get her updates— mostly patients and friends of patients with brain tumors. They exchanged information and research and new treatment options. Liz shortly took a job running communications and social media for a large, advanced care planning organization but would spend her evenings advocating for other patients, mostly at the University of California's Davis Cancer Center.

Soon she was invited to conferences and began speaking about her experience as an "empowered" patient. This then led to an invitation to be part of a documentary about "open-sourcing" patient data. There, Liz met the founders behind OpenNotes, an initiative out of Boston that aims to give patients access to all of their electronic records in real-time.

"I felt a bit like a model because they 'scouted' me, and I was invited to speak about my experience sharing my patient records at a big conference in Austria. By the time I returned back to Sacramento I had a job," she told me, laughing. Indeed, a movement was underway, one that would eventually bubble up and create a larger movement on transparency in healthcare.

When Liz Salmi let go of the life she had envisioned—one that knew nothing of brain cancer, she allowed herself to embrace a new identity: one of an advocate and trailblazer in the OpenNotes movement. But at the same time, the profession of medicine itself had to let go of the iron grip it held on patient data, to open it up, quite literally, and improve the quality of care as a result, even if it meant surrendering some of its power. The irony is that by letting go of that power it became more powerful in another sense—by helping bridge understanding and flatten some of the hierarchy we see in so many industries. And, most crucially, giving patients the information they had the right to have is healing in itself, as it helps reduce anxiety and uncertainty.

Today, the OpenNotes movement has taken hospitals by storm across North America. In Canada, the Toronto General Hospital has signed on to allow patients to have access to their notes in real time. In the U.S., places like Harvard's Massachusetts General Hospital (which is a core partner in OpenNotes) have done the same.

Liz's story is exactly what we saw with Steve Wall, Jessica Harthcock, Ruth, Alua Arthur, and so many others in this book—that often it takes something really drastic in our lives to catalyze a new way of seeing old problems, especially issues that have gone unsolved for decades. And, when applied to healthcare and medicine, this new lens yields new ways to understand healing.

The Western University-based neuroscientist Adrian Owen uses the term "grey zone" in a different way, meaning that in-between state when someone is pronounced "brain-dead" but still exhibits signs of consciousness. When I read his book, *Into the Grey Zone*, I was slightly horrified—I couldn't imagine being in an "in-between state," in a hospital bed, fully aware, as the doctors, nurses, and even my own family presumed I wasn't. But then I realized that's exactly what all of the stories in this book are about. We all find ourselves at the crossroads of any number of dualities, in a type of "grey zone," if you will. Of life and death on the one hand, doctor and patient, well and unwell, to fight or to avoid. To hang on with all our might like a marcescent leaf, or let go as a form of victory (not of hopeless surrender).

Looking back at those early months of the pandemic alone, and *what* and *who* many of us were so attached to in our "pre-pandemic" lives, it's remarkably tragic how much eventually ceased to exist once the year 2020 was up: jobs, loved ones who died, celebrations and trips that were canceled or left unplanned. Even our regular mourning process—a centuries-old rite of passage—had been subject to this same grief: funerals were much different, for instance, often taking place through an iPad screen. We were all navigating this space of transition, shaped by the uncertainties and fears of what lay ahead. For me, the challenge extended beyond external circumstances—it was both a personal and professional reckoning. I had to confront whether my passion for the field would endure or if it was time to let go. In the end, I chose to stand firm, committed to the path I had carved out, determined to see it through with strength and purpose.

7.

As I made my way, for the first time, to visit Klara's grave at the Beechwood Cemetery in Ottawa, I thought back to the stories of many I met through reporting this book. Klara was one of my closest friends in high school at Ashbury College in Ottawa, Canada. She wanted to be a doctor since we were in the tenth grade, working on special projects in cancer research outside of school. As time passed, we drifted apart, choosing different undergraduate colleges (University of Toronto for me, Queen's University for her), but we still kept in touch over text and Skype and would occasionally meet up for coffee. Undergrad was difficult for her—the science courses were challenging, she'd say. I'd agree—it was much tougher than our small private high school had led us to believe. We commiserated that if all else failed, we could go on an adventure—maybe sail somewhere and live on an island.

When I completed my graduate school (Master of Health Science in Global Disease Epidemiology and Control*) in Baltimore and moved back to Toronto in 2008, I applied to medical schools. By then, Klara had already applied and was unsuccessful, so she was in her first year at the University of Leiden in Holland. Her mother was Dutch, so it felt like a reasonable option, except that Klara would need to learn Dutch while also learning the vast amounts of information presented in lectures. Though it was difficult, Klara prevailed in both the language and subject matter. I emailed her to let her know I was interviewing at her old alma mater, Queen's University.

We had a long Skype chat on March 28, 2008, while in the Queen's cafeteria, and she asked me how it went. "I think it went fine, but I am excited about my Toronto interview. Toronto is home," I said. Then, feeling a bit guilty, knowing how tough it was for her to apply to medical school in Canada, I changed the subject and I asked her which food stall was best. She advised the one with the

---

* A mouthful!

paninis. I obliged. We agreed to get dinner and catch up when she was back in Canada: I wanted to know what Holland was like and the kinds of adventures she was up to in Europe. I shared that my Toronto medical school interview had been slated for April 2, and we said goodbye.

On March 31, while prepping for my interview, I received a text message from a mutual friend, Anne. "Did you hear?"

"Hear what?" I texted back. Strangely, my mind went to my own family. Was my family OK? Did Anne know something I didn't?

"About Klara."

It was the grey zone again. I put my phone down for a moment. I didn't want to read any more texts. I went to my laptop—my Skype was still running in the background. Klara's Skype was still "green," as in active. I sent her a message. "Klara?" No answer. I logged onto Facebook and looked up her profile. There was an outpouring of comments on her wall—"R.I.P. you are missed," photos of quotes with candles about memories and death, things like that. It didn't make sense. We had just spoken a few days earlier and had made plans to catch up. I returned to my phone. Three missed calls from Anne; my phone had been on silent. I called Anne back, and she told me.

Klara had been biking in Leiden, having just rented the movie *Ratatouille*, one of her favorites, about a mouse who follows his dreams to be a chef. It was seemingly an analogy or inspiration for her own journey as a Canadian dreaming to be a doctor while learning it all in a foreign country. A driver of a car had looked in the wrong direction at an intersection, turned, and hit Klara while she was on her bike. Anne didn't know if she was wearing a helmet, but those details didn't matter. That information wouldn't bring her back. She was dead. We believe she died instantly, but we would never know for sure. Klara was gone.

The tears took hours to come. I was still in disbelief. I scrolled up to our Skype history and messages. I sent her an email—to this day, I don't know why. Was I hoping she would respond or say it was all just a mistake? Sending a message into the ether like that was all I felt I could do to grasp onto some semblance of connection that had simply vanished in an instant.

That evening, I cried. I began wondering if medicine was even my path—what did I do to deserve the chance that Klara never got? Maybe there's more to life than reaching the next rung of our professional ladders. And Klara was the one who wanted it much more and for much longer. It felt like I had stolen that dream from her, and now that she was dead, I had to give it up, too.

A confluence of emotions tugged at me. The next morning, I emailed the University of Toronto Medical School administrative office. Reading it back now, I'm embarrassed, as it sounds a bit frantic and upset. The sentences weren't even complete—I'm shocked it wasn't used as a screen of some kind to simply renege the interview invitation. I asked to postpone my April 2nd interview. I linked to Klara's obituary, which had since been published, because I worried they would think it was an excuse to have more time to prepare. I received a kind response. "I'm sorry to hear about your friend's death. Of course, our last date is April 16th, so we'll slot you in for that day at 10 am. Take care." I was grateful. This small gesture of kindness from the medical school, the same medical school I would eventually attend, ingrained in me the power of a culture of support.

Klara's memorial was held many days later: it took time for the family to fly to Holland, participate in an investigation, pack up Klara's things, and arrange for the transportation of the body. It took place at our old high school assembly hall, and it was a beautiful service. I left quietly through the back. I couldn't go to the cemetery. It was too much. I said a brief hello to her mother, who was distraught but stoically so, and wrote a check for Klara's memorial fund. I drove back to Toronto, knowing one day when it felt right, I would eventually visit her grave.

That day was in 2018, exactly ten years later, with Chris. The moment I knew I truly loved him was after getting instructions from the cemetery office about the approximate location of Klara's grave. The map looked like Greek to me, so Chris bounded ahead. "I'll find it!" he yelled. Watching him search across the rows and crouch down to read the names, eager to find Klara's, brought me to tears. But we were unsuccessful. There were too many, and it was becoming overwhelming. Chris had to catch his flight to New York, so I drove him to the airport with the plan to return and search on my own.

When I did, it was as though the headstone just appeared, waiting for my return. It was dark grey, with fresh flowers and shells placed on top and underneath. I sat on the damp spring grass and stared into it. It was cleaned in a way that I could see part of my reflection, but it was distorted by the marbling stone and the glare and the engraving of the words:

*Klara Boadway – "courageous clear-eyed one." September 21*st*, 1983 – March 31*st*, 2008.*

I let the tears fall, fiddling with the flowers and the shells. And just sat there. I wondered what she would have to say if she knew what I was facing now and everything that had transpired since our last conversation. I wondered if she knew it would take me a decade to visit her grave and if she knew what that avoidance might have meant. I wondered if she read the email I sent her the day she died. I had many thoughts and things to say but shared them in my mind. Finally, it felt like it was time to leave.

A few years later, I had lunch with Klara's brother, and he shared that he will always remember Klara's tenacity, strength, and singular focus, her ultimately achieving success in a program that was even more challenging than English medical programs. In fact, when she passed away, she was, according to him, "at a high point." Indeed, it was this knowledge of her strength and determination, despite the obstacles in front of her, that I would end up carrying forward on my own path.

Goodbyes aren't always linked with grief. We can grieve without bidding farewell and bid farewell without the grieving process. Sometimes one thing comes first, in other words. I had grieved—beginning that day with Anne's text message, and the memorial, and all the times I had thought about it and imagined her last moments on her bike, with that film about a rat wanting to become a chef, in her shoulder bag. But I hadn't been ready for a goodbye. Visiting her gravesite after the funeral would have been a goodbye. But on that day, 10 years later, it felt like a force pulling me there, towards her. At long last, it was time to let go, to bid farewell to burdens shouldered, plans never fulfilled, and futures never shared. Until we might meet again.

8.

The 19th-century artist William Blake created a series of sketches based on the Biblical Book of Job, which is ultimately a story about how one man comes to terms with loss—of his wealth, his children, and his health—understanding that his grief was secondary to his attachments. While in the first sketch of the series, Job is pictured with his material wealth, Blake intentionally didn't make the last sketch a carbon copy of Sketch 1's abundance, as he likely wanted to reflect Job's newfound wisdom: an understanding that we are more than our attachments. Job became a fundamentally changed man after having gone through such tribulations that would test him, his faith, and his sense of purpose to its very core. Life is indeed unpredictable, and loss is inevitable, and this is echoed in most major religions, especially in Buddhism, which posits that the source of our suffering isn't what happens to us but is rather found in our attachments. Everything is temporary, and the only constant, paradoxically, is this state of change.

Like so many in this book, I realized my challenge was to treat my attachments not simply as the root of suffering but as fuel that, when lost, could propel me forward. I had learned through my own journey, and in large part from my patients and countless others who had crossed my path, that creating meaning from tragedy is a uniquely human form of spiritual alchemy.

A poet as well, Blake also published two famous works of poetry—one called *Songs of Innocence*, published in 1789, and then, after living through the French Revolution, the *Songs of Experience*, published in 1794. The two best-known poems of the series are entitled "The Lamb" and "The Tyger," which, as in the story of Job, contrast innocence and experience with the fundamental changes that occur only after we've lived through tragedy. The lamb effectively *becomes* the tyger—only through its trials. It's another form of resilience, earned in a way that births an entirely different animal. Such transformation could provide another way of looking at what came of Mara the elephant, described in the introduction of this book. Once free from her caged existence, she was no longer angry or threatening. She was at peace. Those who cared for Mara for decades even described her as a totally "different animal" once she was released into the sanctuary.

As difficult as it was, in the midst of a pandemic, burgeoning political uncertainty, and social unrest secondary to society's grappling with systemic racism and discrimination, I was forced to confront my own confusion and anticipation about what lay ahead. Like the story of Job, in which much of the tale focuses on the depth of his suffering, I realized it was possible that, after the painful cycle that was particularly potent in 2020, many of us could emerge with a greater understanding of ourselves and our purpose. And surrender would become a crucial part of that process.

The word "healing," as we know well by now, is derived from the word "whole," so healing is effectively a "return to wholeness"—not the "return to sameness." It's not a rehashing of an old picture or sketch but something new. That's why many of the dying can be healed as they die, as unusual as that is for our minds to put those components together. In the sketches by Blake, it became clear to me that Job's sense of purpose reached a whole new level once he was totally surrendered when he could finally release the attachments he had to his old life to understand his own value and meaning as transcending any one item or person he had attached to. Only then did he understand his part in a wider Universe and cosmos.

Since my grandfather passed away in Sri Lanka, it made me wonder if death was like leaving one room and walking into another, much like the experience of being in a diaspora: leaving one's original homeland for another.*

Similarly, in Claire B. Willis' book *Opening to Grief*, she writes: "You could think of grief as a sacred passage. You are torn from the life you knew before. You are not who you were, and you are not yet who you will become. Like everything else, you are changing. You are, in a very real way, between identities. This experience—profoundly different for each of us—is confusing, agonizing, and potentially life-transforming."

---

* This idea was the basis of a short essay I wrote for Hektoen International's *Journal of Medical Humanities*, which can be found here: https://hekint.org/2017/09/26/death-and-the-diaspora/

When, and only when, we are willing to let go of one identity are we allowed to embrace another one. We eventually must find our way out of the grey zone, and if we choose to do it with grace, we allow it to truly transform every aspect of us.

*

As I walked towards St. James Cemetery in downtown Toronto, I thought back to that day I met Joe, now 12 years ago. He had been the anonymous cadaver in the basement of the Medical Sciences Building at 1 King's College Circle. The woman I had been then was naïve, a bit shocked at what I was about to do—to cut another human so deeply, someone I knew nothing about. The woman I was then was also hopeful and optimistic, almost unconditionally.

Medicine was a calling, certainly, but the profession also felt like home. It felt right and true. And so, when the imperfections and disappointments collected over time, I was forced to re-evaluate whether it was a home to which I could be loyal, irrespective of what I felt or saw with the injustice and harm inflicted on both myself and others, or whether to abandon it all. I suppose I chose a happy medium: to see the goodness within it while at the same time becoming committed to extricating the ills to find a healthy path forward. In other words, do exactly what skilled cancer surgeons do: remove the cancer in a way that leaves the rest of the body unharmed, remembering our duty to "first do no harm." I had learned to heal myself and appreciate my newfound resilience, but in exchange, I had to do my part to help heal that which ails the profession itself.

The Remembrance Ceremony to honor those who willed their bodies to medical science is held every year at the chapel beside St. James Cemetery in downtown Toronto, about two blocks from St. Michael's Hospital. I hadn't attended the one held for my medical school, the one which would have honored Joe. I didn't know anyone in my class who did, and one of our anatomy professors had made his disappointment that only two out of a class of 224 attended very clear to us.

At the time, I couldn't quite understand why: I had thought it was mostly for friends and families of the individual or maybe those classmates who had a particularly difficult emotional time with the dissections. I had thought I was fine, that my friends in the class were fine. Yet the truth, as so often happens with the passage of time, soon became frighteningly clear: we were *not* fine. But we had collectively decided, after our anatomy unit, after weeks of learning through socially acceptable mutilation, that we had crossed the curtain. We had quickly compartmentalized and conditioned ourselves to stop feeling. Because if we didn't, the work ahead would seem much tougher and almost impossibly heartbreaking. The curtain separates, but perhaps it also protects, so we thought. But we had, altogether, reached the wrong understanding.

You see, sometimes, in order to heal, we need to be *within* the curtain *with* the patient: present and "attending" (in the real sense of the word) to their suffering, pain, and illness in order to truly empathize, which then allows us to more accurately understand their condition, and subsequently our own. While Joe couldn't offer that directly, he did so indirectly, as my first "patient," because he invited a curiosity into his story and experience—about what had brought his body onto the metal table of the anatomy lab in the first place. And it's this very curiosity that often holds the key to real healing, even if it is simply a mutual acceptance and letting go.

As I listened to the memorial service, it seemed clear for the first time that all of these lessons were there all along, even in medical school. I was likely too buried in my textbooks and focused on exams to see the big picture, to understand the broader purpose of it all. If healing, then, is a return to wholeness, maybe it is also a return to an experienced form of innocence. An experienced wholeheartedness, perhaps: a transformation that is contingent on something radical enough to shift our entire being from the inside so that it can reflect out magnificently. And if we're lucky, it touches others.

As I walked out of the chapel, my phone buzzed – I was expected to meet a friend nearby for dinner before heading back to pack yet again: my move to New York City would be permanent.

I passed the headstone laid out specifically for the service: it marked the burial place of our first patients. As I made my way out of the chapel grounds, I saw Gingko trees dotted around the cemetery that I hadn't previously noticed. In fact, when I stopped to really look, it seemed they were everywhere. This time, the leaves weren't covering the ground as they had been in Oliver Sacks' essay. Instead, they were whistling in the late summer breeze, a sound my ears could finally hear.

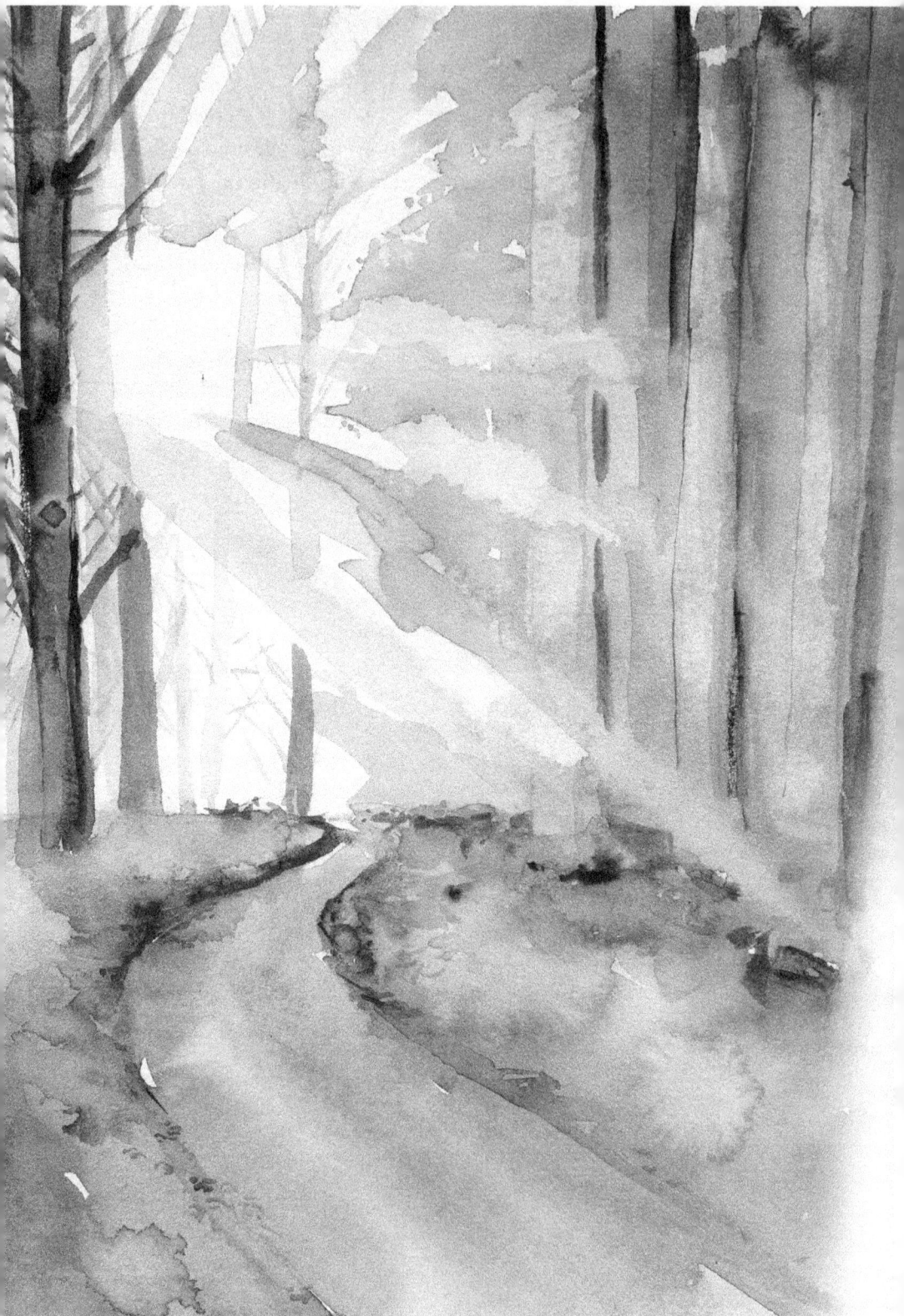

Epilogue

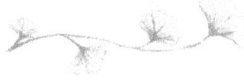

"Those who have a 'why' to leave can tolerate almost any 'how.'"
— Viktor Frankl

As I completed the research for this book, the pandemic's grip began to loosen, revealing the immense sacrifices and challenges faced by healthcare workers, often exacerbated by toxic leadership and cultures. The impact of COVID-19 on healthcare professionals was profound and devastating. At the end of April, eight weeks into the lockdown, Dr. Lorna Breen, an emergency medicine doctor in Manhattan and a friend of my colleague Daniel, ended her life, overwhelmed by the relentless deaths at her hospital during the early days of the pandemic. Her tragic story, which I memorialized in a piece for *Scientific American**, underscored the broader systemic issues plaguing institutionalized medicine.

Dr. Breen's passing during the pandemic provided a critical moment to reflect on the urgent need to address these systemic issues and prevent future tragedies. Years after the death of Chiron, a Centaur in Greek mythology famous for knowledge of medicine, the ancient Greeks came to see suicide as primarily due to malfunction of "humors," the result of the build-up of black bile (melancholia) or yellow bile (mania). The beauty of medical knowledge is that it evolves; so, too, must our understanding. We must take the lessons from as far back as Chiron and as recent as Dr. Breen to understand that environmental factors matter much more than the individual. Dr. Breen's passing during the pandemic offered us a moment to reflect on how best to use

---

* This article, published on May 14 2020, can be found here https://www.scientificamerican.com/blog/observations/during-covid-19-healers-need-healing-too/

our outrage and mourning, as patients and physicians, to finally move out of the clouds of ignorance, willful blindness, and institutional inertia to prevent the same tragedy from repeating itself.

*

In parallel, the murder of Ahmaud Arbery and the false accusation by Amy Cooper highlighted the deep-seated racial injustices that sparked a global reckoning. These events, coupled with the pandemic, forced a collective introspection on the societal structures that perpetuate inequality and oppression. Arbery was hunted down and shot while out running in rural Satilla Shores, Georgia. Then, the case of Amy Cooper, a white, middle-aged woman who used her tears and rage to place a false accusation against a black male birder named Christian Cooper (no relation) in Central Park, New York. Though Christian Cooper had advocated for compassion for Amy, the latter was fired from her job after an investigation and was charged on several accounts. The criminal case against her was eventually dropped in 2021, but as of this writing, she is suing her previous workplace. As for Christian Cooper, he published a book about birding.

Some have argued that all of these events were a "racial epiphany" and not a reckoning. In Martin Luther King Jr.'s 1966 "Letter from Birmingham Jail,"* he likens racism to an abscess to be drained:

> Like a boil that can never be cured so long as it is covered up but must be opened with all its ugliness to the natural medicines of air and light, injustice must be exposed, with all the tension its exposure creates, to the light of human conscience and the air of national opinion before it can be cured.

Ibram X. Kendi would later use a similar analogy in his book *How to be Anti-Racist*, comparing racism to cancer. In medicine, we often break things (like

---

* The full letter can be found here: https://www.csuchico.edu/iege/_assets/documents/susi-letter-from-birmingham-jail.pdf

bones in surgery) or cut things (skin and tissue) to remove something more sinister underneath: what's left is a more resilient body. Breaking something, therefore, isn't bad in and of itself. Another term had emerged, beginning with Amy Cooper, that offered another puzzle piece to understand what I now knew about the role of culture: "Karens," a term coined to refer to entitled older white women who use their privilege to harm others.

I had finally uncovered a key piece of the puzzle: the toxic dynamics I experienced were strikingly similar to the behaviors seen in the Amy Cooper case, where influence was misused, and narratives were manipulated to maintain control. It became clear that the actions were rooted in insecurity, which fueled coordinated efforts to undermine others—particularly women of color by whom they felted professionally or personally threatened—and protect their own standing. While understanding this didn't make it right, it gave me clarity. Their obsession showed through constant gossip—through texts, calls, and emails, sometimes sent in the early morning hours when their attention should have been elsewhere. Recognizing these patterns allowed me to see that their behavior was a reflection of their own fears and limitations, not mine. With this insight, I could finally let go of their grip on my path and move forward with strength and intention.

Karens would remain in the public conversation for months, but the idea was here to stay. In December 2020, an article in *New York Magazine** by writer Allison P. Davis, detailing a similar incident against a Black lawyer by his White female neighbor, described Karens particularly well:

> Was there anything worse to be called in the summer of 2020 than a Karen? An internet term for a complaining White woman who is caught weaponizing her racial privilege, a Karen calls the cops on a person of color for something she perceives to be offensive. Sometimes she exaggerates the situation, sometimes she flat-out lies. The stories Karens tell the police, the world, and themselves go unchallenged because the women are White.

---

* This article, in *New York Magazine,* can be found here: https://www.thecut.com/article/montclair-new-jersey-permit-karen.html

Reading *the New York Times* op-ed* about the Amy Cooper incident by Australian scholar and writer Ruby Hamad, herself a woman of color, lent greater context to this phenomenon. Hamad just came out with a book, *White Tears, Brown Scars*, based on the article she had written in *The Guardian* months earlier**, describing the reasons why White women target and bully women of color, tracing it back throughout centuries of history. It has links to colonialism, where women of color were kept as concubines, which threatened the wives, and it bears its fruits now in many ways. It also helped further explain some of what I had experienced and why all the bullies (aside from one male administrative staff member) fit this description. In her book, Hamad describes that because White women feel oppressed by the White patriarchy, they inflict it on those over which they have power. Brené Brown, in her podcast interview with Austin Channing Brown***, described it as the difference between powerful versus "power over." Channing Brown, who is Black, describes the same phenomenon in her own life. Indeed, I finally had an explanation for what I had experienced.

Malcolm Gladwell's book, *Revenge of the Tipping Point*, discusses inclusion and diversity in organizations. Using the example of "tokens" in Chapter 4, he powerfully argues, based on social science research, that true inclusion is only possible if a minority group makes up at least one-third of the organization. In my hospital, if one-third of the attendings or those in power were women of color (at the time it was less than one-tenth), it would have been far less likely that I would be treated with hostility, as there would be an implied acceptance. The exception to this may be when a minority is protected contractually from hostility—such as being a cofounder or an elected leader of an organization— where their ouster would be legally difficult. Such status would help to inoculate them from mobbing and bullying.

After so many years, integrating this puzzle piece helped spark the very last aspect of my healing because it placed my experience in a wider context. I

---

* This opinion article, in the *New York Times*, can be found here: https://www.nytimes.com/2020/05/27/opinion/amy-cooper-central-park-racism.html

** This article, in *The Guardian*, can be found here: https://www.theguardian.com/commentisfree/2018/may/08/how-white-women-use-strategic-tears-to-avoid-accountability

*** This podcast interview can be found here: https://brenebrown.com/podcast/brene-with-austin-channing-brown-on-im-still-here-black-dignity-in-a-world-made-for-whiteness/

wasn't alone. However, as my wiser self reminded me, being angry is of limited use. That anger must be alchemized into curiosity and compassion, and wise action. That action involved ensuring I was no longer physically and emotionally exposed to their hate, while also pushing for advocacy and accountability. Before accountability comes compassion, much like the compassion Christian Cooper showed Amy.

*

Part of my journey toward advocacy and accountability involved seeing the process through to a resolution that marked a significant personal and symbolic victory. It was the culmination of years of persistence against a system deeply resistant to change, underscoring the need for reform to protect future professionals from toxic environments. While the resolution included some important acknowledgments, the reluctance to address deeper cultural and policy issues became evident.

Inspired by the experiences of others like Ryan Seguin, we had advocated for policies to broaden the definition of harassment, including bullying across genders (for instance, women bullying other women), and to allow swift, fair transitions for those seeking safer environments. Although the resolution we reached acknowledged accountability to some degree, efforts to push for meaningful policy reform were resisted—demonstrating their intent to preserve the status quo that allowed these challenges to persist.

After eight long years, countless tears, and deep personal growth, I had finally reached the end of this chapter. I knew my fight had made a difference, at least for me. The larger battle for systemic change would need to continue, carried forward by others. With this chapter closed and my body strong, new opportunities and paths lay ahead—ones that called for me to integrate the lessons and healing from this long journey. Yet I still needed to integrate my mind more completely.

In January 2023, after six months of intensive internal family systems (IFS), a form of evidence-based therapy to integrate the trauma from my academic hospital experience, my therapist mentioned she had been trained in psychedelic-assisted therapy. There was still a stubborn layer of my trauma that couldn't integrate with therapy alone. It would pop up through various triggers. We agreed that MDMA would help me further integrate what occurred in that one specific unhealthy academic hospital so I could experience fewer triggers and move forward without that anxiety.

The guided MDMA journey occurred in a beautiful space in West London, taking five hours. I saw a side to our existence that felt sublime and felt connected to the larger universe. I integrated many things: too many to describe in these pages, and it made me more open to the use of psychedelics —plant-based and synthetic—for healing from experiences where other tools are of limited effectiveness. As of this writing, both psilocybin (magic mushrooms) and MDMA may be approved by the FDA within the next two years for use in guided therapeutic settings, especially for trauma. If so, I know it has the potential to heal countless others.

*

By the time the research on this book was completed, the role of technology in healthcare had become more prominent, in part accelerated by what the COVID-19 pandemic elucidated about the limits of our healthcare system. Virtual care, through telemedicine, became the norm within existing healthcare clinics and hospitals.

Big Tech companies like Apple, Google, Amazon, and Meta integrated health-focused features into their products, promoting a more holistic approach to wellness. Wearable devices provided valuable biofeedback, enabling individuals to make informed lifestyle changes. These advancements align with the principles of integrative medicine, emphasizing prevention and overall well-being.

In 2015, for the *Huffington Post*, I wrote an article about Apple's healthcare ambitions as it began to enter the world of wellness with its Apple Watch and efforts to collaborate on medical research.* Since then, Apple has been at the forefront of integrating health monitoring into everyday life. The Apple Watch,

---

* That article, published on May 11, 2015, can be found here: https://www.huffpost.com/archive/ca/entry/apple-should-digitize-the-medical-world-with-caution_b_6841298

with its array of health-focused features, exemplifies this commitment. The device tracks physical activity, monitors heart rate, and even detects irregularities such as atrial fibrillation. With the introduction of features like ECG and blood oxygen monitoring, the Apple Watch has become a powerful tool for preventative health care. Moreover, Apple's Health app consolidates data from various health apps and devices, providing users with a comprehensive view of their health metrics. This integration supports a holistic approach by allowing individuals to monitor their physical activity, nutrition, sleep, and mindfulness practices in one place. By empowering users with data, Apple encourages proactive management of their health, aligning with the principles of lifestyle medicine that emphasize prevention and wellness.

Google's contribution to healthcare through technology spans several areas, from information dissemination to advanced artificial intelligence (A.I.). Google Search and YouTube have become primary sources for health information, offering a platform for educational content on integrative and lifestyle medicine. This accessibility democratizes knowledge, enabling individuals to make informed decisions about their health. Google's A.I. capabilities further enhance healthcare through tools like Google Health and DeepMind. Their A.I. algorithms analyze vast amounts of health data to predict disease outbreaks, personalize treatment plans, and even assist in early diagnosis, and at the time of this writing, may help facilitate personal health large language models.* For instance, Google Health's initiatives in developing A.I. for breast cancer screening have shown promising results in improving detection rates. By integrating A.I. into healthcare, Google supports a more precise and personalized approach to health, a cornerstone of root-cause and integrative medicine.

Amazon has entered the healthcare space with initiatives like Amazon Pharmacy and Amazon Care. These services streamline access to medications and healthcare services, making it easier for individuals to manage their health. Amazon Pharmacy delivers prescriptions directly to consumers, often at a lower cost, removing barriers to medication adherence. Their acquisition of One Medical in 2022 allowed them to deliver direct primary care to Prime

---

* Google Health published a paper about this in 2024: https://arxiv.org/abs/2406.06474

members. Amazon Care, a telehealth service, provides virtual consultations and in-person follow-ups, offering a convenient solution for healthcare needs. This service is particularly beneficial for managing chronic conditions and maintaining regular health check-ups, both essential aspects of integrative medicine. By improving accessibility and convenience, Amazon supports continuous and comprehensive healthcare management.

The vast social network provided by Meta (formerly Facebook) offers unique opportunities to support health through community engagement and information sharing. Health-related groups and pages provide platforms for individuals to share experiences, seek advice, and find support. This social support is crucial for mental health and well-being, reinforcing the principle that social factors significantly influence health. Additionally, Meta is beginning to offer preventive health tools that remind users to schedule check-ups and screenings, leveraging social influence to promote healthy behaviors. These reminders can increase compliance with preventative measures, supporting a holistic approach to health maintenance.

ŌURA, known for its Oura Ring, focuses on tracking sleep and recovery, essential components of holistic health. The ring monitors sleep patterns, heart rate variability, and body temperature, providing insights into recovery and readiness. This data helps users optimize their sleep and overall lifestyle, aligning with integrative medicine's focus on balance and preventive care. Oura's emphasis on sleep health highlights the importance of rest and recovery in overall well-being. By providing detailed feedback, more recently through their "Oura Advisor," the Oura Ring empowers individuals to make informed decisions about their lifestyle, promoting a balanced approach to health.

The integration of technology by big tech companies like Apple, Google, Amazon, Meta, and ŌURA is transforming healthcare by advancing root-cause, integrative, and lifestyle medicine approaches. These companies enhance health monitoring, democratize health information, streamline access to healthcare services, foster supportive communities, and emphasize crucial aspects like sleep and recovery.

In addition, on the heels of Big Tech emerged several new healthtech startups positioned to disrupt the healthcare system in the U.S. through business-to-business (B2B) or direct-to-consumer (D2C) ideas. By leveraging their technological prowess, these companies are not only committed to making healthcare more accessible but have also promoted a more comprehensive view of health that encompasses physical, mental, and social well-being. As technology continues to evolve, their role in healthcare will likely expand, further supporting the principles of integrative and lifestyle medicine. It's likely that one D2C company will become a unicorn among the others if they're able to understand the pain points well, leverage an excellent clinician and tech team, deliver an optimal user experience, all which is contingent on high performance and prioritizing employee thriving and wellbeing in their company (which depends on effective leadership and healthy cultures).

The shift towards a more whole-person view of health has the potential to improve outcomes, enhance quality of life, and foster a more proactive approach to wellness. At the time of this writing, I consult for both Big Tech and healthtech startups that work to reverse chronic disease and extend healthspan* through providing root-cause, data-driven insights. Each day is filled with exciting challenges, incredible peers and colleagues, and joy. It means I often say no or back away from cultures or leadership dynamics that seem unsafe or toxic, as I've seen time and again that a toxic culture leads to lower performance and ultimately impacts the company's ability to succeed. My work remains to heal, but through leveraging technology and contributing to companies that value healthy cultures where the team thrives and excels.

Indeed, as this book hopefully made clear, culture is every company or organization's "second product," an intentional production that can fall by the wayside if it is not nourished and tended to with care. A healthy workplace culture, one that helps each employee reach their potential, and thrive professionally and personally, is perhaps more essential for any organization committed to the health of others. It's something that, as a leader, I am committed to every day.

---

* Healthspan is different from lifespan; healthspan refers to the period of one's life that is healthy and free of disease. It reflects 'quality' of life as opposed to 'quantity' of life.

*

Healing is a journey: a dynamic process that moves in fits and bursts, and sometimes in waves so slow that they feel a lot like stagnation. As physicians, returning to wholeness is as essential for ourselves as much as it is for our patients.

Change within a system can take time: sometimes, all we can do is keep our hands on the wheel of our proverbial tugboat and stay steady, as opposed to attempting a sharp steer towards a direction that is not yet available to us. In other words, it's waiting for the tide itself to shift before we allow ourselves to. I felt it had—there were now many more cases like mine at academic hospital centers and elsewhere. The broader understanding of systemic workplace factors and the intersectionality of race and gender had caught up with my experiences and those of many peers. The general understanding of systemic workplace factors involved and the role of bias (and that many perpetrators of harassment against women are women) has also become more widely known. Embracing forgiveness became integral to my healing and the concept of "post-traumatic" growth as part of "earning" resilience and regaining wholeness.

As this book entered the first round of edits, my most impactful mentor as a medical student, whom I earlier have named "Dr. Serge," passed away after a three-year battle with a rare brain tumor. His legacy of compassionate care and excellent teaching, as well as the kind mentoring of hundreds of future doctors, continues to endure and inspire. This book is in part a dedication to him and his impact on the world of healers.

The poet Yung Pueblo penned a piece about the theme of letting go that resonated deeply with me around this time. It is paraphrased below:

> Letting go means not allowing your present happiness to depend
> on past events or future desires. Your task is to stop resisting,
> accept what is, feel fully, and allow yourself to simply be.

My life, and where this story ends (for now), is in New York City: a more permanent move where I am surrounded by people I love, within a place that I love, with a vocation that feels entirely aligned with my heart, mind, and purpose.

Indeed, the journey, though treacherous, was worth it.

I am finally home…and whole.

Resources
for Healing Together

Each one of us is a healer, or someone that needs healing.

FOR PATIENTS

Andrew Weil Center for Integrative Medicine:

- This center provides various free online learning courses, a podcast called "Body of Wonder," and educational materials on integrative health. They also offer specific resources such as an integrative cancer care toolkit and strategies for creating a healing space at home (Andrew Weil Center). awcim.arizona.edu

National Center for Complementary and Integrative Health (NCCIH):

- As part of the U.S. National Institutes of Health, NCCIH offers a wealth of information on complementary and integrative health practices, safety tips, research results, and clinical guidelines. Their website includes topics A-Z, detailed articles on various herbs and supplements, and consumer tips on evaluating health information (NCCIH). nccih.nih.gov

Mayo Clinic Integrative Medicine and Health:

- The Mayo Clinic provides comprehensive information on integrative therapies, such as acupuncture, massage, and yoga. They emphasize the importance of discussing these therapies with your healthcare team to ensure safety and effectiveness. The Mayo Clinic also offers newsletters and updates on the latest research and health tips (Mayo Clinic).   mayoclinic.org

For Current & Future Doctors

Andrew Weil Center for Integrative Medicine:

- The center offers professional training programs, fellowships, and various online courses tailored for healthcare providers. These programs cover integrative medicine principles, practices, and research findings that can be directly applied in patient care.
- Website: Andrew Weil Center for Integrative Medicine   awcim.edu

Institute for Functional Medicine (IFM):

- IFM provides extensive educational resources, including certification programs, clinical practice tools, and webinars focused on functional medicine. Their resources are designed to help practitioners incorporate functional medicine into their practice effectively.
- Website: Institute for Functional Medicine   ifm.org

American Academy of Anti-Aging Medicine (A4M):

- A4M offers a wide range of continuing medical education (CME) courses, certifications, and fellowships in topics related to anti-aging, metabolic, and integrative medicine. They also host annual conferences featuring the latest research and clinical practices in the field.
- Website: American Academy of Anti-Aging Medicine a4m.com

National Center for Complementary and Integrative Health (NCCIH):

- NCCIH provides comprehensive resources for healthcare professionals, including research-based information on various complementary and integrative health practices, clinical guidelines, and tools for patient counseling.

- Website: National Center for Complementary and Integrative Health uhhospitals.org

Mayo Clinic Integrative Medicine and Health:

- Mayo Clinic offers a range of educational materials and clinical practice guidelines for healthcare providers interested in integrative medicine. They also provide access to research updates and expert opinions on integrative health approaches.
- Website: Mayo Clinic Integrative Medicine and Health

University Hospitals Connor Integrative Health Network:

- This network provides educational resources, virtual health talks, and clinical practice tools for healthcare providers to help them integrate holistic approaches into patient care. They offer guidance on various integrative therapies and their clinical applications.
- Website: University Hospitals Connor Integrative Health Network

American Medical Association (AMA) - Steps Forward:

- AMA's Steps Forward program provides numerous toolkits and resources aimed at improving physician well-being. These resources cover topics such as managing stress and burnout, building resilience, and creating a healthy work-life balance.
- Website: AMA Steps Forward   stepsforward.org

Physician Support Line:

- This free, confidential support line is run by volunteer psychiatrists and offers immediate help for physicians in need. It provides a safe space for doctors to discuss their mental health concerns and receive support.
- Website: Physician Support Line physiciansupportline.com

American College of Physicians (ACP) - Physician Well-being and Professional Fulfillment:

- ACP offers a variety of resources, including articles, webinars, and policy papers, focused on improving physician well-being. They cover strategies for reducing burnout and enhancing job satisfaction.
- Website: ACP Physician Well-being   acponline.org

National Academy of Medicine - Action Collaborative on Clinician Well-Being and Resilience:

- This collaborative provides extensive resources, including research papers, toolkits, and case studies, aimed at improving clinician well-being and addressing systemic issues that contribute to burnout.
- Website: National Academy of Medicine Clinician Well-Being nam.edu

Mayo Clinic - Physician Health Center:

- Mayo Clinic offers various programs and resources dedicated to physician health, including workshops, seminars, and wellness coaching. They focus on holistic approaches to maintaining physical and mental health.
- Website: Mayo Clinic Physician Health Center mayoclinic.org

Medscape - Physician Lifestyle and Burnout Report:

- Medscape annually publishes reports on physician lifestyle and burnout, providing insights and data on the current state of physician well-being. These reports also include practical tips and strategies for managing burnout.
- Website: Medscape Physician Lifestyle Report medscape.com

Appendix

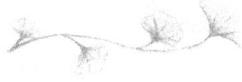

How to Read a Medical Study
By Amitha Kalaichandran, M.D.

*This story was originally published on Feb. 5, 2020
in the* New York Times.

In August 2019, *JAMA Pediatrics*, a widely respected journal, published a study with a contentious result: Pregnant women in Canada who were exposed to increasing levels of fluoride (such as from drinking water) were more likely to have children with lower I.Q. Some media outlets ran overblown headlines, claiming that fluoride exposure actually *lowers* I.Q.

And while academics and journalists quickly pointed out the study's many flaws — that it didn't prove cause and effect; and showed a drop in I.Q. only in boys, not girls — the damage was done. People took to social media, voicing their concerns about the potential harms of fluoride exposure.

We place immense trust in scientific studies, as well as in the journalists who report on them. But deciding whether a study warrants changing the way we live our lives is challenging. Is that extra hour of screen time really devastating? Does feeding processed meat to children increase their risk of cancer?

As a physician and a medical journalist with training in biostatistics and epidemiology, I sought advice from several experts about how parents can gauge the quality of research studies they read about. Here are eight tips to remember the next time you see a story about a scientific study.

1. Wet pavement doesn't cause rain.

Put another way, correlation does not equal causation. This is one of the most common traps that health journalists fall into with studies that have found associations between two things—like that people who drink coffee live longer lives—but which haven't definitively shown that one thing (coffee drinking) causes another (a longer life). These types of studies are typically referred to as observational studies.

When designing and analyzing studies, experts must have satisfactory answers to several questions before determining cause and effect, said Elizabeth Platz, Sc.D., a professor of epidemiology and deputy chair of the Department of Epidemiology at the Johns Hopkins Bloomberg School of Public Health. In smoking and lung cancer studies, for example, researchers needed to show that the chemicals in cigarettes affected lung tissue in ways that resulted in lung cancer and that those changes came after the exposure. They also needed to show that those results were reproducible. In many studies, cause and effect isn't proven after many years, or even decades, of study.

2. Mice aren't men.

Large human clinical studies are expensive, cumbersome, and potentially dangerous to humans. This is why researchers often turn to mice or other animals with human-like physiologies (like flies, worms, rats, dogs, and monkeys) first.

If you spot a headline that seems way overblown, like that aspirin thwarts bowel cancer in mice, it's potentially notable but could take years or even decades (if ever) to test and see the same findings in humans.

3. Study quality matters.

When it comes to study design, not all are created equal. In medicine, randomized clinical trials and systematic reviews are kings. In a randomized clinical trial, researchers typically split people into at least two groups: one that receives or does the thing the study researchers are testing, like a new drug or daily exercise, and another that receives either the current standard of care (like a statin for high cholesterol) or a placebo. To decrease bias, the participant and researcher ideally won't know which group each participant is in.

Systematic reviews are similarly useful in that researchers gather anywhere from five to more than 100 randomized controlled trials on a given subject and comb through them, looking for patterns and consistency among their conclusions. These types of studies are important because they help to show potential consensus in a given body of evidence.

Other types of studies, which aren't as rigorous as the above, include cohort studies (which follow large groups of people over time to look for the development of disease), case-control studies (which first identify the disease, like cancer, and then trace back in time to figure out what might have caused it) and cross-sectional studies (which are usually surveys that try to identify how a disease and exposure might have been correlated with each other, but not which caused the other).

Next on the quality spectrum come case reports (which describe what happened to a single patient) and case series (a group of case reports), which are both lowest in quality, but which often inspire higher quality studies.

4. Statistics can be misinterpreted.

Statistical significance is one of the most common things that confuses the lay reader. When a study or a journalistic publication says that a study's finding was "statistically significant," it means that the results were unlikely to have happened by chance.

But a result that is statistically significant may not be clinically significant, meaning it likely won't change your day-to-day. Imagine a randomized controlled trial that split 200 women with migraines into two groups of 100. One was given a pill to prevent migraines, and another was given a placebo. After six months, 11 women from the pill group and 12 from the placebo group had at least one migraine per week, but the 11 women in the pill group experienced arm tingling as a potential side effect. If women in the pill group were found to be statistically less likely to have migraines than those in the placebo group, the difference might still be too small to recommend the pill for migraines since just one woman out of 100 had fewer migraines. Also, researchers would have to take potential side effects into account.

The opposite is also true. If a study reports that regular exercise helped relieve chronic pain symptoms in 30% of its participants, that might sound like a lot. But if the study included just 10 people, that's only three people helped. This finding may not be statistically significant, but it *could* be clinically important since there are limited treatment options for people with chronic pain, and might warrant a larger trial.

5. Bigger is often better.

Scientists arguably can never fully know the truth about a given topic, but they can get close. And one way of doing that is to design a study that has high power.

"Power is telling us what the chances are that a study will detect a signal, if that signal does exist," John Ioannidis, M.D., a professor of medicine and health research and policy at Stanford Medical School, said via email.

The easiest way for researchers to increase a study's power is to increase its size. A trial of 1,000 people typically has higher power than a trial of 500, and so on. Simply put, larger studies are more likely to help us get closer to the truth than smaller ones.

6. Not all findings apply to you.

If a news article reports that a high-quality study had statistical and clinical significance, the next step might be to determine whether the findings apply to you.

If researchers are testing a hypothetical new drug to relieve arthritis symptoms, they may only include participants who have arthritis and no other conditions. They may eliminate those who take medications that might interfere with the drug they're studying. Researchers may recruit participants by age, gender, or ethnicity. Early studies on heart disease, for instance, were performed primarily on white men.

Each of us is unique, genetically and environmentally, and our lives aren't highly controlled like a study. So, take each study for what it is: information. Over time, it will become clearer whether one conclusion was important enough to change clinical recommendations. Which gets to a related idea.

7. One study is just one study.

If findings from one study were enough to change medical practices and public policies, doctors would be practicing yo-yo medicine, where recommendations would change from day to day. That doesn't typically happen, so when you see a headline that begins or ends with "a study found," it's best to remember that one study isn't likely to shift an entire course of medical practice. If a study is done well and has been replicated, it's certainly possible that it may change medical guidelines down the line. If the topic is relevant to you or your family, it's worth asking your doctor whether the findings are strong enough to suggest that you make different health choices.

8. Not all journals are created equal.

Legitimate scientific journals tend to publish studies that have been rigorously and objectively peer-reviewed, which is the gold standard for scientific research and publishing. A good way to spot a high-quality journal is to look for one with a high impact factor—a number that primarily reflects how often the average article from a given journal has been cited by other articles in a given year. (Keep in mind, however, that lower-impact journals can still publish quality findings.) Most studies published on PubMed, a database of published scientific research articles and book chapters, are peer-reviewed.

Then there are so-called "predatory journals," which aren't produced by legitimate publishers and which will publish almost any study—whether it's been peer-reviewed or not—in exchange for a fee. (Legitimate journals may also request fees, primarily to cover their costs or to publish a study in front of a paywall, but only if the paper is accepted.) Predatory journals are attractive to some researchers who may feel pressure to "publish or perish." It's challenging, however, to distinguish them from legitimate ones because they often sound or look similar. If an article has grammatical errors and distorted images, or if its journal lacks a clear editorial board and physical address, it might be a predatory journal. But it's not always obvious, and even experienced researchers are occasionally fooled.

Reading about a study can be enlightening and engaging, but very few studies are profound enough to base changes to your daily life. When you see the next dramatic headline, read the story—and if you can find it, read the study, too (PubMed or Google Scholar are good places to start). If you have time, discuss the study with your doctor and see if any reputable organizations like the Centers for Disease Control and Prevention, World Health Organization, American Academy of Pediatrics, American College of Cardiology or National Cancer Institute have commented on the matter.

Medicine is not an exact science, and things change every day. In a field of gray, where headlines sometimes try to force us to see things in black-and-white, start with these tips to guide your curiosity. And hopefully, they'll help you decide when—and when not—to make certain health and lifestyle choices for yourself and for your family.

Notes & References

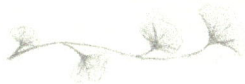

Introduction

1. American Heart Association guidelines for taking statin. "2019 ACC/AHA Guideline on the Primary Prevention of Cardiovascular Disease - American College of Cardiology," American College of Cardiology, March 7, 2019, https://www.acc.org/latest-in-cardiology/ten-points-to-remember/2019/03/07/16/00/2019-acc-aha-guideline-on-primary-prevention-gl-prevention

    *   Patients ages 20-75 years and LDL-C ≥190 mg/dl, use high-intensity statin without risk assessment.
    *   T2DM and age 40-75 years, use moderate-intensity statin and risk estimate to consider high-intensity statins. Risk-enhancers in diabetics include ≥10 years for T2DM and 20 years for type 1 DM, ≥30 mcg albumin/mg creatinine, eGFR <60 ml/min/1.73 m², retinopathy, neuropathy, ABI <0.9. In those with multiple ASCVD risk factors, consider high-intensity statin with aim of lowering LDL-C by 50% or more.
    *   Age >75 years, clinical assessment and risk discussion.
    *   Age 40-75 years and LDL-C ≥70 mg/dl and <190 mg/dl without diabetes, use the risk estimator that best fits the patient and risk-enhancing factors to decide intensity of statin.
        *   Risk 5% to <7.5% (borderline risk). Risk discussion: if risk-enhancing factors are present, discuss moderate-intensity statin and consider coronary CACs in select cases.
        *   Risk ≥7.5-20% (intermediate risk). Risk discussion: use moderate-intensity statins and increase to high-intensity with risk enhancers. Option of CACs to risk stratify if there is uncertainty about risk. If CAC = 0, can avoid statins and repeat CAC in the future (5-10 years), the exceptions being high-risk conditions such as diabetes, family history of premature CHD, and smoking. If CACs 1-100, it is reasonable to initiate moderate-intensity statin for persons ≥55 years. If CAC >100 or 75th percentile or higher, use statin at any age.
        *   Risk ≥20% (high risk). Risk discussion to initiate high-intensity statin to reduce LDL-C by ≥50%.

2. Stress and poor cholesterol metabolism. Susan Bernstein, "Stress and Cholesterol: Is There a Link?," WebMD, July 18, 2023, https://www.webmd.com/cholesterol-management/stress-cholesterol-link.

3. Biomedical model of disease. National Academies Press (US), "Biomedical Model Definition," Biomedical Models and Resources - NCBI Bookshelf, 1998, https://www.ncbi.nlm.nih.gov/books/NBK230283/.

4. My project was about the use of complementary health approaches in children and found 61.7% of parents used these approaches for their child, with vitamins and minerals being the most common treatment. Amitha Kalaichandran et al., "Use And Perceived Effectiveness of Complementary Health Approaches in Children," *Paediatrics & Child Health* 23, no. 1 (December 8, 2017): 12–19, https://academic.oup.com/pch/article/23/1/12/4706299.

5. NYT Mara the elephant: Sofía López Mañán and Brooke Jarvis, "How to Move Your Elephant During a Pandemic," *The New York Times*, August 10, 2020, https://www.nytimes.com/2020/08/09/science/coronavirus-elephants-wildlife-zoo.html.

6. Elephant God Ganesh/Ganesha: Wendy Doniger, "Ganesha | Meaning, Symbolism, & Facts," Encyclopedia Britannica, May 28, 2024, https://www.britannica.com/topic/Ganesha.

7. Rumi: wound is where light enters you from a poem "A Quote by Rumi (Jalal ad-Din Muhammad ar-Rumi)," n.d., https://www.goodreads.com/quotes/103315-the-wound-is-the-place-where-the-light-enters-you.

8. Wendell Berry's essay The Body and the Earth. Wendell Berry, "THE BODY AND THE EARTH - ProQuest," n.d., https://www.proquest.com/openview/eec40fc4de5 98d90f35784b4df08920a/1?pq-origsite=gscholar&cbl=1820904.

9. US Healthcare spending. "Historical | CMS," n.d., https://www.cms.gov/data-research/statistics-trends-and-reports/national-health-expenditure-data/historical#:~:text=U.S.%20health%20care%20spending%20grew,spending%20accounted%20for%2017.7%20percent.

10. Canada Healthcare spending: "Topic: Healthcare Expenditure in Canada," Statista, January 10, 2024, https://www.statista.com/topics/11061/healthcare-expenditure-in-canada/#topicOverview.

11. UK healthcare spending: James Cooper, "Healthcare Expenditure, UK Health Accounts - Office for National Statistics," April 27, 2020, https://www.ons.gov.uk/peoplepopulationandcommunity/healthandsocialcare/healthcaresystem/bulletins/ukhealthaccounts/2018.

12. Japan healthcare spending: "Japan Health Expenditure as a Share of GDP, 1960-2023 - knoema.com," Knoema, June 2, 2024, https://knoema.com/atlas/Japan/Health-expenditure-as-a-share-of-GDP.

13. Wellness coined by Sir Archibald Johnson in the 1500s "I bossed God...for my daughter wealnesse". John S. Morrill, "Archibald Johnston, Lord Warriston | Covenanter, Presbyterian, Edinburgh," Encyclopedia Britannica, April 15, 2024, https://www.britannica.com/biography/Archibald-Johnston-Lord-Warriston. Amitha Kalaichandran, "Staying Mindful in Quarantine," Thrive Global, April 21, 2020, https://community.thriveglobal.com/staying-mindful-in-quarantine/.

14. John W Travis, 1975 Hopkins, Wellness resource center in Mill valley – described wellness. 1979 interview with Dan Rather, Travis described it. "Wellness," *The New York Times*, April 16, 2010, https://www.nytimes.com/2010/04/18/magazine/18FOB-onlanguage-t.html.

15. Halbert Dunn, chief of the US National Office of Vital Statistics wrote that environment should 'encourage you to live to the very full'. Halbert L. Dunn, "High-Level Wellness for Man and Society," *American Journal of Public Health and the Nation's Health* 49, no. 6 (June 1, 1959): 786–92, https://ajph.aphapublications.org/doi/abs/10.2105/AJPH.49.6.786.

Chapter 1: Healing Stories

1. Description of Match Day: Nina Bai, "Match Day 101: How Does the Medical Residency Match Work?," Scope, March 13, 2024, https://scopeblog.stanford.edu/2024/03/13/match-day-medical-school-residency/.

2. Joshua Foer, "Walker Library of the History of Human Imagination," *Atlas Obscura*, June 2, 2024, https://www.atlasobscura.com/places/walker-library-of-the-history-of-human-imagination.

3. "The Flayed Angel," c.1745 by Jacques Fabien Gautier dAgoty. MeisterDrucke, n.d. https://www.meisterdrucke.uk/fine-art-prints/Jacques-Fabien-Gautier-dAgoty/821765/The-Flayed-Angel%2C-c.1745.html.

4. "On the Physicians" by Hippocrates was published in sometime around 420-370 BCE. and described the ideal characteristics of physicians as honest, considerate, and beyond corruption. A key set of lines became the basis of the Hippocratic Oath: "I will never do harm to anyone…I will give no deadly medicine if asked…All that may come to my knowledge in the exercise of my profession or in daily commerce…I will keep to myself, holding such things shameful to be spoken about, and will never reveal," "Health Care Practices in Ancient Greece: The Hippocratic Ideal." PubMed Central (PMC). 2014. https://www.ncbi.nlm.nih.gov/pmc/articles/PMC4263393/.

5. The Editors of Encyclopaedia Britannica. "Chiron | Centaur, Healer, Teacher." Encyclopedia Britannica, April 12, 2024. https://www.britannica.com/topic/Chiron-Greek-mythology.

6. The Editors of Encyclopaedia Britannica. "Asclepius | Definition, Myth, & Facts." Encyclopedia Britannica, April 12, 2024. https://www.britannica.com/topic/Asclepius.

7. Enrico De Divitiis, Paolo Cappabianca, and Oreste De Divitiis, "The 'Schola Medica Salernitana': The Forerunner of The Modern University Medical Schools," Neurosurgery/Neurosurgery Online 55, no. 4 (October 1, 2004): 722–45, https://pubmed.ncbi.nlm.nih.gov/15458581/.

8. Charles B. Drucker, "Surgery Issue: Ambroise Paré and the Birth of the Gentle Art of Surgery." PubMed Central (PMC). December 1, 2008. https://www.ncbi.nlm.nih.gov/pmc/articles/PMC2605308/.

9. William Osler and his quote "The good physician treats the disease; the great physician treats the patient who has the disease" is described in context here: Robert M. Centor, "To Be a Great Physician, You Must Understand the Whole Story." PubMed Central (PMC). 2007. https://www.ncbi.nlm.nih.gov/pmc/articles/PMC1924990/.

10. Roger Irving Lee, a World War I medic (https://history.rcplondon.ac.uk/inspiring-physicians/roger-irving-lee) who served as the president of the American Medical Association in 1945, left behind a remarkable understanding of the medical profession, and the doctor's role within it, in his 1944 essay. Roger I. Lee, "Are Doctors People?" published in the *New England Journal of Medicine* October 12, 1944. https://www.nejm.org/doi/abs/10.1056/NEJM194410122311502.

11. Mikhail Bulgakov's *A Country Doctor's Notebook*, published in 1925, which is an unusual meld of autobiography and fiction. Mikhail Bulgakov, *"A Country Doctor's Notebook"* 1925. https://www.goodreads.com/work/quotes/2709608.

12. "Narrative medicine" was coined by Rita Charon. Marguerite Holloway, "When Medicine Meets Literature." Scientific American. February 20, 2024. https://www.scientificamerican.com/article/when-medicine-meets-liter/.

13. Melanie Thernstrom, "The Writing Cure." The New York Times, April 18, 2004. https://www.nytimes.com/2004/04/18/magazine/the-writing-cure.html.

14. James W. Pennebaker, Expressive Writing in Psychological Science. Perspectives on Psychological Science, 13(2), 226-229. https://journals.sagepub.com/doi/10.1177/1745691617707315.

15. In Untamed, Glennon Doyle poignantly writes that "the moral arc of our life bends toward meaning, especially if we bend it that way with all our damn might." "Untamed by Glennon Doyle." n.d. https://untamedbook.com/.

Chapter 2: From Cell to Body

1. Dr. Serge, a pseudonym, was my first medical school mentor, my attending on general internal medicine.

2. Homeless people often seek medical care, often up to four times a year. "QuickStats: Rate* of Emergency Department Visits,† by Homeless Status§ — National Hospital Ambulatory Medical Care Survey, United States, 2010–2021," *Morbidity and Mortality Weekly Report* 72, no. 42 (October 20, 2023): 1153, https://www.cdc.gov/mmwr/volumes/72/wr/mm7242a6.htm?s_cid=mm7242a6_w. "Policy Brief: How Hospital Discharge Data Can Inform State Homelessness Policy," Public Policy Institute of California, May 1, 2024, https://www.ppic.org/publication/policy-brief-how-hospital-discharge-data-can-inform-state-homelessness-policy.

3. "Silver in Wound Care—Friend or Foe?: A Comprehensive Review," *Plastic and Reconstructive Surgery. Global Open* 7, no. 8 (August 1, 2019): e2390, https://journals.lww.com/prsgo/fulltext/2019/08000/silver_in_wound_care_friend_or_foe___a.28.aspx.

4. Joshua J. Mark and Trustees of the British Museum, "Gula," *World History Encyclopedia*, December 8, 2022, https://www.worldhistory.org/Gula/.

5. Egyptologist Edwin Smith purchased a papyrus from Luxor in the late 1800s which described ancient Egyptian medical treatments that included sutures for wounds and topical honey for infections. But it also went further: another papyrus, dated some 3500 years ago, included spells to ward off spirits, harnessed through amulets. "The Edwin Smith Papyrus, the Oldest Surgical Treatise : History of Information," n.d., https://www.historyofinformation.com/detail.php?id=1352.

6. Galen's book, ("On Medical Substances") was a tome detailing the use of opium, herbs, and alcohol for pain relief during procedures, treatments that became commonplace. It is paralleled in *Dioscorides De materia medica*. Lijuan Lin, "Dioscorides and Galen in the Syriac Tradition: A Reconsideration of Three Passages About Herbs in an Anonymous Syriac Pharmacological Book," *Journal of Semitic Studies* 68, no. 2 (May 12, 2023): 473–99, https://academic.oup.com/jss/article-abstract/68/2/473/7161091.

7. Dark Ages birthed many untrained medical providers and charlatans peddling practices like witchcraft, it also ushered in the creation of early hospitals and aspects of the modern-day medical exam, like taking a pulse and noting a patient's breathing. Bloodletting and using leeches, was popularized during this time, with the idea that sickness was secondary to too much blood circulating. The role of poetry, prayer, and music also reached prominence. Cornell University Press, "Product Details - Cornell University Press," November 4, 2021, https://www.cornellpress.cornell.edu/book/9780801406973/witchcraft-in-the-middle-ages/#bookTabs=1.

8. Ibn Sina, one of the most famous doctors of the Islamic Golden Age, had a particular interest in bridging using metals for healing. Ibn Sina authored two books—*Kitab al-Shifa* ("The Book of Healing") as well as the *Al Qanun fi al-Tibb* ("The Canon of Medicine")—which detailed both mineral and plant-derived healing methods that would go on to influence medicine for the next 500 years. "Ibn Sina [Avicenna] (Stanford Encyclopedia of Philosophy)," September 15, 2016, https://plato.stanford.edu/entries/ibn-sina/.

9. In his *Kitab al-Mansouri fi al-Tibb* ("The Book on Medicine Dedicated to al-Mansur"), Iranian physician Al-Rhazi described approaches to treatment, such as diet and hygiene, while outlining the components of diagnosis, therapy and surgery. Importantly, Al-Rhazi was one of the first to recognize that some diseases did *not* have a cure, and that doctors shouldn't be blamed for this. He relied on herbs, minerals, and mercury-containing drugs and was an early proponent of sutures and casting to heal wounds and bones. "Kunnāsh al-Manṣūrī," The Library of Congress, n.d., https://www.loc.gov/item/2008401689/.

10. Of the "Alchemists," a group known for changing metals like lead into gold, as well as promoting a "universal remedy" to cure all diseases, the most famous would be a predecessor of Al-Rhazi and Ibn Sina, Jabbir ibn Hayyan, an Iraqi chemist who would grind mercury, sulfur, and gold to use as ointments and potions. Alchemy was so popular that it would dominate during the time of the Crusades in the 11th and 12th centuries. In Europe, leaders like Albertus Magnus combined it with Christian prayer as a way to "clean the soul and heal," which lost favor after the advent of

the scientific method. Jabir Ibn Hayyan, "Jabir Ibn Hayyan: The Father of Arab Chemistry," *Unknown*, 721, https://www.qmul.ac.uk/spcs/media/school-of-physical-and-chemical-sciences/Jabir-Ibn-Hayyan-JP.pdf.

11. Michał K. Owecki, "Theodor Schwann (1810–1882)," *Journal of Neurology* 268, no. 12 (June 2, 2021): 4921–22, https://www.ncbi.nlm.nih.gov/pmc/articles/PMC8563666/.

12. Andrzej Grzybowski and Krzysztof Pietrzak, "Robert Remak (1815–1865)," *Journal of Neurology* 260, no. 6 (November 28, 2012): 1696–97, https://www.ncbi.nlm.nih.gov/pmc/articles/PMC3675270/.

13. Father of modern pathology, Rudolph Virchow, in *Omnis cellula e cellula*," aimed to sort out Schwann's faulty third premise. Theodore M. Brown and Elizabeth Fee, "Rudolf Carl Virchow," *American Journal of Public Health* 96, no. 12 (December 1, 2006): 2104–5, https://www.ncbi.nlm.nih.gov/pmc/articles/PMC1698150/.

14. In the 1860s Louis Pasteur was researching diseases in silkworms, finding that microbes were the source. Kendall A. Smith, "Louis Pasteur, the Father of Immunology?," *Frontiers in Immunology* 3 (January 1, 2012), https://www.ncbi.nlm.nih.gov/pmc/articles/PMC3342039/.

15. Based in Germany, Pasteur's rival, Robert Koch, was 20 years younger and a rising star in both microbiology and medicine. He also studied anthrax and inoculated rodents with diseased spleens of farm animals. Koch then purified the microbes in a laboratory culture. In 1880, after moving to Berlin, he developed his "Koch's postulates" to summarize how microbes cause disease. Later on, in 1905, his work on isolating the organism responsible for tuberculosis was awarded the Nobel prize. Lloyd Grenfell Stevenson, "Robert Koch | German Bacteriologist & Nobel Laureate," Encyclopedia Britannica, May 23, 2024, https://www.britannica.com/biography/Robert-Koch.

16. Cellular injury may be due to many things: chemical agents such as chemotherapy (which is therapeutic, when applied to cancer cells), heat (for instance radiation from the sun's ultraviolet light), blunt force that breaks the tissues (like a knife wound), infectious organisms (like viruses), and auto-immune factors which attack the cell as though it were a foreign invader. Margaret A. Miller and James F. Zachary, "Mechanisms and Morphology of Cellular Injury, Adaptation, and Death," in *Elsevier eBooks*, 2017, 2-43. e19, https://www.ncbi.nlm.nih.gov/pmc/articles/PMC7171462/

17. there are also ways, albeit fewer, that cells can repair themselves. Often the body will remove the damaged cell through the spleen (which acts as a filter for damaged cells along with modulating the number of white cells, red cells, and platelets circulating in the blood), but the body often first attempts to fix the cell through DNA repair. For larger tissues, it may regenerate parenchyma cells to help bridge the damage left by the faulty cells or through flexible stromal cells, which support the damaged cells. Aubrey D. N. J. De Grey and Michael Rae, "Cellular Repair Processes," in *Springer eBooks*, 2019, 1–10, https://www.researchgate.net/publication/348944207_Cellular_Repair_Processes.

18. Seminal paper by Wallace Marshall, a biochemist and biophysicist at UCSF, published in *Science* in 2017. With his colleague Sindy Tang, they compared the cell to a spacecraft. So, when a hole is punched through, they must repair by stopping the run-off of cytoplasm (the liquid stuff inside the cell) and then subsequently regenerating the damaged parts. They also distinguished between 'wound healing' and 'regeneration.' Sindy K. Y. Tang and Wallace F. Marshall, "Self-repairing Cells: How Single Cells Heal Membrane Ruptures and Restore Lost Structures," *Science* 356, no. 6342 (June 9, 2017): 1022–25, https://www.science.org/doi/10.1126/science.aam6496.

19. Years after the structure of DNA was elucidated by Francis Crick and Jim Watson, DNA was found to be inherently unstable and subject to damage by radiation such as ionizing radiation and the sun's ultraviolet radiation. At the cellular level, DNA damage is the most crucial to understand. DNA repair was discovered by accident by an American scientist named Albert Kelner in what is now known as the Cold Spring Harbor laboratory in upstate New York. Errol C. Friedberg, "A History of the DNA Repair and Mutagenesis Field," *DNA Repair* 33 (September 1, 2015): 35–42, https://pubmed.ncbi.nlm.nih.gov/26151545/

20. Errol Friedberg, a South-African-American professor Emeritus from University of Texas SouthWestern. He wrote a review about the history of DNA repair, so was eager to simplify the overall mechanism for me: "Two DNA molecules line up next to each other, and the damaged one exchanges its strand so it becomes normal again," Friedberg told me. Errol C. Friedberg, "A History of the DNA Repair and Mutagenesis Field," *DNA Repair* 33 (September 1, 2015): 35–42, https://pubmed.ncbi.nlm.nih.gov/26151545/

21. More recently, the DNA repair field gained immense ground through a new discovery called Crispr-Cas9, which was discovered at the same time by two labs: one in Europe and one at the University of California Berkeley. When I spoke with Sam Sternberg in 2015 about it, he was just finishing his post-doctoral work in that lab. His supervisor was none other Jennifer Doudna, one of the co-recipients (with Emmanuelle Charpentier) of the 2020 Nobel Prize in Chemistry. Sternberg now runs his own lab out of Columbia University. CRISPR stands for "Clustered Regularly Interspaced Short Palindromic Repeats," which are areas of DNA that are widespread in microbes such as bacteria. It was first found in 1987 in *E.Coli*, but it took twenty years – not until in 2007 — for scientists to discover protein-coding genes called "Cas" (CRISPR-associated) in milk-fermenting bacteria. It was then found to produce RNA that could go on to detect viral DNA through pairing with them, cutting that DNA in half, subsequently destroying the virus. The precise molecular components for this DNA cutting reaction was named "CRISPR-Cas9." Amitha Kalaichandran, "This Discovery Takes Us a Step Closer to Curing Genetic Diseases," *HuffPost* (blog), April 2, 2017, https://www.huffpost.com/archive/ca/entry/this-discovery-takes-us-a-step-closer-to-curing-genetic-diseases_b_9326478. Tianxiang Li et al., "CRISPR/Cas9 Therapeutics: Progress and Prospects," *Signal Transduction and Targeted Therapy* 8, no. 1 (January 16, 2023), https://www.nature.com/articles/s41392-023-01309-7

22. CRISPR-Cas9 succeeded as a genome editing tool inside human cells almost immediately, and is now being used to tackle eliminating certain genetic diseases (like Cystic Fibrosis). "New CRISPR/Cas9 Technique Corrects Cystic Fibrosis in Cultured Human Stem Cells," ScienceDaily, August 21, 2021, https://www.sciencedaily.com/releases/2021/08/210809105908.htm.

23. Once the foundation of cellular repair was established, the field of 'regenerative medicine' was born. Coined in 1992, the field was used as part of the work by Leland Kaiser, who envisioned the use of technology to regenerate organ systems. In 2010, President Barack Obama relaxed the regulations on stem cell work which helped facilitate stem cell treatment for spinal cord injury in 2010 by the Geron Corporation. "International Online Medical Council (IOMC) | Medical Research," n.d., https://www.iomcworld.org/medical-journals/academic-journals-in-regenerative-medicine-37817.htmlhttps://ir.geron.com/investors/press-releases/press-release-details/2009/Geron-Receives-FDA-Clearance-to-Begin-Worlds-First-Human-Clinical-Trial-of-Embryonic-Stem-Cell-Based-Therapy/default.aspx. Note: trial was halted for financial reasons in 2014: Christopher Thomas Scott and David Magnus, "Wrongful Termination: Lessons From the Geron Clinical Trial," *Stem Cells Translational Medicine* 3, no. 12 (October 8, 2014): 1398–1401, https://pubmed.ncbi.nlm.nih.gov/25298371/

24. In 1968, a controversial paper in *Science* showed that axolotl heads could be transplanted onto the torso of another, and both organisms still somehow lived. N. J. De Both, "Transplantation of Axolotl Heads," *Science* 162, no. 3852 (October 25, 1968): 460–61, https://www.science.org/doi/10.1126/science.162.3852.460.

25. Tatiana Sandoval-Guzmán and Joshua D Currie, "The Journey of Cells Through Regeneration," *Current Opinion in Cell Biology* 55 (December 1, 2018): 36–41, https://pubmed.ncbi.nlm.nih.gov/30031323/. "The Currie Lab @ WFU," The Currie Lab @ WFU, n.d., https://www.currie-regenerationlab.com/

26. Karen Echeverri's analogy is humorous and powerful. Marine Biological Laboratory, "Scientists identify gene partnerships that promote spinal cord regeneration" March 6, 2019, https://phys.org/news/2019-03-scientists-gene-partnerships-spinal-cord.amp.

27. In early 2019, a controversial study using stem cells to treat spinal cord injuries was announced, yet the work around this hadn't actually been published. A journalist's article in *Nature*, however, reported that the study involved 113 participants received stem cells that were obtained from their own bone marrow, and all but one regained some of their movement and sensation. Michele Trott Ph.D., "Japan Approves Stem Cell Therapy for Spinal Cord Injuries," *Biopharma From Technology Networks*, February 22, 2019, https://www.technologynetworks.com/biopharma/news/japan-approves-stem-cell-therapy-for-spinal-cord-injuries-315803.

28. Cleveland Clinic Medical Professional, "Neuropsychological Testing and Assessment," Cleveland Clinic, n.d., https://my.clevelandclinic.org/health/diagnostics/4893-neuropsychological-testing-and-assessment.

29. Nithyani Anandakugan, "The Sri Lankan Civil War and Its History, Revisited in 2020," Harvard International Review, April 30, 2021, https://hir.harvard.edu/sri-lankan-civil-war/

30. At Northwestern University in Chicago, in partnership with the University of California, San Diego (UC San Diego), scientists have designed a way to insert a bioactivated, biodegradable 'nanomaterial' that alters the body's natural inflammatory response into a signal that allows healing. "Stephen Miller, Nanoparticle Therapy for Allergy and Inflammation: Innovation and New Ventures - Northwestern University," n.d., https://www.invo.northwestern.edu/technologies/invo-spotlights/featured-innovators/stephen-miller.html.

31. In March 2019 scientists out of the Wake Forest Institute for Regenerative Medicine (WFIRM) presented their 'mobile skin bioprinting system' which allows two layers of skin to be 'printed' right onto the wound. Mohammed Albanna et al., "In Situ Bioprinting of Autologous Skin Cells Accelerates Wound Healing of Extensive Excisional Full-Thickness Wounds," Scientific Reports 9, no. 1 (February 12, 2019), https://www.nature.com/articles/s41598-018-38366-w.

32. In 2016 Ortiz Catalan's group published a seminal article in the Lancet, which took 14 patients (all but one were based in Sweden) and guided them through 12 augmented reality (AR) and virtual reality (VR) sessions that incorporated gaming to "retrain" this phantom limb. After that pilot study, Ortiz Catalan and his team expanded the work to include multiple other centers around the world as part of a multicenter trial. He was involved in shifting a major paradigm. Mirror therapy is thought to work through the visual system – our minds 'see' a real limb instead of space, where a limb has been amputated, and attempt to move it, which then decreases the pain signals fired to that area. Publishing his work in 2020, Ortiz Catalan's group discovered something else: the treatment works without needing the visual system. Instead, it's the sense of movement itself. Max Ortiz-Catalan et al., "Phantom Motor Execution Facilitated by Machine Learning and Augmented Reality as Treatment for Phantom Limb Pain: A Single Group, Clinical Trial in Patients With Chronic Intractable Phantom Limb Pain," Lancet 388, no. 10062 (December 1, 2016): 2885–94, https://www.thelancet.com/journals/lancet/article/PIIS0140-6736(16)31598-7/abstract.

Chapter 3: Surroundings

1. Paul Barach, a physician scientist, wrote in a 2008 paper: "One of the greatest ironies of modern medicine is that the very environments created to heal are the cause of countless injuries, illnesses and death to the vulnerable population they were created to serve." Some researchers, such as Jonas Rehn and Kai Schuster out of Germany, suggest that the placebo effect may also be part of why hospital design seems to have a healing effect. In their 2017 study they found that patients self-rated behavior change as more likely if they were provided care in a more modern clinic space. This is termed the 'design placebo.' Jonas Rehn and Kai Schuster, "Clinic Design as Placebo—Using

Design to Promote Healing and Support Treatments," *Behavioral Sciences* 7, no. 4 (November 9, 2017): 77, https://pubmed.ncbi.nlm.nih.gov/29120378/

2. Reimagine Well dared to think about the issue differently. At that hospital, children needing chemotherapy are brought into a special infusion room – called an Infusionarium™. "Reimagine Well | Evolving the Patient Journey," n.d., https://reimaginewell.com/

3. Florence Nightingale was a pioneer, among the first to attribute differences in mortality to hospital design. Steven Lockley, "What Florence Nightingale Can Teach Us About Architecture and Health," Scientific American, February 20, 2024, https://www.scientificamerican.com/article/what-florence-nightingale-can-teach-us-about-architecture-and-health/

4. The concept of using design elements specifically to promote health is dubbed "salutogenic architecture", (a term popularized in the mid-1990s) which runs against the chaos of ill health. HealthManagement.org, "The Therapeutic Benefits of Salutogenic Hospital Design," n.d., https://healthmanagement.org/c/hospital/issuearticle/the-therapeutic-benefits-of-salutogenic-hospital-design. Jan A. Golembiewski, "Salutogenic Architecture in Healthcare Settings," in *Springer eBooks*, 2016, 267–76, https://www.researchgate.net/publication/307513474_Salutogenic_Architecture_in_Healthcare_Settings.

5. In a paper published in *Science* in April 1984, aptly entitled "View through a window may influence recovery from surgery," Roger Ulrich described his surprising findings. Roger S. Ulrich, "View Through a Window May Influence Recovery from Surgery," *Science* 224, no. 4647 (April 27, 1984): 420–21, https://pubmed.ncbi.nlm.nih.gov/6143402/

6. According to a commissioned, but unpublished, report Ulrich contributed to, several in-hospital deaths secondary to this outbreak followed [Ulrich, personal correspondence 2020].

7. Now, in the United States, the Centers for Disease Prevention and Control have strict regulations for hospital ventilation systems, specifically that air should be refreshed in the patient's room at least 12 times an hour. "Prevention Strategies for Seasonal Influenza in Healthcare Settings | CDC," n.d., https://www.cdc.gov/flu/professionals/infectioncontrol/healthcaresettings.htm.

8. Sir James Dyson also funded a unique hospital called the Dyson Centre for Neonatal Care, located in Bath, England, which incorporates light-colored wood and greenery, a pebbled garden, and a serious investment in soundproof materials. The result is a facility said to be eight decibels quieter neonatal intensive care unit (NICU) it replaced. RUHX official NHS charity of the Royal United Hospital / RUH Bath, "Dyson Centre for Neonatal Care | RUHX | Official NHS Charity of RUH Bath," RUHX, August 10, 2022, https://ruhx.org.uk/having-an-impact/our-campaigns-and-projects/bath-nicu/. Amy Frearson and Amy Frearson, "The Dyson Centre for Neonatal Care by Feilden Clegg Bradley Studios," *Dezeen*, May 8, 2015, https://

www.dezeen.com/2011/08/08/the-dyson-centre-for-neonatal-care-by-feilden-clegg-bradley-studios/

9. Ulrich penned an essay in the *Lancet* in 2006 about evidence-based healthcare architecture, in which he highlights the damage done by noisy healthcare environments: Roger Ulrich et al., "Evidence-based Health-care Architecture," *The Lancet*, vol. 368, 2006, https://www.thelancet.com/pdfs/journals/lancet/PIIS0140-6736(06)69921-2.pdf.

10. Design principles, specifically layout and flow, affect teamwork in hospitals specifically that attention to healthcare design, specifically layout and accessibility, improved teamwork and communication. Arsalan Gharaveis, D. Kirk Hamilton, and Debajyoti Pati, "The Impact of Environmental Design on Teamwork and Communication in Healthcare Facilities: A Systematic Literature Review," *HERD* 11, no. 1 (October 12, 2017): 119–37, https://pubmed.ncbi.nlm.nih.gov/29022368/

11. I expanded upon this concept in an article for *The New York Times*, on "Design Thinking,". Amitha Kalaichandran, "Design Thinking for Doctors and Nurses," *The New York Times*, August 3, 2017, https://www.nytimes.com/2017/08/03/well/live/design-thinking-for-doctors-and-nurses.html.

12. Evidence-based design is described in an excellent paper by Stichler. Jaynelle F. Stichler, "State of the Science in Healthcare Design," *HERD* 10, no. 2 (December 19, 2016): 6–12, https://journals.sagepub.com/doi/10.1177/1937586716676552.

13. Bridgepoint and it's design is described here: "The Surprising Science Behind Evidence-based Hospital Design," Healthy Debate, accessed February 17, 2021, https://healthydebate.ca/2014/07/topic/evidence-based-hospital-design/

14. Outdoor Care Retreat in Oslo. Mindbodygreen, "This Hospital in a Norwegian Forest Is Taking Nature Is the Best Medicine to the Next Level," January 20, 2019, https://www.mindbodygreen.com/articles/this-hospital-is-taking-nature-is-the-best-medicine-to-the-next-level.

15. Serena del Mar hospital in Colombia. "Serena Del Mar Hospital," n.d., https://www.safdiearchitects.com/projects/serena-del-mar-hospital.

16. International Well Being Institute. "International WELL Building Institute," n.d., https://resources.wellcertified.com/articles/telling-the-well-core-story/. In 2014, they created the WELL Building Standard™ to rate buildings based on their ability to facilitate health and wellness. In 2019 the institute was featured by *Fast Company* as one of the most innovative wellness companies for 2019. "International WELL Building Institute," n.d., https://www.wellcertified.com/about-iwbi/. "The World's Most Innovative Companies 2019: Wellness Honorees | Fast Company," Fast Company, January 1, 2000, https://www.fastcompany.com/most-innovative-companies/2019/sectors/wellness.

17. Prouty garden in Boston. Deborah Franklin, "How Hospital Gardens Help Patients Heal," Scientific American, February 20, 2024, https://www.scientificamerican.com/article/nature-that-nurtures/.

18. NYU horticultural therapy at the Rusk Rehabilitation Center. "Horticultural Therapy for Adults," NYU Langone Health, n.d., https://nyulangone.org/locations/rusk-rehabilitation/rehabilitation-support-services-for-adults/horticultural-therapy-for-adults.

19. Shinrin Yoku is the Japanese term for "forest bathing," and I wrote about it for NYT. Amitha Kalaichandran MD, "Take a Walk in the Woods. Doctor's Orders.," *The New York Times*, July 16, 2018, https://www.nytimes.com/2018/07/12/well/take-a-walk-in-the-woods-doctors-orders.html.

20. Toshiya Ochiai, who is (at the time of writing) currently the CEO of Japan-based International Society of Nature and Forest Medicine. "INFOM | International Society of Nature and Forest Medicine," (C)INFOM. All Rights Reserved., n.d., http://infom.org/

21. Time in nature, specifically in lush forests, can decrease stress and blood pressure, improve heart-rate variability (the variation of time between each heartbeat, which may reflect high stress when variability isn't constant), and lower cortisol, while boosting one's mood. Angel Bauer and Nicole D. White, "Time in Nature: A Prescription for the Prevention or Management of Hypertension," *American Journal of Lifestyle Medicine* 17, no. 4 (March 25, 2023): 476–78, https://www.ncbi.nlm.nih.gov/pmc/articles/PMC10328205. Bum-Jin Park et al., "Physiological Effects of Forest Recreation in a Young Conifer Forest in Hinokage Town, Japan," *Silva Fennica* 43, no. 2 (January 1, 2009), https://www.researchgate.net/publication/255496496_Physiological_Effects_of_Forest_Recreation_in_a_Young_Conifer_Forest_in_Hinokage_Town_Japan. Bum Jin Park et al., "The Physiological Effects of Shinrin-yoku (Taking in the Forest Atmosphere or Forest Bathing): Evidence From Field Experiments in 24 Forests Across Japan," *Environmental Health and Preventive Medicine* 15, no. 1 (May 2, 2009): 18–26, https://pubmed.ncbi.nlm.nih.gov/19568835/. Chorong Song, Harumi Ikei, and Yoshifumi Miyazaki, "Physiological Effects of Nature Therapy: A Review of the Research in Japan," *International Journal of Environmental Research and Public Health/ International Journal of Environmental Research and Public Health* 13, no. 8 (August 3, 2016): 781, https://pubmed.ncbi.nlm.nih.gov/27527193/. Jo Barton and Jules Pretty, "What Is the Best Dose of Nature and Green Exercise for Improving Mental Health? A Multi-Study Analysis," *Environmental Science & Technology* 44, no. 10 (May 15, 2010): 3947–55, https://pubmed.ncbi.nlm.nih.gov/20337470/

22. Richard Louv's term "nature deficit disorder," which more formally is termed "Attention Restoration Theory," refers to how nature can restore executive function in the brain. Sara L. Warber et al., "Addressing 'Nature-Deficit Disorder': A Mixed Methods Pilot Study of Young Adults Attending a Wilderness Camp," *Evidence-Based Complementary and Alternative Medicine* 2015 (January 1, 2015): 1–13, https://www.ncbi.nlm.nih.gov/pmc/articles/PMC4695668/. Richard Louv, "Books - Richard Louv," n.d., https://richardlouv.com/books/

23. Emi Morita et al., "No Association Between the Frequency of Forest Walking and Blood Pressure Levels or the Prevalence of Hypertension in a Cross-sectional Study of a Japanese Population," *Environmental Health and Preventive Medicine* 16, no. 5 (January 6, 2011): 299–306, https://www.ncbi.nlm.nih.gov/pmc/articles/PMC3156837/. Diana E Bowler et al., "A Systematic Review of Evidence for the Added Benefits to Health of Exposure to Natural Environments," *BMC Public Health* 10, no. 1 (August 4, 2010), https://bmcpublichealth.biomedcentral.com/articles/10.1186/1471-2458-10-456. In Sook Lee et al., "Effects of Forest Therapy on Depressive Symptoms Among Adults: A Systematic Review," *International Journal of Environmental Research and Public Health/International Journal of Environmental Research and Public Health* 14, no. 3 (March 20, 2017): 321, https://pubmed.ncbi.nlm.nih.gov/28335541/. Hannah Hoag, "This Is Your Brain on Trees: Why Is Urban Nature so Good for Our Minds, and What Happens When a Pandemic Isolates Us From It?," *The Globe and Mail*, April 22, 2021, https://www.theglobeandmail.com/canada/article-this-is-your-brain-on-trees-why-is-urban-nature-so-good-for-our-minds/

24. In Peter Crane's 2015 book on the Gingko tree, he underscores that the species almost went extinct at the end of the last ice age, but eventually made its way to Japan in the 13th century, where it flourished. After the Hiroshima bombing, which scorched people, buildings and trees, thousands of Gingkos mysteriously survived by regenerating from the inside: while the bark was burnt, the inside was not. Yale University Press, "Book Details - Yale University Press," February 5, 2024, https://yalebooks.yale.edu/book/9780300213829/ginkgo/

25. Emma Betuel, "Hiroshima A-Bomb: Ginkgo Trees That Survived the Blast Still Grow," Inverse, August 6, 2018, https://www.inverse.com/article/47833-hiroshima-gingko-trees-atomic-bomb.

26. As Oliver Sacks wrote in the *New Yorker* in 2014, not long before his death, they also miraculously shed their leaves almost on the same day. Oliver Sacks, "Night of the Ginkgo," *The New Yorker*, November 17, 2014, https://www.newyorker.com/magazine/2014/11/24/night-ginkgo.

27. In other words, the area was both a 'food swamp,' the term used for areas with copious fast food options and convenience stores and a 'food desert,' the term used for an area with little to no access to nutritious food. Amber Charles Alexis, "What Are Food Deserts? All You Need to Know," Healthline, June 14, 2021, https://www.healthline.com/nutrition/food-desert.

28. A 2018 article published in *Lancet Planetary Health* reported on a cross-sectional study of 122,993 participants with major depressive disorder in the United Kingdom. The researchers described the protective effect of residential greenness on depression, which was even greater among women, those under 60, and among residents in poorer neighborhoods. Chinmoy Sarkar, Chris Webster, and John Gallacher, "Residential Greenness and Prevalence of Major Depressive Disorders: A Cross-sectional, Observational, Associational Study of 94 879 Adult UK Biobank Participants," "the

Lancet. Planetary Health 2, no. 4 (April 1, 2018): e162–73, https://www.thelancet.com/journals/lanplh/article/PIIS2542-5196(18)30051-2/fulltext.

29. The most famous study to evaluate social and physical environments in neighborhoods was perhaps the Jackson Heart Study led by Samson Gebreab. Samson Y. Gebreab et al., "Neighborhood Social and Physical Environments and Type 2 Diabetes Mellitus in African-Americans: The Jackson Heart Study," *Health and Place/Health & Place (Online)* 43 (January 1, 2017): 128–37, https://pubmed.ncbi.nlm.nih.gov/28033588/

30. R. S. Piccolo et al., "Cohort Profile: The Boston Area Community Health (BACH) Survey," *International Journal of Epidemiology* 43, no. 1 (December 5, 2012): 42–51, https://pubmed.ncbi.nlm.nih.gov/23220718/

31. Amitha Kalaichandran, "What to Know About the Negative Health Effects of Separating Kids and Parents," ABC News, June 20, 2018, https://abcnews.go.com/Health/negative-health-effects-separating-kids-parents/story?id=55974081. Jason Hanna, "'Crying Girl' Picture Near US Border Wins World Press Photo of the Year," CNN, April 12, 2019, https://edition.cnn.com/2019/04/12/us/crying-girl-john-moore-immigration-photo-of-the-year/index.html.

32. Karen Hughes et al., "The Effect of Multiple Adverse Childhood Experiences on Health: A Systematic Review and Meta-analysis," ~the Lancet. Public Health 2, no. 8 (August 1, 2017): e356–66, https://pubmed.ncbi.nlm.nih.gov/29253477/

33. While at ABC News, I interviewed the director of Harvard's Center on the Developing Child, Dr. Jack Shonkoff. "Jack P. Shonkoff, M.D. - Center Director," Center on the Developing Child at Harvard University, April 16, 2021, https://developingchild.harvard.edu/people/jack-shonkoff/

34. The research is clear, from the landmark 1998 study in the *American Journal of Preventative Medicine* by Felitti and colleagues: in that study a questionnaire was mailed to over 13,000 adults to look at seven categories of ACEs – Vincent J Felitti et al., "Relationship of Childhood Abuse and Household Dysfunction to Many of the Leading Causes of Death in Adults," *American Journal of Preventive Medicine* 14, no. 4 (May 1, 1998): 245–58, https://pubmed.ncbi.nlm.nih.gov/9635069/

35. A Cleveland intervention, called "Healthy Eating & Active Living" (HEAL), which used neighborhood-based lifestyle interventions, including improving food affordability and access through neighborhood gardens and community kitchens, and free exercise classes, engaged the community to improve their social and physical environment. Vedette R. Gavin et al., "If We Build It, We Will Come: A Model for Community-Led Change to Transform Neighborhood Conditions to Support Healthy Eating and Active Living," *American Journal of Public Health* 105, no. 6 (June 1, 2015): 1072–77, https://www.ncbi.nlm.nih.gov/pmc/articles/PMC4431080/

36. And a similar Baltimore program, the "B'More Healthy Communities for Kids" (BHCK) multi-level intervention. Joel Gittelsohn et al., "B'More Healthy Communities for Kids: Design of A Multi-level Intervention for Obesity Prevention for Low-income African-American Children," *BMC Public Health* 14, no. 1 (September 11, 2014), https://pubmed.ncbi.nlm.nih.gov/25209072/

37. Oliver Sacks, as quoted from Everything in its Place by Oliver Sacks, and used by permission of the Oliver Sacks Foundation.

Chapter 4: Network Effects

1. Ogimi historically has the most centenarians per square mile of anywhere on Earth. "Stephaniehuber," n.d., https://www.buzzworthy.com/okinawans-live-until-100/

2. Referred to as traditional Chinese medicine (TCM), it is a therapeutic system described by Huang-di Nei'Jing as addressing the role of yin qi (female energy) and yang qi (male energy). Acupuncture, a central aspect of TCM, aims to correct for stagnant qi, which was believed to be responsible for most ailments. F Yu et al., "Traditional Chinese Medicine and Kampo: A Review From the Distant Past for the Future," *Journal of International Medical Research* 34, no. 3 (May 1, 2006): 231–39, https://pubmed.ncbi.nlm.nih.gov/16866016/

3. Physician Zhang Zhongjing (150-219 CE) and the Chinese surgeon Hua T'o, are described here: https://www.britannica.com/biography/Hua-Tuo ; https://en.wikipedia.org/wiki/Zhang_Zhongjing

4. Serenbe is a... a wellness community. "Bloomberg - Are You a Robot?," March 16, 2018, https://www.bloomberg.com/news/articles/2018-03-16/the-allure-of-serenbe-atlanta-s-suburban-utopia.

5. Richard Fausset, "Ahmaud Arbery Shooting: What to Know About the Trial and More," *The New York Times*, August 8, 2022, https://www.nytimes.com/article/ahmaud-arbery-shooting-georgia.html.

6. Biophilic design. "14 Patterns of Biophilic Design," September 12, 2014, https://www.terrapinbrightgreen.com/reports/14-patterns/

7. Nicholas Kristof, "Opinion | Let's Wage a War on Loneliness," *The New York Times*, November 9, 2019, https://www.nytimes.com/2019/11/09/opinion/sunday/britain-loneliness-epidemic.html.

8. *The Okinawa Program*, "The Okinawa Program by Bradley J. Willcox, D. Craig Willcox, Makoto Suzuki: 9780609807507 | PenguinRandomHouse.com: Books," PenguinRandomHouse.com, March 12, 2002, https://www.penguinrandomhouse.com/books/190921/the-okinawa-program-by-bradley-j-willcox-md-d-craig-willcox-phd-and-makoto-suzuki-md-foreword-by-andrew-weil-md/

9. Together by Dr. Vivek Murthy," Drvivekmurthy, n.d., https://www.vivekmurthy.com/together-book.

10. A.Regula Herzog, Mary Beth Ofstedal, and Laura M Wheeler, "Social Engagement and Its Relationship to Health," *Clinics in Geriatric Medicine* 18, no. 3 (August 1, 2002): 593–609, https://pubmed.ncbi.nlm.nih.gov/12424874/. Yoram Barak, Sharon Leitch, and Paul Glue, "The Great Escape. Centenarians' Exceptional Health," *Aging Clinical and Experimental Research* 33, no. 3 (June 2, 2020): 513–20, https://link.springer.com/article/10.1007/s40520-020-01552-w.

11. Maija Reblin and Bert N Uchino, "Social and Emotional Support and Its Implication for Health," *Current Opinion in Psychiatry* 21, no. 2 (March 1, 2008): 201–5, https://www.ncbi.nlm.nih.gov/pmc/articles/PMC2729718/

12. Ayfer Peker and Süreyya Karaöz, "The Effects of Social Support and Hope in the Healing of Diabetic Foot Ulcers Treated With Standard Care," *Population Health Management* 20, no. 6 (December 1, 2017): 507, https://pubmed.ncbi.nlm.nih.gov/28387580/

13. One of the most interesting studies to look at this was out of Auckland in 2017, co-authored by University of Auckland researcher, Elizabeth Broadbent, who has been studying this association for 15 years. She and her team looked at social closeness on how well skin recovered after it was punctured. They found that it did have a beneficial effect, and was also accompanied by self-reported decrease in stress. Hayley Robinson et al., "The Effects of Psychological Interventions on Wound Healing: A Systematic Review of Randomized Trials," *British Journal of Health Psychology* 22, no. 4 (July 3, 2017): 805–35, https://pubmed.ncbi.nlm.nih.gov/28670818/

14. In 1991 two sociologists named Richard Nisbett and Lee Ross wrote what's perhaps the seminal social psychology textbook called "The Person and the Situation," arguing that most of our behaviour—what we deem as personality—is actually subject to our environments. "APA PsycNet," n.d., https://psycnet.apa.org/record/1991-97382-000.

15. Institute for Quality and Efficiency in Health Care (IQWiG), "Depression: Learn More – What Is Burnout?," InformedHealth.org - NCBI Bookshelf, June 18, 2020, https://www.ncbi.nlm.nih.gov/books/NBK279286/

16. "Lost Connections: Uncovering the Real Causes of Depression," Goodreads, n.d., https://www.goodreads.com/book/show/34921573-lost-connections.

17. Occam's razor: the most unified explanation, which is often the simplest, is the most likely to be correct. Brian Duignan, "Occam's Razor | Origin, Examples, & Facts," Encyclopedia Britannica, May 27, 2024, https://www.britannica.com/topic/Occams-razor.

18. Osteogenesis Imperfecta. I wrote about this case diagnosis in 2018 for *Discover* magazine. Amitha Kalaichandran, "Eye of the Beholder," Discover Magazine, April 18, 2020, https://www.discovermagazine.com/health/eye-of-the-beholder.

19. Batten Disease (known colloquially as "childhood dementia"), subtype CLN2 is also known as neuronal ceroid lipofuscinosis (NCL) type 2, and forms part of a broader group of NCL diseases. CLN2 specifically refers to the build-up of protein waste in the cell organelles called lysosomes which produce enzymes to break down this waste. Children with CLN2 have a genetic mutation that prevents the production of these enzymes. As such, it's like trash building up in a home with no garbage truck able to pick it up each week. Over time, the home becomes non-functional, as the waste predominates, impacting activities. Children with CLN2 then lose the parts of their brain involved movement, cognition, and speech. The treatment is enzyme replacement, ideally, early on. Patrick J. Silva and Nancy K. Sweitzer, "Chimeric

Cohorts and Consortia Can Power and Scale Precision Medicine," in *Elsevier eBooks*, 2024, 264–82, https://www.sciencedirect.com/topics/medicine-and-dentistry/batten-disease.

20. Jean M. Twenge, "Have Smartphones Destroyed a Generation?," *The Atlantic*, July 8, 2022, https://www.theatlantic.com/magazine/archive/2017/09/has-the-smartphone-destroyed-a-generation/534198/

21. Lydia Denworth, "Social Media Has Not Destroyed a Generation," Scientific American, February 20, 2024, https://www.scientificamerican.com/article/social-media-has-not-destroyed-a-generation/

22. 2020, a documentary called *The Social Dilemma*. "The Social Dilemma," The Social Dilemma, March 14, 2022, https://www.thesocialdilemma.com/

23. Later, a damning Wall Street Journal investigation report about Facebook, and what internal researchers knew about the harms to adolescents, suggests the picture is complex (Facebook, for their part, responded with a counterargument from their Head of Research). Georgia Wells, Jeff Horwitz, and Deepa Seetharaman, "Facebook Knows Instagram Is Toxic for Teen Girls, Company Documents Show," *WSJ*, September 14, 2021, https://www.wsj.com/articles/facebook-knows-instagram-is-toxic-for-teen-girls-company-documents-show-11631620739. Pratiti Raychoudhury Vice President Research Head Of and Meta, "What Our Research Really Says About Teen Well-Being and Instagram," *Meta*, September 30, 2021, https://about.fb.com/news/2021/09/research-teen-well-being-and-instagram/

24. Jena Hilliard, "Social Media Addiction: Recognize the Signs," Addiction Center, April 30, 2024, https://www.addictioncenter.com/drugs/social-media-addiction/

Chapter 5: Mind Medicine

1. Mindfulness-based stress reduction, or "MBSR," from its creator, Jon Kabat-Zinn. Sarah Angela Kriakous et al., "The Effectiveness of Mindfulness-Based Stress Reduction on the Psychological Functioning of Healthcare Professionals: A Systematic Review," *Mindfulness* 12, no. 1 (September 24, 2020): 1–28, https://www.ncbi.nlm.nih.gov/pmc/articles/PMC7511255/

2. Dr. Saki Santorelli. For several decades they had been running an 8-week MBSR program at the University of Massachusetts and surrounding hospitals for patients with chronic pain—and Kabat-Zinn had been publishing his studies in this field. The Center for Mindfulness in Medicine, Healthcare, and Society and Jon Kabat-Zinn, Mindfulness-Based Stress Reduction (MBSR): Standards of Practice, ed. Saki F. Santorelli (Center for Mindfulness in Medicine, Health Care & Society, 2014), https://mindfulness.au.dk/fileadmin/mindfulness.au.dk/Artikler/Santorelli_mbsr_standards_of_practice_2014.pdf. Jon Kabat-Zinn, Leslie Lipworth, and Robert Burney, "The Clinical Use of Mindfulness Meditation for the Self-regulation of Chronic Pain," *Journal of Behavioral Medicine* 8, no. 2 (June 1, 1985): 163–90, https://pubmed.ncbi.nlm.nih.gov/3897551/

3. One of Santorelli's and Kabat-Zinn's first studies together looked at the potential benefits of MBSR for anxiety. There, 22 participants who met diagnostic criteria for an anxiety disorder received weekly MBSR training for one month, and then monthly for three months, and found that anxiety as well as depression scores were reduced and remained reduced at follow-up after three years time (regardless of whether they continued their practice). It appears that, in the brain, the impact of an 8-week MBSR course can mimic the brain function seen in those who have meditating for years. Changes are seen in the amygdala specifically. J Kabat-Zinn et al., "Effectiveness of a Meditation-based Stress Reduction Program in the Treatment of Anxiety Disorders," ~the œAmerican *Journal of Psychiatry* 149, no. 7 (July 1, 1992): 936–43, https://pubmed.ncbi.nlm.nih.gov/1609875/.

4. Rinske A. Gotink et al., "8-week Mindfulness Based Stress Reduction Induces Brain Changes Similar to Traditional Long-term Meditation Practice – a Systematic Review," *Brain and Cognition* 108 (October 1, 2016): 32–41, https://www.researchgate.net/publication/305391293_8-week_Mindfulness_Based_Stress_Reduction_induces_brain_changes_similar_to_traditional_long-term_meditation_practice_-_A_systematic_review.

5. Madhav Goyal et al., "Meditation Programs for Psychological Stress and Well-being," *JAMA Internal Medicine* 174, no. 3 (March 1, 2014): 357, https://www.ncbi.nlm.nih.gov/pmc/articles/PMC4142584/

6. Erica M.S. Sibinga et al., "School-Based Mindfulness Instruction: An RCT," *Pediatrics* 137, no. 1 (January 1, 2016), https://pubmed.ncbi.nlm.nih.gov/26684478/

7. Xiang Zhou et al., "Effects of Mindfulness-based Stress Reduction on Anxiety Symptoms in Young People: A Systematic Review and Meta-analysis," *Psychiatry Research* 289 (July 1, 2020): 113002, https://pubmed.ncbi.nlm.nih.gov/32438210/. Erica M.S. Sibinga et al., "Mindfulness-Based Stress Reduction for Urban Youth," ~the œJournal *of Alternative and Complementary Medicine/Journal of Alternative and Complementary Medicine* 17, no. 3 (March 1, 2011): 213–18, https://pubmed.ncbi.nlm.nih.gov/21348798/

8. Mindfulness-based meditation more broadly, even if it isn't as structured as MBSR, has been linked to many health benefits, everything from improving the immune system. David S. Black and George M. Slavich, "Mindfulness Meditation and the Immune System: A Systematic Review of Randomized Controlled Trials," *Annals of the New York Academy of Sciences* 1373, no. 1 (January 21, 2016): 13–24, https://pubmed.ncbi.nlm.nih.gov/26799456/

9. Seong-Hi Park and Kuem Sun Han, "Blood Pressure Response to Meditation and Yoga: A Systematic Review and Meta-Analysis," ~the Journal of Alternative and Complementary Medicine/Journal of Alternative and Complementary Medicine 23, no. 9 (September 1, 2017): 685–95, https://pubmed.ncbi.nlm.nih.gov/28384004/

10. Goyal, M., Singh, S., Sibinga, E. M., Gould, N. F., Rowland-Seymour, A., Sharma, R., ... & Haythornthwaite, J. A. (2014). Meditation programs for psychological stress

and well-being: A systematic review and meta-analysis. *JAMA Internal Medicine*, 174(3), 357-368.

11. Wang Lq et al., "A Randomized Controlled Trial of a Mindfulness-based Intervention Program for People With Schizophrenia: 6-month Follow-up," December 1, 2016, https://doaj.org/article/eae803333ad84ae5876ab4c749124c57.

12. A systematic review and meta-analysis of 16 studies (1,268 people with schizophrenia) published in 2019 hospitalizations decreased, though symptoms were not as impacted. Seena Fazel et al., "Schizophrenia and Violence: Systematic Review and Meta-Analysis," *PLoS Medicine* 6, no. 8 (August 11, 2009): e1000120, https://journals.plos.org/plosmedicine/article?id=10.1371/journal.pmed.1000120.

13. Jens Einar Jansen et al., "Acceptance- and Mindfulness-based Interventions for Persons With Psychosis: A Systematic Review and Meta-analysis," Schizophrenia Research 215 (January 1, 2020): 25–37, https://www.researchgate.net/publication/337541580_Acceptance-_and_mindfulness-based_interventions_for_persons_with_psychosis_A_systematic_review_and_meta-analysis

14. Kerem Böge et al., "Mindfulness-Based Interventions for In-Patients With Schizophrenia Spectrum Disorders—A Qualitative Approach," Frontiers in Psychiatry 11 (June 26, 2020), https://www.frontiersin.org/journals/psychiatry/articles/10.3389/fpsyt.2020.00600/full

15. Kerem Böge et al., "Mindfulness-Based Interventions for In-Patients With Schizophrenia Spectrum Disorders—A Qualitative Approach," *Frontiers in Psychiatry* 11 (June 26, 2020), https://www.frontiersin.org/journals/psychiatry/articles/10.3389/fpsyt.2020.00600/full.

16. Meditation is not without its controversies. In some cases, it can actually be triggering, and thus harmful, for some individuals with PTSD. Troy Erstling, "What I Wish I Knew Before Vipassana - Troy Erstling - Medium," *Medium*, April 12, 2024, https://medium.com/@troyerstling/what-i-wish-i-knew-before-vipassana-a214ff054d40.

17. Willoughby B Britton, "Can Mindfulness Be Too Much of a Good Thing? The Value of a Middle Way," *Current Opinion in Psychology* 28 (August 1, 2019): 159–65, https://www.sciencedirect.com/science/article/pii/S2352250X18301453.

18. There have been some case reports of psychosis induced by mindfulness meditation, and though extremely rare, this side effect featured prominently in a 2021 article in *Harper's* magazine, and on occasion, the *type* of meditation can be controversial. David Kortava, "Lost in Thought," Harper's Magazine, July 24, 2023, https://harpers.org/archive/2021/04/lost-in-thought-psychological-risks-of-meditation/

19. Transcendental Meditation (TM) is a form of silent, mantra-based meditation developed by Maharishi Mahesh Yogi in the 1950s. It involves the use of a specific mantra, or sound, which is silently repeated during the meditation session. The practice is typically done for 20 minutes twice a day while sitting comfortably with the eyes closed. Sangeeta P. Joshi et al., "Efficacy of Transcendental Meditation to Reduce Stress Among Health Care Workers," *JAMA Network Open* 5, no. 9 (September 19, 2022): e2231917, https://pubmed.ncbi.nlm.nih.gov/36121655/

20. TM may improve anxiety according to a 2006 Cochrane review, but it may not be substantially different from other relaxation therapies; heterogeneity within studies remains an issue, which means it's hard to compare them side to side. For instance, the impact on blood pressure may not be significant. Notably, a Cochrane review on TM for cardiovascular disease prevention, by Louise Hartley and colleagues from RTI Health Solutions, was withdrawn after questions were raised about the study analysis. Thawatchai Krisanaprakornkit et al., "Meditation Therapy for Anxiety Disorders," Review, by The Cochrane Collaboration, *Cochrane Database of Systematic Reviews*, 2009, https://transformationalchange.pbworks.com/f/meditation+therapy_cochrane.pdf. Louise Hartley et al., "Transcendental Meditation for the Primary Prevention of Cardiovascular Disease," *Cochrane Library* 2019, no. 6 (November 15, 2017), https://pubmed.ncbi.nlm.nih.gov/29140556/

21. "If you practice TM long enough, you really can fly," some have said. Claims like this have led to a lawsuit in 1986; films like *David Wants to Fly*, which aimed to expose the dark side of the movement, and a recent book called *Greetings from Utopia Park* by Claire Hoffman. "WashingtonPost.com: The Cult Controversy," n.d., https://www.washingtonpost.com/wp-srv/national/longterm/cult/trans_med/main.htm.

22. Steven Hassan, "Meditation, Yes! But Please Be Careful and Do Your Homework Regarding Transcendental Meditation (TM).," Freedom of Mind Resource Center, March 22, 2024, https://freedomofmind.com/meditation-yes-but-please-be-careful-and-do-your-homework-regarding-transcendental-meditation-tm/

23. Dr. Daniel Kohen, of the University of Massachusetts, was leading me through a classic hypnosis exercise as part of the National Pediatric Hypnosis Training Institute conference. "Home | National Pediatric Hypnosis Training Institute," NPHTI, n.d., https://www.nphti.org/

24. In 2014, Kohen published a review of clinical hypnosis in pediatrics and the positive effects on everything from headaches, to pain and sleep. Daniel Kohen and Pamela Kaiser, "Clinical Hypnosis With Children and Adolescents—What? Why? How?: Origins, Applications, and Efficacy," *Children* 1, no. 2 (August 12, 2014): 74–98, https://www.ncbi.nlm.nih.gov/pmc/articles/PMC4928724/

25. Hypnosis may also be used as an immune system suppressor and pain modulator in breast cancer patients before, and even to a degree during, surgery. "Human Verification," n.d., https://app.dimensions.ai/details/publication/pub.1007520776.

26. Dr. David Spiegel from Stanford University describes hypnosis as a "state of highly focused attention [combined with] dissociation of competing thoughts and sensations toward the periphery of awareness and enhanced response to social cues." Spiegel has found that hypnosis works on specific brain areas that deal with attention and emotional control, while also allowing that people vary in their ability to be hypnotized, as suggestibility is a key component. There are specific areas of the brain—the dorsolateral prefrontal cortex and the dorsal anterior cingulate cortex, specifically—which may be downregulated during hypnosis to alleviate anxiety or pain. Indeed, the evidence suggests that medical hypnosis can help in the clinical context,

specifically if it's led by an experienced facilitator. David Spiegel, "Tranceformatins: Hypnosis in Brain and Body," Special Article, *Depression and Anxiety* 30 (2013): 342–52, https://med.stanford.edu/content/dam/sm/nbc/documents/journalclub/2023/ Tranceformation_AandD.pdf.

27. Before his death in November 2020, Alex Trebek, long-time host of the popular television quiz show *Jeopardy*, credited his "optimistic mindset" with why he believed he would recover from stage-four pancreatic cancer. Merrit Kennedy, "Alex Trebek Says He's Seeing 'Mind-Boggling' Positive Results in Cancer Fight," *NPR*, May 29, 2019, https://www.npr.org/2019/05/29/727849422/alex-trebek-says-hes-seeing-mind-boggling-positive-results-in-cancer-fight

28. Lauren C. Howe et al., "Changing Patient Mindsets About Non–Life-Threatening Symptoms During Oral Immunotherapy: A Randomized Clinical Trial," *Journal of Allergy and Clinical Immunology. In Practice/˜the œJournal of Allergy and Clinical Immunology. In Practice* 7, no. 5 (May 1, 2019): 1550–59, https://www.jaci-inpractice.org/article/ S2213-2198(19)30075-3/abstract.

29. Alia J Crum, Kari A Leibowitz, and Abraham Verghese, "Making Mindset Matter," *BMJ. British Medical Journal*, February 15, 2017, j674, https://www.bmj.com/ content/356/bmj.j674.

30. Roy C. Ziegelstein and Sara D. Miller, "Just a Spoonful of Sugar." *Journal of the American College of Cardiology* 48, no. 11 (December 1, 2006): 2223–24, https://pubmed.ncbi. nlm.nih.gov/17161250/

31. "Ted Jack Kaptchuk," Global Health and Social Medicine, December 1, 2020, https://ghsm.hms.harvard.edu/faculty-staff/ted-jack-kaptchuk.

32. Adriaan Louw et al., "Sham Surgery in Orthopedics: A Systematic Review of the Literature," *Pain Medicine*, July 11, 2016, pnw164, https://academic.oup.com/ painmedicine/article/18/4/736/2924731.

33. Kaptchuk and others have commented on the ethics of such trials. F. G Miller and T. J Kaptchuk, "Sham Procedures and the Ethics of Clinical Trials," *Journal of the Royal Society of Medicine* 97, no. 12 (December 1, 2004): 576–78, https://www.ncbi.nlm.nih. gov/pmc/articles/PMC1079669/

34. Ted J Kaptchuk et al., "Components of Placebo Effect: Randomised Controlled Trial in Patients With Irritable Bowel Syndrome," *BMJ. British Medical Journal* 336, no. 7651 (April 3, 2008): 999–1003, https://pubmed.ncbi.nlm.nih.gov/18390493/

35. In 2020, Kaptchuk's team found that providing a placebo to a patient can reduce opioid usage by 30% in post-lower back surgery pain management, and that MRI may uncover brain areas involved in placebo effect. Claudia Carvalho et al., "Open-label Placebo for Chronic Low Back Pain: A 5-year Follow-up," *Pain* 162, no. 5 (November 30, 2020): 1521–27, https://pubmed.ncbi.nlm.nih.gov/33259459/.

36. Dan-Mikael Ellingsen et al., "Dynamic Brain-to-brain Concordance and Behavioral Mirroring as a Mechanism of the Patient-clinician Interaction," *Science Advances* 6, no. 43 (October 23, 2020), https://www.science.org/doi/10.1126/sciadv.abc1304.

37. In an interview for NPR's "The Hidden Brain," Kaptchuk was careful to also point out that florid deception is not necessary (which he also wrote about) as the placebo effect can still work. Shankar Vedantam, "A Dramatic Cure," *NPR*, April 29, 2019, https://www.npr.org/transcripts/718227789

38. Claudia Carvalho et al., "Open-label Placebo for Chronic Low Back Pain: A 5-year Follow-up," *Pain* 162, no. 5 (November 30, 2020): 1521–27, https://pubmed.ncbi.nlm. nih.gov/33259459/. Teri W. Hoenemeyer et al., "Open-Label Placebo Treatment for Cancer-Related Fatigue: A Randomized-Controlled Clinical Trial," *Scientific Reports* 8, no. 1 (February 9, 2018), https://www.nature.com/articles/s41598-018-20993-y. Yiqi Pan et al., "Open-label Placebos for Menopausal Hot Flushes: A Randomized Controlled Trial," *Scientific Reports* 10, no. 1 (November 18, 2020), https://www.nature. com/articles/s41598-020-77255-z.

39. Evers, A. W. M., Colloca, L., Blease, C., Annoni, M., Atlas, L. Y., Benedetti, F., Bingel, U., Büchel, C., Carvalho, C., Colagiuri, B., Crum, A. J., Enck, P., Gaab, J., Geers, A. L., Howick, J., Jensen, K. B., Kirsch, I., Meissner, K., Napadow, V., Peerdeman, K. J., Raz, A., Rief, W., Vase, L., Wager, T. D., Wampold, B. E., Weimer, K., Wiech, K., Kaptchuk, T. J., Klinger, R., & Kelley, J. M. (2018). Implications of placebo and nocebo effects for clinical practice: Expert consensus. *Psychotherapy and Psychosomatics, 87*(4), 204-210. https://doi.org/10.1159/000490354

40. Entertainment Tonight, "Alex Trebek Was 'At Peace' During His Final Days," November 9, 2020, https://www.youtube.com/watch?v=g6NLTCnRb9o.

41. Yoga is a word derived from the Sanskrit word "Yuj" meaning "yolk" or "join," so it effectively means "union" of the mind and body. "MEA | Search Result," Ministry of External Affairs, Government of India, n.d., https://www.mea.gov.in/search-result. htm?25096/Yoga:_su_origen,_historia_y_desarrollo.

42. EMDR stands for Eye Movement Desensitization and Reprocessing, and has evidence for trauma, suggesting the connection between the eyes and brain (and mind). Francine Shapiro, "The Role of Eye Movement Desensitization and Reprocessing (EMDR) Therapy in Medicine: Addressing the Psychological and Physical Symptoms Stemming From Adverse Life Experiences," ˜the Permanente Journal/Permanente Journal 18, no. 1 (March 1, 2014): 71–77, https://www.ncbi.nlm.nih.gov/pmc/ articles/PMC3951033/

43. In recent years several academics have explored the impact of yoga on healing: from the impact on reducing depressive symptoms in adults and children, to blood pressure improvement. "Yoga for Health: What the Science Says," NCCIH, n.d., https:// www.nccih.nih.gov/health/providers/digest/yoga-for-health-science.

44. A Cochrane review of yoga for breast cancer patients found it reduced fatigue and improved health-related quality of life compared to education or psychosocial interviews, but that similar results were achieved with any regular exercise. Holger Cramer et al., "Yoga for Improving Health-related Quality of Life, Mental Health and Cancer-related Symptoms in Women Diagnosed With Breast Cancer," *Cochrane Library* 2017, no. 1 (January 3, 2017), https://www.cochrane.org/CD010802/BREASTCA_ yoga-women-diagnosis-breast-cancer.

45. There is also moderate evidence for yoga in kids with ADHD – i.e. improvements in attentiveness and impulsivity. Xue Luo, Xu Huang, and Shuang Lin, "Yoga and Music Intervention Reduces Inattention, Hyperactivity/Impulsivity, and Oppositional Defiant Disorder in Children's Consumer With Comorbid ADHD and ODD," *Frontiers in Psychology* 14 (September 20, 2023), https://www.frontiersin.org/journals/psychology/articles/10.3389/fpsyg.2023.1150018/full.

46. There is evidence just for breathwork, for instance, but breathwork is also taught in diving and in the military, so teasing this out from any other effects of yoga is problematic. Shanna McGoldrick and Shanna McGoldrick, "How Scuba Diving Can Boost Mental Health and Mindfulness, and Lower Stress – It's All That Deep Breathing, and the Undersea Wonders," *South China Morning Post*, December 8, 2019, https://www.scmp.com/lifestyle/health-wellness/article/3040909/how-scuba-diving-can-boost-mental-health-and-mindfulness.

47. Anxiety and depression can also induce an inflammatory response that can impact other aspects of physical health—especially heart health. Chieh-Hsin Lee and Fabrizio Giuliani, "The Role of Inflammation in Depression and Fatigue," *Frontiers in Immunology* 10 (July 19, 2019), https://www.ncbi.nlm.nih.gov/pmc/articles/PMC6658985/.

48. "Depression, Anxiety and Stress Linked to Poor Heart Health in Two New Studies," American Heart Association, n.d., https://newsroom.heart.org/news/depression-anxiety-and-stress-linked-to-poor-heart-health-in-two-new-studies.

49. Healthline: Elea Carey, "How Are Cholesterol and Stress Connected?," Healthline, March 29, 2020, https://www.healthline.com/health/high-cholesterol/does-stress-affect-cholesterol#stress-and-cholesterol.

50. Research professor and bestselling author Brené Brown has shared that leaders, in order to lead effectively, must *care* for those they lead. Simply put, if a leader looks at their subordinates with envy, animosity, anger or hatred, leading effectively becomes near impossible. "Dare to Lead | Leaders Must Invest a Reasonable Amount of Time Attending to Fears and Feelings. - Brené Brown," Brené Brown, November 14, 2023, https://brenebrown.com/art/dare-to-lead-leaders-must-either-invest-a-reasonable-amount-of-time.

51. "Man's Search for Meaning by Viktor E. Frankl - Teacher's Guide: 9780807000007 - PenguinRandomHouse.com: Books," PenguinRandomhouse.com, February 18, 2014, https://www.penguinrandomhouse.com/books/206272/mans-search-for-meaning-by-viktor-e-frankl/9780807000007/teachers-guide/

Chapter 6: Nourished

1. The Napa program, Healthy Kitchens, Health Lives, is run by a physician named David Eisenberg, who is based at Harvard Medical School. "Healthy Kitchens, Healthy Lives," Healthy Kitchens, Healthy Lives, n.d., https://www.healthykitchens.org/

2. Culinary medicine is defined as "a new evidence-based field in medicine that blends the art of food and cooking with the science of medicine." John La Puma, "What Is

Culinary Medicine and What Does It Do?," *Population Health Management* 19, no. 1 (February 1, 2016): 1–3, https://www.ncbi.nlm.nih.gov/pmc/articles/PMC4739343/

3. D J Jenkins et al., "Glycemic Index of Foods: A Physiological Basis for Carbohydrate Exchange," ˜the American Journal of Clinical Nutrition 34, no. 3 (March 1, 1981): 362–66, https://pubmed.ncbi.nlm.nih.gov/6259925/

4. David J. A. Jenkins et al., "Effect of a Low–Glycemic Index or a High–Cereal Fiber Diet on Type 2 Diabetes," *JAMA* 300, no. 23 (December 17, 2008): 2742, https://pubmed.ncbi.nlm.nih.gov/19088352/

5. Later, Jenkins adapted these principles to the Portfolio diet which is a vegetarian diet high in fiber and plant-based cholesterols called sterols… I followed the evidence that foods with soluble fiber reduce cholesterol by binding it. David Jenkins, "In Depth: The Portfolio Diet," n.d., http://www.lipidgeneticsclinic.ca/pdf/2015%2009%20 22%20The%20Portfolio%20Diet.pdf. Harvard Health, "11 Foods That Lower Cholesterol," March 26, 2024, https://www.health.harvard.edu/heart-health/11-foods-that-lower-cholesterol.

6. D J A Jenkins et al., "Does Conventional Early Life Academic Excellence Predict Later Life Scientific Discovery? An Assessment of the Lives of Great Medical Innovators," *QJM* 114, no. 6 (June 26, 2020): 381–89, https://pubmed.ncbi.nlm.nih.gov/32589722/

7. Ventana Al Conocimiento, "James Lind and Scurvy: The First Clinical Trial in History? | OpenMind," OpenMind, July 27, 2018, https://www.bbvaopenmind.com/en/science/leading-figures/james-lind-and-scurvy-the-first-clinical-trial-in-history/

8. Jeremy Hugh Baron, "Evolution of Clinical Research: A History Before and Beyond James Lind," *Perspectives in Clinical Research* 3, no. 4 (January 1, 2012): 149, https://www.ncbi.nlm.nih.gov/pmc/articles/PMC3530985/

9. Most prominently, Type 2 diabetes, which is a lifestyle disease, can be reversed through diet, primarily by adding in more complex carbohydrates and fiber. Harvard Health, "Healthy Lifestyle Can Prevent Diabetes (and Even Reverse It)," October 20, 2023, https://www.health.harvard.edu/blog/healthy-lifestyle-can-prevent-diabetes-and-even-reverse-it-2018090514698.

10. N Wright et al., "The BROAD Study: A Randomised Controlled Trial Using a Whole Food Plant-based Diet in the Community for Obesity, Ischaemic Heart Disease or Diabetes," *Nutrition & Diabetes* 7, no. 3 (March 20, 2017): e256, https://www.ncbi.nlm.nih.gov/pmc/articles/PMC5380896/

11. Ayurvedic medicine is a form of traditional medicine that hails from India. "Ayurvedic Medicine: In Depth," NCCIH, n.d., https://www.nccih.nih.gov/health/ayurvedic-medicine-in-depth.

12. "Ojas: A Cookbook - Little Green," Little Green, February 3, 2020, https://littlegreen.me/product/ojas-a-cookbook/

13. "The Longevity Diet - Valter Longo," Valter Longo, August 2, 2020, https://www.valterlongo.com/the-longevity-diet/

14. Ontario, Canada, where an 11-year old cancer patient – "J.J." — with acute lymphoblastic leukemia (ALL), was eating an extreme diet from a group based in Florida. Ian Mitchell, Juliet R Guichon, and Sam Wong, "Caring for Children, Focusing on Children," *Paediatrics & Child Health* 20, no. 6 (August 1, 2015): 293–95, https://www.ncbi.nlm.nih.gov/pmc/articles/PMC4578466/

15. An angry op-ed in *StatNews* entitled 'No food isn't medicine,' attempted to course-correct the influence of these harmful diet approaches, but was overly simplistic and reductionist, Dylan MacKay, "Hey, Hippocrates: Food Isn'T Medicine. It's Just Food," *STAT*, August 4, 2017, https://www.statnews.com/2017/08/07/food-medicine-hippocrates/

16. Amitha Kalaichandran , Shuang Esther Shan The Canadian Press, "Nutrition a Challenge for Many Cancer Patients Navigating the 'Cancer-specific' Diet," *Toronto Star*, February 28, 2017, https://www.thestar.com/news/world/nutrition-a-challenge-for-many-cancer-patients-navigating-the-cancer-specific-diet/article_24616ee5-6f30-5fa2-9487-454ac8ee08a2.html.

17. In 1994, at the age of 26, Longo found an issue with a paper published in the 1950s, which was still influencing the work of many researchers. It described the lifespan of yeast, but measured aging by counting the number of daughter cells generated by the mother cell – assuming if the mother produced 25 daughter cells it would mean it reached a lifespan of 25. K.A. Steinkraus, M. Kaeberlein, and B.K. Kennedy, "Replicative Aging in Yeast: The Means to the End," *Annual Review of Cell and Developmental Biology* 24, no. 1 (November 1, 2008): 29–54, https://www.ncbi.nlm.nih.gov/pmc/articles/PMC2730916/

18. Mona Wanda Schmidt et al., "Effects of Intermittent Fasting on Quality of Life Tolerance of Chemotherapy in Patients With Gynecological Cancers: Study Protocol of a Randomized-controlled Multi-center Trial," *Frontiers in Oncology* 13 (July 19, 2023), https://www.ncbi.nlm.nih.gov/pmc/articles/PMC10396395/

19. Remembering that a hallmark of cancer, as per a famous paper authored by Douglas Hanahan and Robert Weinberg in *Cell* (1980 but updated in 2011), includes cells unresponsive to anti-growth signals. Douglas Hanahan and Robert A. Weinberg, "Hallmarks of Cancer: The Next Generation," *Cell* 144, no. 5 (March 1, 2011): 646–74, https://pubmed.ncbi.nlm.nih.gov/21376230/

20. Stefanie De Groot et al., "Fasting Mimicking Diet as an Adjunct to Neoadjuvant Chemotherapy for Breast Cancer in the Multicentre Randomized Phase 2 DIRECT Trial," *Nature Communications* 11, no. 1 (June 23, 2020), https://www.nature.com/articles/s41467-020-16138-3.

21. Physician-writer Siddhartha Mukherjee has explored other ways diet might benefit cancer patients. His lab looked at low-carbohydrate ketogenic diets in combination with a cancer drug, effectively to decrease the amount of insulin released. For some cancers they tested, tumor growth seemed to be hindered by diet alone – but for other cancers, like leukemia, the cancer grew faster on the diet but was kept at bay with the combination of diet and drug. Hannah Devlin, "Top Oncologist to Study Effect of

Diet on Cancer Drugs," *The Guardian*, July 6, 2018, https://www.theguardian.com/science/2018/jul/06/top-oncologist-to-study-effect-of-diet-on-cancer-drugs.

22. A review published in the December 2019 issue of the *New England Journal of Medicine* suggested that researchers like Longo and Mukherjee could be on to something: "Evidence is accumulating that eating in a 6-hour period and fasting for 18 hours can trigger a metabolic switch from glucose-based to ketone-based energy, with increased stress resistance, increased longevity, and a decreased incidence of diseases, including cancer and obesity." Rafael De Cabo and Mark P. Mattson, "Effects of Intermittent Fasting on Health, Aging, and Disease," *New England Journal of Medicine* 381, no. 26 (December 26, 2019): 2541–51, https://www.nejm.org/doi/full/10.1056/NEJMra1905136.

23. Newmark's book, "ADHD Without Drugs," can be found here: https://www.goodreads.com/book/show/8677234-adhd-without-drugs---a-guide-to-the-natural-care-of-children-with-adhd.

24. "Attention Deficit Hyperactivity Disorder (ADHD)," n.d., https://www.aap.org/en/patient-care/attention-deficit-hyperactivity-disorder-adhd/

25. Farsad-Naeimi Et Al 2020 - Sugar Consumption, Sugar Sweetened Beverages and Attention Deficit Hyperactivity Disorder: A Systematic Review and Meta-analysis," n.d., https://www.fabresearch.org/viewItem.php?id=13566&listId=988&categoryId=&navPageId=989

26. Sara N. Bleich and Kelsey A. Vercammen, "The Negative Impact of Sugar-sweetened Beverages on Children's Health: An Update of the Literature," BMC Obesity 5, no. 1 (February 20, 2018), https://bmcobes.biomedcentral.com/articles/10.1186/s40608-017-0178-9.

27. M Zheng et al., "Sugar-sweetened Beverages Consumption in Relation to Changes in Body Fatness Over 6 and 12 Years Among 9-year-old Children: The European Youth Heart Study," European Journal of Clinical Nutrition 68, no. 1 (November 27, 2013): 77–83, https://www.nature.com/articles/ejcn2013243.

28. Felice N. Jacka et al., "A Randomised Controlled Trial of Dietary Improvement for Adults With Major Depression (the 'SMILES' Trial)," *BMC Medicine* 15, no. 1 (January 30, 2017), https://bmcmedicine.biomedcentral.com/articles/10.1186/s12916-017-0791-y

29. Well over 95% of the neurotransmitter serotonin, which is responsible for regulating appetite, moods, pain experience, and sleep is made in the gastrointestinal tract. Natalie Terry and Kara Gross Margolis, "Serotonergic Mechanisms Regulating the GI Tract: Experimental Evidence and Therapeutic Relevance," in *Handbook of Experimental Pharmacology*, 2016, 319–42, https://www.ncbi.nlm.nih.gov/pmc/articles/PMC5526216/#:~:text=Serotonin%20(5%2Dhydroxytryptamine%3B%205,%2C%20paracrine%2C%20and%20endocrine%20actions

30. More generally, the field of "nutritional psychiatry" is gaining ground as it recognizes that our mood responds to the fuel we feed our brains. Eva Selhub MD, "Nutritional

Psychiatry: Your Brain on Food," Harvard Health, September 18, 2022, https://www.health.harvard.edu/blog/nutritional-psychiatry-your-brain-on-food-201511168626

31. Marco Colizzi, Antonio Lasalvia, and Mirella Ruggeri, "Prevention and Early Intervention in Youth Mental Health: Is It Time for a Multidisciplinary and Trans-diagnostic Model for Care?," International Journal of Mental Health Systems 14, no. 1 (March 24, 2020), https://ijmhs.biomedcentral.com/articles/10.1186/s13033-020-00356-9.

32. Patrick D McGorry and Cristina Mei, "Early Intervention in Youth Mental Health: Progress and Future Directions," Evidence-Based Mental Health 21, no. 4 (October 23, 2018): 182–84, https://mentalhealth.bmj.com/content/21/4/182.

33. Margaret M Barry et al., "A Systematic Review of the Effectiveness of Mental Health Promotion Interventions for Young People in Low and Middle Income Countries," BMC Public Health 13, no. 1 (September 11, 2013), https://bmcpublichealth.biomedcentral.com/articles/10.1186/1471-2458-13-835.

34. Akash Kumar et al., "Gut Microbiota in Anxiety and Depression: Unveiling the Relationships and Management Options," Pharmaceuticals 16, no. 4 (April 9, 2023): 565, https://www.ncbi.nlm.nih.gov/pmc/articles/PMC10146621/

35. Sundus Khalid, Claire M. Williams, and Shirley A. Reynolds, "Is There an Association Between Diet and Depression in Children and Adolescents? A Systematic Review," British Journal of Nutrition 116, no. 12 (December 28, 2016): 2097–2108, https://www.cambridge.org/core/journals/british-journal-of-nutrition/article/is-there-an-association-between-diet-and-depression-in-children-and-adolescents-a-systematic-review/D7CCDB619E786B8B34940D87E344C179.

36. Siyu Wang et al., "From Gut to Brain: Understanding the Role of Microbiota in Inflammatory Bowel Disease," Frontiers in Immunology 15 (March 21, 2024), https://www.frontiersin.org/journals/immunology/articles/10.3389/fimmu.2024.1384270/full

37. Akash Kumar et al., "Gut Microbiota in Anxiety and Depression: Unveiling the Relationships and Management Options," Pharmaceuticals 16, no. 4 (April 9, 2023): 565, https://www.mdpi.com/1424-8247/16/4/565.

38. The production of neurotransmitters like serotonin—which leads us away from feelings of depression—is influenced by these good bacteria functioning well. Foods rich in probiotics (like yogurt) and fermented foods (miso, fermented olives, kombucha and kimchi, all of which are rich in probiotics) both promote gut health. Changing one's diet more broadly (the Mediterranean Diet, for example) can also help make the gut more conducive to flourishing of good bacteria, and lead two to three-times reduction in depression. Cleveland Clinic Medical Professional, "Probiotics," Cleveland Clinic, n.d., https://my.clevelandclinic.org/health/treatments/14598-probiotics. Giuseppe Merra et al., "Influence of Mediterranean Diet on Human Gut Microbiota," Nutrients 13, no. 1 (December 22, 2020): 7, https://www.ncbi.nlm.nih.gov/pmc/articles/PMC7822000/

39. Bryant Terry, the resident chef at the Museum of the African Diaspora in San Francisco. "MoAD Chef-in-Residence — Bryant Terry," Bryant Terry, n.d., https://www.bryant-terry.com/moad-chef-in-residence.
40. Terry's 2015 TedMED talk about veganism and political change cites the 1969 "free breakfast for children program" run by the Black Panthers and primarily served poor Black children. TEDMED, "Stirring up Political Change From the Kitchen," August 16, 2016, https://www.youtube.com/watch?v=cL8e9xM9zoA.
41. Dariush Mozaffarian, Jerold Mande, and Renata Micha, "Food Is Medicine—The Promise and Challenges of Integrating Food and Nutrition Into Health Care," JAMA Internal Medicine 179, no. 6 (June 1, 2019): 793, https://jamanetwork.com/journals/jamainternalmedicine/article-abstract/2730764
42. .University of California San Francisco, "The UCSF Guide to Healthy and Happy Eating | UCSF Magazine," The UCSF Guide to Healthy and Happy Eating | UCSF Magazine, September 15, 2020, https://www.ucsf.edu/news/2019/06/414696/ucsf-guide-healthy-and-happy-eating.
43. And while supplements are a divisive topic, the best overview is from Annals of Internal Medicine. In summary, there is evidence for some, not for others, and it's a balance of assessment of quality, evidence, and cost. Safi U. Khan et al., "Effects of Nutritional Supplements and Dietary Interventions on Cardiovascular Outcomes," Annals of Internal Medicine 171, no. 3 (July 9, 2019): 190, https://www.acpjournals.org/doi/10.7326/M19-0341.

Chapter 7: Faith, Spirit, Magic...Woo?
1. The tweet came from a woman in Los Angeles named Kaye Steinsapir, a 43-year old lawyer and mother of three. "x.com," X (Formerly Twitter), n.d., https://twitter.com/KayeEllen17/status/1355981636211408898?s=20.
2. "Bernadette Soubirous," Bienvenue Au Sanctuaire Notre-Dame De Lourdes, September 16, 2022, https://www.lourdes-france.org/en/bernadette-soubirous/
3. On May 10, 1948, Jeanne Fretel arrived at Lourdes in a comatose state as a result of tuberculosis peritonitis. After being given some Eucharist (the disc shaped wafer used in Christian mass), Jeanne woke from her coma and declared herself cured. The Catholic church recognized her recovery in 1950 to be a genuine miracle. "Five Miracles in History," Sky HISTORY TV Channel, n.d., https://www.history.co.uk/article/five-miracles-in-history.
4. Since Jeanne, the church has documented almost 70 miracles in Lourdes as of 2017, and in 2014 a group of scientists and doctors from Lyon and Maryland reviewed hundreds of these cases and concluded that some simply defy scientific explanation. B. Francois, E. M. Sternberg, and E. Fee, "The Lourdes Medical Cures Revisited," Journal of the History of Medicine and Allied Sciences 69, no. 1 (July 27, 2012): 135–62, https://pubmed.ncbi.nlm.nih.gov/22843835/
5. In 2024, the Pope deemed Carlo Acutis the first millennial saint, due to his ability to heal. Alexandra E. Petri, "Pope Francis Clears Way for Carlo Acutis to Become

First Millennial Saint," *The New York Times*, May 24, 2024, https://www.nytimes.com/2024/05/23/world/europe/carlo-acutis-saint-catholic.html.

6. C.S. Lewis, who is perhaps most known for writing the Chronicles of Narnia, wrote a treatise on faith-based miracles called simply *Miracles: A Preliminary Study*, in which he interrogates the possibility of miracles, a key part of Christian faith (most crucially in the Corinthians Book 1 15:13-14). C.S. Lewis Institute, "C.S. Lewis on Miracles: Why They Are Possible And Significant - C.S. Lewis Institute," May 27, 2022, https://www.cslewisinstitute.org/resources/c-s-lewis-on-miracles-why-they-are-possible-and-significant/

7. A 2012 *New York Times* article describes a concept called "Thin Places," which refers to "locales where the distance between heaven and earth collapses and we're able to catch glimpses of the divine, or the transcendent or, as I like to think of it, the Infinite Whatever." https://www.nytimes.com/2012/03/11/travel/thin-places-where-we-are-jolted-out-of-old-ways-of-seeing-the-world.html.

8. And in her book by the same name Jordan Kisner writes: *"thin places' comes from Celtic folklore: that 'the barrier between the physical world and the spiritual world wears thin and become porous."* n+1 Shop, "Thin Places, by Jordan Kisner," n.d., https://shop.nplusonemag.com/products/thin-places-by-jordan-kisner.

9. I saw a white rabbit...and took a photo for Instagram. ☺

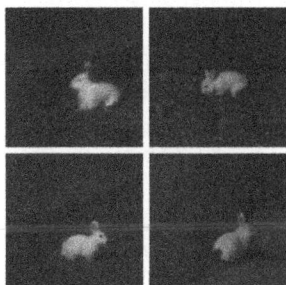

10. Clarissa Romez et al., "Case Report of Instantaneous Resolution of Juvenile Macular Degeneration Blindness After Proximal Intercessory Prayer," *Explore* 17, no. 1 (January 1, 2021): 79–83, https://pubmed.ncbi.nlm.nih.gov/32234287/.

11. Clarissa Romez, David Zaritzky, and Joshua W. Brown, "Case Report of Gastroparesis Healing: 16 Years of a Chronic Syndrome Resolved After Proximal Intercessory Prayer," *Complementary Therapies in Medicine* 43 (April 1, 2019): 289–94, https://pubmed.ncbi.nlm.nih.gov/30935546/.

12. L Leibovici, "Effects of Remote, Retroactive Intercessory Prayer on Outcomes in Patients With Bloodstream Infection: Randomised Controlled Trial," *BMJ. British Medical Journal* 323, no. 7327 (December 22, 2001): 1450–51, https://pubmed.ncbi.nlm.nih.gov/11751349/

13. Herbert Benson et al., "Study of the Therapeutic Effects of Intercessory Prayer (STEP) in Cardiac Bypass Patients: A Multicenter Randomized Trial of Uncertainty

and Certainty of Receiving Intercessory Prayer," *American Heart Journal/"the %American Heart Journal* 151, no. 4 (April 1, 2006): 934–42, https://pubmed.ncbi.nlm.nih.gov/16569567/

14. More prominently, a Cochrane review from 2009 examined the question of intercessory prayer and found no beneficial effect compared with no prayer. The study, however, also caught a wave of criticism for failing to "live up to the high standards required of Cochrane reviews." Leanne Roberts, Irshad Ahmed, and Andrew Davison, "Intercessory Prayer for the Alleviation of Ill Health," *Cochrane Library*, April 15, 2009, https://pubmed.ncbi.nlm.nih.gov/19370557/

15. Christina Puchalski In her book, *Making Healthcare Whole.* "Making Health Care Whole: Integrating Spirituality Into Patient Care," Goodreads, n.d., https://www.goodreads.com/book/show/9685244-making-health-care-whole

16. "Clinical FICA Tool," GWish | GW School of Medicine and Health Sciences, n.d., https://gwish.smhs.gwu.edu/programs/transforming-practice-health-settings/clinical-fica-tool.

17. Elizabeth Gilbert's *"Eat, Pray, Love"*. "Eat, Pray, Love," Goodreads, n.d., https://www.goodreads.com/book/show/19501.Eat_Pray_Love.

18. Tirth Dave et al., "Sushruta: The Father of Indian Surgical History," *Plastic and Reconstructive Surgery. Global Open* 12, no. 4 (April 1, 2024): e5715, https://www.ncbi.nlm.nih.gov/pmc/articles/PMC11000756/

19. Reiki is a form of therapeutic touch with spiritual origins. The history of Reiki originates in Japan, as a founded by spiritual aspirant, Mikao Usui in the early 1920s. "Where Does Reiki Come From? | Taking Charge of Your Wellbeing," Taking Charge of Your Wellbeing, n.d., https://www.takingcharge.csh.umn.edu/where-reiki-from.

20. Over 800 hospitals in the U.S., including the likes of Johns Hopkins Hospital and Massachusetts General Hospital now offer Reiki and therapeutic touch. Linda Fehrs Lmt, "Hospital-Based Reiki and Documentation | Massage Professionals Update," Massage Professionals Update, February 5, 2024, https://www.integrativehealthcare.org/mt/hospital-based-reiki-and-documentation.

21. Maxime Billot et al., "Reiki Therapy for Pain, Anxiety and Quality of Life," *BMJ Supportive & Palliative Care*, April 4, 2019, bmjspcare-001775, https://spcare.bmj.com/content/9/4/434.

22. David E. McManus, "Reiki Is Better Than Placebo and Has Broad Potential as a Complementary Health Therapy," *Journal of Evidence-Based Complementary & Alternative Medicine* 22, no. 4 (September 5, 2017): 1051–57, https://pubmed.ncbi.nlm.nih.gov/28874060/

23. "Braving the Wilderness - Brené Brown," Brené Brown, July 13, 2023, https://brenebrown.com/book/braving-the-wilderness/

24. Laura Lynne Jackson: *The Light Between Us.* "Book: The Light Between Us," Laura Lynne Jackson, May 17, 2024, https://lauralynnejackson.com/book-the-light-between-us/

25. 2018 YouTube talk with Jackson and Mark Epstein. Rubin Museum of Art, "Psychic Medium Laura Lynne Jackson + Dr. Mark Epstein," February 23, 2018, https://www.youtube.com/watch?v=I7oJ67l_N_Q.

26. Jackson's work with the Forever Family Foundation. Forever Family Foundation, "Forever Family Foundation," n.d., https://www.foreverfamilyfoundation.org/site/page/28.

27. Barrett Swanson's *Atavist* article on Lily Dale. Barrett Swanson and Barrett Swanson, "Lost in Summerland," The Atavist Magazine, January 30, 2024, https://magazine.atavist.com/lost-in-summerland-lily-dale-psychics-mediums-spiritualism/

28. Netflix *Surviving Death*. "Surviving Death: Now Streaming on Netflix - Division of Perceptual Studies," Division of Perceptual Studies, February 2, 2024, https://med.virginia.edu/perceptual-studies/dops-media/surviving-death-now-streaming-on-netflix/

29. Jim Tuckers book *Return to Life*. "Return to Life | Dr. Jim B. Tucker," n.d., https://www.jimbtucker.com/return-to-life/

30. The Bible's Philippians 4:13: *"I can do all things through Christ who strengthens me"* reflects this. "Philippians 4:13 (NIV)," Bible Gateway, n.d., https://www.biblegateway.com/passage/?search=Philippians%204%3A13&version=NIV.

31. Hindu spiritual text, the Upanishads, provides a wealth of wisdom, insight, and metaphor.

32. Joshua J. Mark and Don Kennedy, "Upanishads," *World History Encyclopedia*, July 18, 2022, https://www.worldhistory.org/Upanishads/

33. "Indian Philosophy," Google Books, n.d., https://books.google.com/books?id=cBNbDwAAQBAJ&pg=PA58&lpg=PA58&dq.

Chapter 8: Movement

1. Katie Maguire and Katie Maguire, "Barry Jay's Inspiring Journey From Addict to Barry's Bootcamp Founder," Well+Good, November 9, 2022, https://www.wellandgood.com/barry-jays-inspiring-journey-from-addict-to-barrys-bootcamp-founder/

2. Lisa S. Gorham et al., "Involvement in Sports, Hippocampal Volume, and Depressive Symptoms in Children," *Biological Psychiatry. Cognitive Neuroscience and Neuroimaging* 4, no. 5 (May 1, 2019): 484–92, https://www.sciencedirect.com/science/article/abs/pii/S2451902219300254?via%3Dihub.

3. Molly C. Easterlin et al., "Association of Team Sports Participation With Long-term Mental Health Outcomes Among Individuals Exposed to Adverse Childhood Experiences," *JAMA Pediatrics* 173, no. 7 (July 1, 2019): 681, https://pubmed.ncbi.nlm.nih.gov/31135890/

4. A 2013 Cochrane review of 37 trials, which found exercise as effective as medication for depression, though the few number of trials included was a limitation. Gary M Cooney et al., "Exercise for Depression," *Cochrane Library* 2013, no. 9 (September 12, 2013), https://pubmed.ncbi.nlm.nih.gov/24026850/

5. Kassia S Weston, Ulrik Wisløff, and Jeff S Coombes, "High-intensity Interval Training in Patients With Lifestyle-induced Cardiometabolic Disease: A Systematic Review and Meta-analysis," *British Journal of Sports Medicine* 48, no. 16 (October 21, 2013): 1227–34, https://bjsm.bmj.com/content/48/16/1227.

6. Yaoshan Dun et al., "High-intensity Interval Training Improves Metabolic Syndrome and Body Composition in Outpatient Cardiac Rehabilitation Patients With Myocardial Infarction," *Cardiovascular Diabetology* 18, no. 1 (August 14, 2019), https://www.ncbi.nlm.nih.gov/pmc/articles/PMC6694483/.

7. "Study in Mice Helps Explain How Exercise Protects Against Heart Disease | NHLBI, NIH," NHLBI, NIH, November 17, 2019, https://www.nhlbi.nih.gov/news/2019/study-mice-helps-explain-how-exercise-protects-against-heart-disease.

8. Ramires Alsamir Tibana and Nuno Manuel Frade De Sousa, "Are Extreme Conditioning Programmes Effective and Safe? A Narrative Review of High-intensity Functional Training Methods Research Paradigms and Findings," *BMJ Open Sport & Exercise Medicine* 4, no. 1 (November 1, 2018): e000435, https://pubmed.ncbi.nlm.nih.gov/30498574/.

9. Dana G Smith, "More Than Endorphins: The Brain Benefits of Exercise | Elemental," *Medium*, December 9, 2021, https://elemental.medium.com/this-is-what-exercise-does-to-your-brain-7068b6a1af81. "How Can Exercise Affect Hearing Loss? | Connect Hearing," n.d., https://www.connecthearing.com.au/blog/hearing-and-hearing-loss/exercise-hearing-loss/.

10. Monalisha Sahu and Josyula G Prasuna, "Twin Studies: A Unique Epidemiological Tool," *Indian Journal of Community Medicine/Indian Journal of Community Medicine* 41, no. 3 (January 1, 2016): 177, https://www.ncbi.nlm.nih.gov/pmc/articles/PMC4919929/

11. Fraizer Rehab Institute in Kentucky, led by Dr. Susan Harkema, who is a leader in this area. "Susan Harkema, Ph.D. — Kentucky Spinal Cord Injury Research Center," n.d., https://louisville.edu/kscirc/basic-research/faculty-1/susan-harkema.

12. Jessica Harthcock and Utilize Health (utilizehealth.com), of which she serves as Co-Founder and Chief Executive Officer. "Utilize Health – Better Care Together," n.d., https://www.utilizehealth.com/.

13. Kathy Ehrich Dowd, "Michael Phelps Opens up About ADHD Struggles," *Sports Illustrated*, November 5, 2019, https://www.si.com/olympics/2017/04/28/michael-phelps-opens-about-adhd-struggles-teacher-told-me-id-never-amount-anything.

14. "John Ratey M.D. - Books," n.d., http://www.johnratey.com/Books.php.

15. Afton M. Bierlich et al., "An Evaluation of the German Version of the Sensory Perception Quotient From an Expert by Experience Perspective," *Frontiers in Psychology* 15 (February 29, 2024), https://www.frontiersin.org/journals/psychology/articles/10.3389/fpsyg.2024.1252277/full.

16. Other high-quality reviews – from Chile to Denmark to Israel -- have reported that short-term aerobic exercise can improve ADHD symptoms. Yaira Barranco-Ruiz et al., "Interventions Based on Mind–Body Therapies for the Improvement of Attention-

Deficit/Hyperactivity Disorder Symptoms in Youth: A Systematic Review," *Medicina* 55, no. 7 (June 30, 2019): 325, https://www.mdpi.com/1648-9144/55/7/325.

17. Feilong Zhu et al., "Comparative Effectiveness of Various Physical Exercise Interventions on Executive Functions and Related Symptoms in Children and Adolescents With Attention Deficit Hyperactivity Disorder: A Systematic Review and Network Meta-analysis," *Frontiers in Public Health* 11 (March 24, 2023), https://www.frontiersin.org/journals/public-health/articles/10.3389/fpubh.2023.1133727/full.

18. Urbina, S., Suarez-Manzano, S., Pozo-Cruz, B. D., & Pozo-Cruz, J. D. (2015). Acute and chronic effect of physical activity on cognition and behaviour in young people with ADHD: A systematic review of intervention studies. *International Journal of Behavioral Nutrition and Physical Activity*, 12(1), 1-15. https://ijbnpa.biomedcentral.com/articles/10.1186/s12966-020-00959-y

19. Xie, Y., Gao, X., Song, Y., Zhu, X., Chen, M., Yang, L., & Ren, Y. (2021). Effectiveness of physical activity intervention on ADHD symptoms: A systematic review and meta-analysis. *Frontiers in Psychiatry*, 12, 706625. https://www.frontiersin.org/journals/psychiatry/articles/10.3389/fpsyt.2021.706625/full

20. Mark L. Wolraich et al., "Clinical Practice Guideline for the Diagnosis, Evaluation, and Treatment of Attention-Deficit/Hyperactivity Disorder in Children and Adolescents," *Pediatrics* 144, no. 4 (October 1, 2019), https://www.ncbi.nlm.nih.gov/pmc/articles/PMC7067282/

21. E. Wesley Ely, "The ABCDEF Bundle: Science and Philosophy of How ICU Liberation Serves Patients and Families," *Critical Care Medicine* 45, no. 2 (February 1, 2017): 321–30, https://www.ncbi.nlm.nih.gov/pmc/articles/PMC5830123/

22. John P. Kress et al., "Daily Interruption of Sedative Infusions in Critically Ill Patients Undergoing Mechanical Ventilation," *New England Journal of Medicine* 342, no. 20 (May 18, 2000): 1471–77, https://www.nejm.org/doi/full/10.1056/NEJM200005183422002.

23. Over the subsequent years, additional research showed that sedation has its own side effects like cognitive issues, which are often memory deficits. Katherine Rowe and Simon Fletcher, "Sedation in the Intensive Care Unit," *Continuing Education in Anaesthesia, Critical Care & Pain* 8, no. 2 (April 1, 2008): 50–55, https://academic.oup.com/bjaed/article/8/2/50/338650.

24. Lara Dhingra et al., "Cognitive Effects and Sedation," *Pain Medicine* 16, no. suppl 1 (October 1, 2015): S37–43, https://pubmed.ncbi.nlm.nih.gov/26461075/

25. Eddy Fan et al., "Physical Complications in Acute Lung Injury Survivors," *Critical Care Medicine* 42, no. 4 (April 1, 2014): 849–59, https://www.ncbi.nlm.nih.gov/pmc/articles/PMC3959239/

26. Beth Wieczorek et al., "PICU up!: Impact of a Quality Improvement Intervention to Promote Early Mobilization in Critically Ill Children*," *Pediatric Critical Care Medicine* 17, no. 12 (December 1, 2016): e559–66, https://journals.lww.com/pccmjournal/Abstract/2016/12000/PICU_Up___Impact_of_a_Quality_Improvement.21.aspx.

27. Erwin Ista et al., "Mobilization Practices in Critically Ill Children: A European Point Prevalence Study (EU PARK-PICU)," *Critical Care* 24, no. 1 (June 24, 2020), https://ccforum.biomedcentral.com/articles/10.1186/s13054-020-02988-2.

28. Kalaichandran, Amitha. "When Exercise Comes to the Hospital's Intensive Care Unit," https://undark.org/2020/01/22/exercise-hospital-icu/

Chapter 9: System Overdrive

1. Brené Brown discusses "common enemy intimacy," where a sense of community forms, through mutual agreement, around a person who is perceived as a threat. Galen Emanuele, "Common Enemy Intimacy & Relating to Others Through Negativity." Team Culture & Leadership Keynotes, November 24, 2020, https://galenemanuele.com/blog/relate-negativity.

2. William O. Cooper et al., "Association of Coworker Reports About Unprofessional Behavior by Surgeons With Surgical Complications in Their Patients," *JAMA Surgery* 154, no. 9 (September 1, 2019): 828, https://jamanetwork.com/journals/jamasurgery/article-abstract/2736337.

3. Other research shows that even witnessing incivility or bullying can negatively impact performance—I'd noticed this among my co-residents. Daniel Katz et al., "Exposure to Incivility Hinders Clinical Performance in a Simulated Operative Crisis," *BMJ Quality & Safety* 28, no. 9 (May 31, 2019): 750–57, https://qualitysafety.bmj.com/content/28/9/750.

4. "'Leadership Shapes Culture': Addressing Doctor Burnout, Depression Must Start at the Top, Doctors Say | CBC Radio," CBC, October 22, 2018, https://www.cbc.ca/radio/thecurrent/the-current-for-october-18-2018-1.4867922/leadership-shapes-culture-addressing-doctor-burnout-depression-must-start-at-the-top-doctors-say-1.4867926.

5. Amitha Kalaichandran MD, "In America, Becoming a Doctor Can Prove Fatal," BostonGlobe.Com, March 15, 2019, https://www.bostonglobe.com/ideas/2019/03/15/america-becoming-doctor-can-prove-fatal/u3x4xfPC9VR2zSCnKArgYM/story.html.

6. I pitched the *Boston Globe* a story about bullying and abuse in residency programs in North America. "Med School Bullying Takes a New Form," *BostonGlobe.Com*, March 18, 2019, https://www.bostonglobe.com/opinion/letters/2019/03/18/med-school-bullying-takes-new-form/iRQImyJAeRz9r1x3rPYtvN/story.html.

7. Mark Shapiro MD, "Amitha Kalaichandran on Bullying in Medicine," Apple Podcasts, April 10, 2019, https://podcasts.apple.com/gb/podcast/amitha-kalaichandran-on-bullying-in-medicine/id993287419?i=1000434660400.

8. Lawrence R. Huntoon, "Tactics Characteristic of Sham Peer Review," *Journal of American Physicians and Surgeons*, season-03 2009, 64, https://www.jpands.org/vol14no3/huntoon.pdf.

9. David Yamada, "Workplace Bullying, Mobbing, and Abuse – Page 2 – Minding the Workplace," Minding the Workplace, n.d., https://newworkplace.wordpress.com/category/workplace-bullying-mobbing-and-abuse/page/2/.

10. David Yamada, "'Puppet Master' Bullying Vs. Genuine Mobbing at Work," Minding the Workplace, November 22, 2014, https://newworkplace.wordpress.com/2012/01/23/puppet-master-bullying-vs-genuine-mobbing-at-work/

11. Jennifer Freyd. "What Is DARVO?," n.d., https://dynamic.uoregon.edu/jjf/defineDARVO.html.

12. David Yamada, "Workplace Bullying, DARVO, and Aggressors Claiming Victim Status," Minding the Workplace, March 7, 2019, https://newworkplace.wordpress.com/2019/03/07/workplace-bullying-darvo-and-aggressors-claiming-victim-status/

13. Uché Blackstock, "Why Black Doctors Like Me Are Leaving Faculty Positions in Academic Medical Centers," STAT, May 4, 2021, https://www.statnews.com/2020/01/16/black-doctors-leaving-faculty-positions-academic-medical-centers/

14. Elisabeth Mahase, "Bawa-Garba: 'At Rock Bottom I Had to Remember Why I Wanted to Be a Doctor,'" BMJ. British Medical Journal, June 7, 2019, l4130, https://www.bmj.com/content/365/bmj.l4130.

15. Dereck W. Paul et al., "Beyond a Moment — Reckoning With Our History and Embracing Antiracism in Medicine," New England Journal of Medicine 383, no. 15 (October 8, 2020): 1404–6, https://www.nejm.org/doi/full/10.1056/NEJMp2021812.

16. Robin Klein et al., "Association of Gender With Learner Assessment in Graduate Medical Education," JAMA Network Open 3, no. 7 (July 16, 2020): e2010888, https://jamanetwork.com/journals/jamanetworkopen/fullarticle/2768342.

17. Emily Lawler, elawler@mlive.com, "Michigan to Require All Medical Professionals to Undergo Implicit Bias Training," Mlive, March 6, 2023, https://www.mlive.com/public-interest/2020/07/michigan-to-require-all-medical-professionals-to-undergo-implicit-bias-training.html.

18. Kemi M. Doll and Charles R. Thomas, "Structural Solutions for the Rarest of the Rare — Underrepresented-Minority Faculty in Medical Subspecialties," New England Journal of Medicine/˜the œNew England Journal of Medicine 383, no. 3 (July 16, 2020): 283–85, https://www.nejm.org/doi/full/10.1056/NEJMms2003544.

19. Gabrielle Horne, "Physician, Heal Thyself: The Potential Crisis of Conscience in Canadian Medicine," The Globe and Mail, May 31, 2019, https://www.theglobeandmail.com/opinion/article-physician-heal-thyself-the-potential-crisis-of-conscience-in/. TEDx Talks, "Using Medical Research Tools to Survive Workplace Bullying | Gabrielle Horne | TEDxDalhousieU," April 12, 2019, https://www.youtube.com/watch?v=qUI8aJONrM8.

20. "Gabrielle Horne - Successful Legal Battle Over Workplace Bullying," Gabrielle Horne, October 19, 2020, http://www.gabriellehorne.com/

21. Eve Seguin wrote in *University Affairs* in 2016, *"Mobbing is social murder* and, by definition, people cannot survive their own murder. "Academic Mobbing, or How to Become Campus Tormentors — University Affairs," University Affairs, February 6, 2019, https://universityaffairs.ca/opinion/in-my-opinion/academic-mobbing-become-campus-tormentors/

22. Robin Klein et al., "Gender Bias in Resident Assessment in Graduate Medical Education: Review of the Literature," Journal of General Internal Medicine 34, no. 5 (April 16, 2019): 712–19, https://www.ncbi.nlm.nih.gov/pmc/articles/PMC6502889/

23. Tiffany Champagne-Langabeer and Andrew L. Hedges, "Physician Gender as a Source of Implicit Bias Affecting Clinical Decision-making Processes: A Scoping Review," BMC Medical Education 21, no. 1 (March 19, 2021), https://bmcmededuc.biomedcentral.com/articles/10.1186/s12909-021-02601-2

24. Carl Kelly, a family medicine resident at University of British Columbia. "Disabled Doctor: Just How Much Should Damage to Dignity Cost?," *CBC*, September 27, 2015, https://www.cbc.ca/news/canada/british-columbia/disabled-doctor-just-how-much-should-damage-to-dignity-cost-1.3245372

25. In 2018 on Twitter, a woman named Ruth McCrea tagged me in a story on CBC radio on bullying in medicine and hospitals, in which she detailed a horrific experience with her daughter, Minimosa (Mini) at the children's hospital I had been training in. As of 2024, the tweet was pulled down, but Mini's obituary remains: https://ottawacitizen.remembering.ca/obituary/minimosa-mccrea-1071876823

26. In May 2019, a landmark investigation by Ellen Gabler in the *New York Times* exposed a troubling situation at North Carolina Children's Hospital. Ellen Gabler, "Doctors Were Alarmed: 'Would I Have My Children Have Surgery Here?,'" *The New York Times,* June 18, 2019, https://www.nytimes.com/interactive/2019/05/30/us/children-heart-surgery-cardiac.html.

27. "Moral Distress, Moral Residue, and the Crescendo Effect," PubMed, n.d., https://pubmed.ncbi.nlm.nih.gov/20120853/

28. Amy Edmondson, "The Fearless Organization: Creating Psychological Safety in the Workplace for Learning, Innovation, and Growth - Book - Faculty & Research - Harvard Business School," n.d., https://www.hbs.edu/faculty/Pages/item.aspx?num=54851.

29. "The Fearless Organization," n.d., https://fearlessorganizationscan.com/the-fearless-organization.

30. A C Edmondson, "Learning From Failure in Health Care: Frequent Opportunities, Pervasive Barriers," BMJ Quality & Safety 13, no. suppl_2 (December 1, 2004): ii3–9, https://www.ncbi.nlm.nih.gov/pmc/articles/PMC1765808/

31. Leslie A Curry et al., "Influencing Organisational Culture to Improve Hospital Performance in Care of Patients With Acute Myocardial Infarction: A Mixed-methods Intervention Study," *BMJ Quality & Safety* 27, no. 3 (November 3, 2017): 207–17, https://pubmed.ncbi.nlm.nih.gov/29101292/.

32. Erika Linnander et al., "Changing Hospital Organisational Culture for Improved Patient Outcomes: Developing and Implementing the Leadership Saves Lives Intervention," *BMJ Quality & Safety* 30, no. 6 (July 16, 2020): 475–83, https://qualitysafety.bmj.com/content/30/6/475.

33. American College of Physicians, "Impact of Race on the Professional Lives of Physicians of African Descent Annals of Internal Medicine, n.d., https://www.acpjournals.org/doi/abs/10.7326/0003-4819-146-1-200701020-00008?journalCode=aim.

34. Melanie F. Molina et al., "Addressing the Elephant in the Room: Microaggressions in Medicine," *Annals of Emergency Medicine* 76, no. 4 (October 1, 2020): 387–91, https://pubmed.ncbi.nlm.nih.gov/32456801/.

35. F. Perry Wilson, "Harassment of Medical Students Common, Directed at Most Vulnerable," The Methods Man, February 26, 2020, https://www.methodsman.com/blog/med-school-harassment.

36. Sundiatu Dixon-Fyle et al., "Diversity Wins: How Inclusion Matters," McKinsey & Company, May 19, 2020, https://www.mckinsey.com/featured-insights/diversity-and-inclusion/diversity-wins-how-inclusion-matters.

37. Jesse Feith, Montreal Gazette, "Indigenous Woman Records Slurs by Hospital Staff Before Her Death," *Montrealgazette*, September 30, 2020, https://montrealgazette.com/news/local-news/indigenous-woman-who-died-at-joliette-hospital-had-recorded-staffs-racist-comments.

38. Jeffrey Braithwaite et al., "Association Between Organisational and Workplace Cultures, and Patient Outcomes: Systematic Review," *BMJ Open* 7, no. 11 (November 1, 2017): e017708, https://bmjopen.bmj.com/content/7/11/e017708.

39. Mirjam Körner et al., "Relationship of Organizational Culture, Teamwork and Job Satisfaction in Interprofessional Teams," *BMC Health Services Research* 15, no. 1 (June 23, 2015), https://pubmed.ncbi.nlm.nih.gov/26099228/

40. Jenny W. Rudolph, Daniel B. Raemer, and Robert Simon, "Establishing a Safe Container for Learning in Simulation," *Simulation in Healthcare* 9, no. 6 (December 1, 2014): 339–49, https://journals.lww.com/simulationinhealthcare/abstract/2014/12000/establishing_a_safe_container_for_learning_in.2.aspx.

41. Supply and Demand restaurant, Ottawa. "Supply & Demand – Foods & Raw Bar," n.d., https://www.supplyanddemandfoods.ca/

42. Danny Meyer, "Setting the Table," n.d., https://www.harpercollins.com/products/setting-the-table-danny-meyer?variant=32122420363298.

43. Douglas A. Mata et al., "Prevalence of Depression and Depressive Symptoms Among Resident Physicians," JAMA 314, no. 22 (December 8, 2015): 2373, https://jamanetwork.com/journals/jama/fullarticle/2474424

44. Liselotte N. Dyrbye et al., "Association of Clinical Specialty With Symptoms of Burnout and Career Choice Regret Among US Resident Physicians," JAMA 320, no. 11 (September 18, 2018): 1114, https://jamanetwork.com/journals/jama/article-abstract/2702870

45. Resident Doctors of Canada, "2018 National Resident Survey," 2018, https://residentdoctors.ca/wp-content/uploads/2018/10/National-Resident-Survey-2018-R8.pdf

46. "Harvard Macy Institute - Blog - Burnout: Addressing the Epidemic in Medical Trainees," n.d., https://harvardmacy.org/blog/burnout-addressing-the-epidemic-in-medical-trainees.

47. Steven Hassan, Freedom of Mind Resource Center, "Combating Cult Mind Control - Freedom of Mind Resource Center," March 14, 2024, https://freedomofmind.com/combating-cult-mind-control/.

48. George Wright, "Nxivm: 'Why I Joined a Cult - and How I Left,'" April 13, 2019, https://www.bbc.com/news/world-47900242.

49. The *Harvard Business Review* underscored the importance of obtaining unfiltered feedback. "The Wrong Ways to Strengthen Culture," Harvard Business Review, August 14, 2019, https://hbr.org/2019/07/the-wrong-ways-to-strengthen-culture.

50. A Kalaichandran and J Sukhera. "For The Sake of Doctors and Patients, We Must Fix Hospital Culture," The BMJ, July 24, 2019, https://blogs.bmj.com/bmj/2019/07/12/for-the-sake-of-doctors-and-patients-we-must-fix-hospital-culture/

51. Kate Aubusson, "Third Major Sydney Hospital Unit Banned From Training Junior Doctors," The Sydney Morning Herald, June 19, 2019, https://www.smh.com.au/national/nsw/third-major-sydney-hospital-unit-banned-from-training-junior-doctors-20190619-p51z9m.html.

52. Suicide of Ryan Seguin. Kevan Lu and Justin Schellenberg, "Canadian Federation of Medical Students," December 14, 2019, https://www.cfms.org/news/2019/12/14/cfms-letter-of-condolence-to-medical-students-in-mourning-of-ryan-seguin.

Chapter 10: Plant Medicine

1. Ayuhuasca is a psychoactive plant combination of *Banisteriopsis caapi* and *Psychotria viridis*, usually served as a drink. The chemical constituents which are β-carboniles and N,N dimethyltryptamine (DMT). Daniel F. Jiménez-Garrido et al., "Effects of Ayahuasca on Mental Health and Quality of Life in Naïve Users: A Longitudinal and Cross-sectional Study Combination," *Scientific Reports* 10, no. 1 (March 5, 2020), https://www.nature.com/articles/s41598-020-61169-x.

2. Psilocybin is the medicinal component of the 'magic mushroom'. Dev B Goel and Sarju Zilate, "Potential Therapeutic Effects of Psilocybin: A Systematic Review," *Curēus*, October 12, 2022, https://www.ncbi.nlm.nih.gov/pmc/articles/PMC9650681/

3. Thomas Chan case in Canada represented a landmark ruling. Leah McLaren, a Canadian journalist, took a deep dive here, for Macleans magazine in 2020: https://macleans.ca/society/life/thomas-chan-supreme-court/

4. Amitha Kalaichandran, "How We Can Help Prevent Children From Dying in Hot Cars," *Washington Post*, August 15, 2019, https://www.washingtonpost.com/opinions/

how-we-can-help-prevent-children-from-dying-in-hot-cars/2019/08/13/b49a016c-be0d-11e9-a5c6-1e74f7ec4a93_story.html.

5. Amitha Kalaichandran, "An Explainer of a New Marijuana-based Pharmaceutical Drug Approved by FDA," ABC News, June 27, 2018, https://abcnews.go.com/Health/explainer-marijuana-based-pharmaceutical-drug-approved-fda/story?id=56167305.

6. "Young Men at Highest Risk of Schizophrenia Linked With Cannabis Use," National Institutes of Health (NIH), May 4, 2023, https://www.nih.gov/news-events/news-releases/young-men-highest-risk-schizophrenia-linked-cannabis-use-disorder.

7. Haden founded MAPS Canada, and served as its executive director for 10 years. "Brief Bio – Mark Haden," n.d., https://markhaden.com/?page_id=7.

8. 20 year hiatus since 1994 on psychedelic research, Michael Pollan described this in detail in his excellent Harper's essay from 1997, Opium Made Easy. Michael Pollan, "Opium, Made Easy," Harper's Magazine, June 17, 2021, https://harpers.org/archive/1997/04/opium-made-easy/

9. MDMA, and its use for psychiatric purposes are described in this thorough review: Sarah Tedesco et al., "The Efficacy of MDMA (3,4-Methylenedioxymethamphetamine) for Post-traumatic Stress Disorder in Humans: A Systematic Review and Meta-Analysis," Curēus, May 17, 2021, https://www.ncbi.nlm.nih.gov/pmc/articles/PMC8207489/

10. Collin M. Reiff et al., "Psychedelics and Psychedelic-Assisted Psychotherapy: Clinical Implications," Am J Psychiatry, 2020, https://adaa.org/sites/default/files/Psychedelics%20and%20Psychedelic-Assisted%20Psychotherapy%20AJP%202020.pdf.

11. Joost J. Breeksema et al., "Psychedelic Treatments for Psychiatric Disorders: A Systematic Review and Thematic Synthesis of Patient Experiences in Qualitative Studies," CNS Drugs 34, no. 9 (August 17, 2020): 925–46, https://pubmed.ncbi.nlm.nih.gov/32803732/

12. Both MDMA and psilocybin could potentially offer a "single dose, rapid effect model" for treatment-resistant mental illness. Hartej Gill et al., "The Emerging Role of Psilocybin and MDMA in the Treatment of Mental Illness," Expert Review of Neurotherapeutics 20, no. 12 (September 30, 2020): 1263–73, https://pubmed.ncbi.nlm.nih.gov/32954860/

13. Other reviews published since have emphasized the promise of MDMA (for PTSD specifically) and psilocybin (for depression and end-of-life anxiety), even though the FDA failed to grant approval for MDMA use in 2024. Erwin Krediet et al., "Reviewing the Potential of Psychedelics for the Treatment of PTSD," International Journal of Neuropsychopharmacology 23, no. 6 (March 14, 2020): 385–400, https://academic.oup.com/ijnp/article/23/6/385/5805249. Mason Marks et al., "Introducing Psychedelics to End-of-life Mental Healthcare," Nature Mental Health 1, no. 12 (November 8, 2023): 920–22, https://www.nature.com/articles/s44220-023-00166-1.

14. Anees Bahji et al., "Efficacy of 3,4-methylenedioxymethamphetamine (MDMA)-assisted Psychotherapy for Posttraumatic Stress Disorder: A Systematic Review and Meta-analysis," Progress in Neuro-Psychopharmacology & Biological Psychiatry 96 (January

1, 2020): 109735, https://pubmed.ncbi.nlm.nih.gov/31437480/. Ben Sessa, Laurie Higbed, and David Nutt, "A Review of 3,4-methylenedioxymethamphetamine (MDMA)-Assisted Psychotherapy," *Frontiers in Psychiatry* 10 (March 20, 2019), https://www.frontiersin.org/journals/psychiatry/articles/10.3389/fpsyt.2019.00138/full.

15. R. L. Carhart-Harris et al., "Psilocybin With Psychological Support for Treatment-resistant Depression: Six-month Follow-up," *Psychopharmacology/Psychopharmacologia* 235, no. 2 (November 8, 2017): 399–408, https://www.ncbi.nlm.nih.gov/pmc/articles/PMC5813086/

16. Rosalind Watts et al., "Patients' Accounts of Increased 'Connectedness' and 'Acceptance' After Psilocybin for Treatment-Resistant Depression," *Journal of Humanistic Psychology* 57, no. 5 (June 19, 2017): 520–64, https://journals.sagepub.com/doi/abs/10.1177/0022167817709585. Robin L Carhart-Harris et al., "Psilocybin for Treatment-resistant Depression: fMRI-measured Brain Mechanisms," *Scientific Reports* 7, no. 1 (October 13, 2017), https://www.ncbi.nlm.nih.gov/pmc/articles/PMC5640601/. "Home - DOSED - Award-winning Films Plus Bonus Features," DOSED, April 26, 2024, https://www.dosedmovie.com/

17. Robin Carhart-Harris et al., "Trial of Psilocybin Versus Escitalopram for Depression," *New England Journal of Medicine/˜the œNew England Journal of Medicine* 384, no. 15 (April 15, 2021): 1402–11, https://www.nejm.org/doi/full/10.1056/NEJMoa2032994.

18. Alan K. Davis et al., "Effects of Psilocybin-Assisted Therapy on Major Depressive Disorder," *JAMA Psychiatry* 78, no. 5 (May 1, 2021): 481, https://jamanetwork.com/journals/jamapsychiatry/fullarticle/2772630.

19. Rachel Yehuda et al., "Holocaust Exposure Induced Intergenerational Effects on FKBP5 Methylation," *Biological Psychiatry* 80, no. 5 (September 1, 2016): 372–80, https://www.biologicalpsychiatryjournal.com/article/S0006-3223(15)00652-6/fulltext.

20. Eric Vermetten and Rachel Yehuda, "MDMA-assisted Psychotherapy for Posttraumatic Stress Disorder: A Promising Novel Approach to Treatment," *Neuropsychopharmacology* 45, no. 1 (August 27, 2019): 231–32, https://pubmed.ncbi.nlm.nih.gov/31455855/

21. Paul Conti, "Trauma: The Invisible Epidemic: How Trauma Works and How We Can Heal From It | Paperback," Barnes & Noble, n.d., https://www.barnesandnoble.com/w/trauma-paul-conti/1138594984.

22. Gabrielle Agin-Liebes and Alan K. Davis, "Psilocybin for the Treatment of Depression: A Promising New Pharmacotherapy Approach," in *Current Topics in Behavioral Neurosciences*, 2021, 125–40, https://www.ncbi.nlm.nih.gov/pmc/articles/PMC10072288/#R14

23. Tudor Florea et al., "Oxytocin: Narrative Expert Review of Current Perspectives on the Relationship With Other Neurotransmitters and the Impact on the Main Psychiatric Disorders," *Medicina* 58, no. 7 (July 11, 2022): 923, https://www.ncbi.nlm.nih.gov/pmc/articles/PMC9318841/.

24. Sandee LaMotte, "How Love Sparks Better Heart Health," CNN, February 14, 2019, https://edition.cnn.com/2019/02/14/health/love-heart-health/index.html.

25. "In Flanders Fields by John McCrae | Poetry Foundation," Poetry Foundation, n.d., https://www.poetryfoundation.org/poems/47380/in-flanders-fields.

26. Arthur Gale, "Sacklers Sacked but Purdue Still Caused Opioid Epidemic," PubMed Central (PMC), April 1, 2022, https://www.ncbi.nlm.nih.gov/pmc/articles/PMC9339402/

27. Amy Sue Biondich and Jeremy David Joslin, "Coca: The History and Medical Significance of an Ancient Andean Tradition," *Emergency Medicine International* 2016 (January 1, 2016): 1–5, https://www.ncbi.nlm.nih.gov/pmc/articles/PMC4838786/

28. United States General Accounting Office, "The Crack Cocaine Epidemic: Health Consequences and Treatment," January 30, 1991, https://www.gao.gov/assets/hrd-91-55fs.pdf.

29. Drug dependency and addiction used to be differentiated. In medical school we learned the DSM-IV distinction, where dependency required tolerance and withdrawal symptoms, while addiction requires a change in behavior secondary to brain alterations due to the substance which causes heavier focus on obtaining the substance. The DSM-V doesn't include that distinction, and the scientific community much prefers the more umbrella term "substance use disorder," to define addiction or dependence on a substance like drug or alcohol. Charles O'Brien, "Addiction and Dependence in DSM-V," *Addiction* 106, no. 5 (October 6, 2010): 866–67, https://www.ncbi.nlm.nih.gov/pmc/articles/PMC3812919/

30. Amitha Kalaichandran, "Can Police Help Solve the Opioid Epidemic?," The Walrus, July 28, 2017, https://thewalrus.ca/can-police-help-solve-the-opioid-epidemic/

31. David M Schiff et al., "A Police-Led Addiction Treatment Referral Program in Massachusetts," *New England Journal of Medicine* 375, no. 25 (December 22, 2016): 2502–3, https://www.nejm.org/doi/full/10.1056/NEJMc1611640#t=article.

32. David Armstrong and Evan Allen — Boston Globe, "The Addict Brokers: Middlemen Profit as Desperate Patients Are 'Treated Like Paychecks,'" *STAT*, July 25, 2023, https://www.statnews.com/2017/05/28/addict-brokers-opioids/

33. Wood, S. (2016). Letter to the editor: Critique of detoxification approaches. *New England Journal of Medicine*, 375(4), 389-390.

34. David M Schiff, Mari-Lynn Drainoni, and David Rosenbloom, "Addiction Treatment Referral Through Local Police," *New England Journal of Medicine/~the æNew England Journal of Medicine* 376, no. 10 (March 9, 2017): 999, https://www.nejm.org/doi/full/10.1056/NEJMc1700537?af=R&rss=currentIssue#t=article.

35. Dr. Gabor Maté, In the Realm of Hungry Ghosts. https://drgabormate.com/book/in-the-realm-of-hungry-ghosts/

36. Tim Ferriss, "Dr. Gabor Maté — New Paradigms, Ayahuasca, and Redefining Addiction (#298)," The Blog of Author Tim Ferriss, May 23, 2024, https://tim.blog/2018/02/20/gabor-mate/

37. The pivotal role of trauma was best described in a 2021 book by Bruce Perry and Oprah, called *What Happened to You*, (Macmillan 2021) as it underscores how both early childhood events and later life events can radically impact our responses to both

abnormal and normal situations. https://us.macmillan.com/books/9781250223210/whathappenedtoyou.

Chapter 11: Rest to Recover

1. Amitha Kalaichandran MD, "Protecting Sleep in the Hospital, for Both Patients and Doctors," *The New York Times*, June 8, 2019, https://www.nytimes.com/2019/06/04/well/mind/sleep-hospital-patients-doctors-fatigue.html.

2. Katherine Price Snedaker, Pink Concussions, n.d., https://www.pinkconcussions.com/

3. Natasha Desai et al., "Factors Affecting Recovery Trajectories in Pediatric Female Concussion," *Clinical Journal of Sport Medicine* 29, no. 5 (September 1, 2019): 361–67, https://pubmed.ncbi.nlm.nih.gov/31460948/

4. Tracey Covassin, C. Buz Swanik, and Michael L. Sachs, "Sex Differences and the Incidence of Concussions Among Collegiate Athletes," PubMed Central (PMC), September 1, 2003, https://www.ncbi.nlm.nih.gov/pmc/articles/PMC233178/

5. M Aubry et al., "Summary and Agreement Statement of the First International Conference on Concussion in Sport, Vienna 2001," *British Journal of Sports Medicine* 36, no. 1 (February 1, 2002): 6–7, https://pubmed.ncbi.nlm.nih.gov/11867482/.

6. Noah D. Silverberg and Grant L. Iverson, "Is Rest After Concussion 'The Best Medicine?,'" *Journal of Head Trauma Rehabilitation* 28, no. 4 (July 1, 2013): 250–59, https://pubmed.ncbi.nlm.nih.gov/22688215/.

7. Danny George Thomas et al., "Benefits of Strict Rest After Acute Concussion: A Randomized Controlled Trial," *Pediatrics* 135, no. 2 (February 1, 2015): 213–23, https://pubmed.ncbi.nlm.nih.gov/25560444/

8. The work of Dr. John Leddy, an orthopedic surgeon at the University of Buffalo (he created the Buffalo Concussion Treadmill Test), was pivotal to shifting the dogma around rest. John J Leddy, Mohammad N Haider, and Barry S Willer, Buffalo Concussion Treadmill Test (BCTT) – Instruction Manual, n.d., https://cdn-links.lww.com/permalink/jsm/a/jsm_2020_01_28_haider_19-313_sdc1.pdf.

9. Anne M. Grool et al., "Association Between Early Participation in Physical Activity Following Acute Concussion and Persistent Postconcussive Symptoms in Children and Adolescents," *JAMA* 316, no. 23 (December 20, 2016): 2504, https://pubmed.ncbi.nlm.nih.gov/27997652/.

10. John J. Leddy et al., "Early Subthreshold Aerobic Exercise for Sport-Related Concussion," *JAMA Pediatrics* 173, no. 4 (April 1, 2019): 319, https://pubmed.ncbi.nlm.nih.gov/30715132/

11. "Dr. Michael Grandner," n.d., https://www.michaelgrandner.com/about.html.

12. "Meeta Singh MD," Meeta Singh MD, n.d., https://www.meetasinghmd.com/

13. "About – Dr. Amy Bender," n.d., http://www.sleepintowin.com/about/

14. Cheri D. Mah et al., "The Effects of Sleep Extension on the Athletic Performance of Collegiate Basketball Players," *Sleep* 34, no. 7 (July 1, 2011): 943–50, https://www.ncbi.nlm.nih.gov/pmc/articles/PMC3119836/.

15. Baxter Holmes, "NBA Schedule Alert! Games Your Team Will Lose in 2018-19 - ESPN," *ESPN*, October 30, 2018, https://www.espn.in/nba/story/_/id/25117649/nba-schedule-alert-games-your-team-lose-2018-19.

16. Boston Celtics head coach Joe Mazzulla on the importance of sleep, rest, and HRV. The entire interview, with Dr Leah Lagos, is worth the listen. https://www.youtube.com/watch?v=EJRhBLNXH_0

17. Jonathan Charest and Michael A. Grandner, "Sleep and Athletic Performance," *Sleep Medicine Clinics* 15, no. 1 (March 1, 2020): 41–57, https://europepmc.org/article/med/32005349.

18. Ashley A. Brauer et al., "Sleep and Health Among Collegiate Student Athletes," *Chest* 156, no. 6 (December 1, 2019): 1234–45, https://journal.chestnet.org/article/S0012-3692(19)33467-1/abstract.

19. David A Kalmbach et al., "Poor Sleep Is Linked to Impeded Recovery From Traumatic Brain Injury," *Sleep* 41, no. 10 (July 24, 2018), https://academic.oup.com/sleep/article/41/10/zsy147/5057802.

20. Keith A. Scorza and Wesley Cole, "Current Concepts in Concussion: Initial Evaluation and Management," AAFP, April 1, 2019, https://www.aafp.org/pubs/afp/issues/2019/0401/p426.html.

21. Carol DeMatteo et al., "Concussion Management for Children Has Changed: New Pediatric Protocols Using the Latest Evidence," *Clinical Pediatrics* 59, no. 1 (October 18, 2019): 5–20, https://journals.sagepub.com/doi/10.1177/0009922819879457.

22. Ginger Yang's work is described here: "Study Finds Adolescents With Concussion May Benefit From More Activity Earlier," n.d., https://www.nationwidechildrens.org/newsroom/news-releases/2024/02/yang_pommering_concussionstudy.

23. David A Kalmbach et al., "Poor Sleep Is Linked to Impeded Recovery From Traumatic Brain Injury," *Sleep* 41, no. 10 (July 24, 2018), https://pubmed.ncbi.nlm.nih.gov/30053263/

24. Cara F. Levitch et al., "The Impact of Sleep on the Relationship Between Soccer Heading Exposure and Neuropsychological Function in College-Age Soccer Players," *Journal of the International Neuropsychological Society* 26, no. 7 (February 26, 2020): 633–44, https://www.cambridge.org/core/journals/journal-of-the-international-neuropsychological-society/article/abs/impact-of-sleep-on-the-relationship-between-soccer-heading-exposure-and-neuropsychological-function-in-collegeage-soccer-players/C59A60AFC50F6911187A65B37E74C495.

25. Meeta Singh et al., "From the National Basketball Association to the National Hockey League: A Parallel Problem Exists," *Journal of Clinical Sleep Medicine* 17, no. 4 (April 1, 2021): 863–64, https://pubmed.ncbi.nlm.nih.gov/33538689/

26. Meeta Singh et al., "Urgent Wake up Call for the National Basketball Association," *Journal of Clinical Sleep Medicine* 17, no. 2 (February 1, 2021): 243–48, https://www.ncbi.nlm.nih.gov/pmc/articles/PMC7853218/

27. Joseph Goldstein and Jesse McKinley, "Manhattan Woman Is First Confirmed Coronavirus Case in State," *The New York Times*, March 5, 2020, https://www.nytimes.com/2020/03/01/nyregion/new-york-coronvirus-confirmed.html.

28. Mussa, "Race Was a Factor in uOttawa Carding Incident, Report Finds," *CBC*, May 20, 2020, https://www.cbc.ca/news/canada/ottawa/race-was-a-factor-in-u-of-o-carding-incident-report-finds-1.5575998. "Students Call for Systemic Change in Wake of N-word Controversy at University of Ottawa | CBC Radio," CBC, October 23, 2020, https://www.cbc.ca/radio/thecurrent/the-current-for-oct-23-2020-1.5772694/students-call-for-systemic-change-in-wake-of-n-word-controversy-at-university-of-ottawa-1.5774034.

29. Ahmar Khan, "2 Medical Experts Allege Harassment, Bullying, Exploitation at U of O," *CBC*, August 12, 2021, https://www.cbc.ca/news/canada/ottawa/harassment-bullying-allegations-university-of-ottawa-international-medical-experts-1.6136229?fbclid=IwAR3TMuvu4BFqe4xITmU77oDlwHj4p9TsjUqfV7IQDIA-2MyNRkdgYBiboX-8.

30. It was then when I was reminded of the quote by David Whyte, which applied not just to me, but to all of us during what would feel like an immensely challenging year with so much loss: *"Courage is the measure of our heartfelt participation with life, with another, with a community, a work; a future. To be courageous is not necessarily to go anywhere or do anything except to make conscious those things we already feel deeply and then to live through the unending vulnerabilities of those consequences."* David Whyte, "Courage," Grateful.org, November 30, 2022, https://grateful.org/resource/courage-david-whyte/

31. Gerald Imber, is one worth reading yourself – it's a good one, so get comfy. "Genius on the Edge: The Bizarre Double Life of Dr. William Halsted," n.d., https://www.goodreads.com/book/show/6949655-genius-on-the-edge.

32. "Was The Right Lesson Learned From Libby Zion? : Emergency Medicine News," LWW, n.d., https://journals.lww.com/em-news/fulltext/2005/05000/was_the_right_lesson_learned_from_libby_zion_.35.aspx

33. Steven W. Lockley et al., "Effect of Reducing Interns' Weekly Work Hours on Sleep and Attentional Failures," *New England Journal of Medicine* 351, no. 18 (October 28, 2004): 1829–37, https://www.nejm.org/doi/full/10.1056/NEJMoa041404.

34. Glenn Rosenbluth et al., "I-PASS Handoff Program: Use of a Campaign to Effect Transformational Change," *Pediatric Quality & Safety* 3, no. 4 (July 1, 2018): e088, https://www.ncbi.nlm.nih.gov/pmc/articles/PMC6135553/

35. The most infamous handover period happens on July 1, known as the "July Effect," when new residents and medical students begin, and though this link remains controversial – January 20th in Presidential terms may be the equivalent. The Joint Commission, n.d., https://www.jointcommission.org/-/media/deprecated-unorganized/imported-assets/tjc/system-folders/blogs/tst_hoc_persp_08_12pdf.pdf?db=web&hash=BA7C8CDB4910EF6633F013D0BC08CB1C.

36. American College of Physicians, "'July Effect': Impact of the Academic Year-End Changeover on Patient Outcomes: A Systematic Review: Annals of Internal Medicine: Vol 155, No 5," Annals of Internal Medicine, n.d., https://www.acpjournals.org/doi/10.7326/0003-4819-155-5-201109060-00354.

37. Emily Hughes, "July Effect? Maybe Not," *CMAJ. Canadian Medical Association Journal* 189, no. 32 (August 13, 2017): E1050–51, https://www.ncbi.nlm.nih.gov/pmc/articles/PMC5555760/

38. Amy J. Starmer et al., "Changes in Medical Errors After Implementation of a Handoff Program," *New England Journal of Medicine* 371, no. 19 (November 6, 2014): 1803–12, https://www.nejm.org/doi/full/10.1056/nejmsa1405556.

39. Jennifer K. O'Toole et al., "I-PASS Mentored Implementation Handoff Curriculum: Implementation Guide and Resources," *MedEdPORTAL*, August 3, 2018, https://www.ncbi.nlm.nih.gov/pmc/articles/PMC6342372/

40. Clare Anderson et al., "Self-reported Drowsiness and Safety Outcomes While Driving After an Extended Duration Work Shift in Trainee Physicians," *Sleep* 41, no. 2 (December 22, 2017), https://pubmed.ncbi.nlm.nih.gov/29281091/.

41. Denis Campbell, "NHS Hospitals Bring in Sleep Pods to Help Tired Staff Take a Break," *The Guardian*, February 3, 2020, https://www.theguardian.com/society/2020/feb/03/nhs-hospitals-bring-in-sleep-pods-to-help-tired-staff-take-a-break

42. Dr. Matthew Walker's perspective was described in my article for the *Times*. Amitha Kalaichandran MD, "Protecting Sleep in the Hospital, for Both Patients and Doctors," *The New York Times*, June 8, 2019, https://www.nytimes.com/2019/06/04/well/mind/sleep-hospital-patients-doctors-fatigue.html.

53. Cameron S. McAlpine et al., "Sleep Modulates Haematopoiesis and Protects Against Atherosclerosis," Nature 566, no. 7744 (February 1, 2019): 383–87, https://www.nature.com/articles/s41586-019-0948-2

54. George Michalopoulos, "Association of Sleep Quality and Mucosal Healing in Patients With Inflammatory Bowel Disease in Clinical Remission," Annals of Gastroenterology, January 1, 2018, https://www.ncbi.nlm.nih.gov/pmc/articles/PMC5825951/

43. Wells, "Gregg Popovich Weighs in on Debate About Resting NBA Players," *Bleacher Report*, September 29, 2017, https://bleacherreport.com/articles/2700072-gregg-popovich-weighs-in-on-debate-about-resting-nba-players.

44. "League Debating Benefits of 'DNP-Rest' - Baltimore Sun," n.d., https://digitaledition.baltimoresun.com/tribune/article_popover.aspx?guid=1af73d64-693f-48d6-a304-5b3fa1cbff5a.

45. "Heat's Pat Riley Rails Against Players Resting During NBA Season: 'It's Become a Travesty' - CBSSports.com," CBSSports.com, n.d., https://www.cbssports.com/nba/news/heats-pat-riley-rails-against-players-resting-during-nba-season-its-become-a-travesty/

46. Zito Madu, "The NBA Needs Players to Be Healthy, but Is Against Them Resting," *SBNation.Com*, March 22, 2017, https://www.sbnation.com/2017/3/22/15012220/nba-rest-players-lebron-james-gregg-popovich.

47. The Greek tragedy of Milo of Croton: Milo of Croton, a renowned wrestler from ancient Greece, is celebrated not only for his extraordinary strength but also for his tragic and somewhat ironic death. According to legend, Milo attempted to split a tree with his bare hands, demonstrating his immense strength. However, the wedges

holding the tree apart slipped, trapping his hands. Unable to free himself, Milo was left vulnerable and was subsequently devoured by wolves (or, in some versions of the story, lions). This story is often cited as a cautionary tale about the limits of human strength and the dangers of hubris. Milo's death symbolizes the idea that even the strongest individuals are not invincible and that pushing oneself beyond natural limits can lead to dire consequences. Cody Copeland. The Bizarre Death of Milo of Croton. February 10, 2021. https://www.grunge.com/331467/the-bizarre-death-of-milo-of-croton/

48. Bbc Sport, "Simone Biles Says 'I Have to Focus on My Mental Health' After Pulling Out of Team Final," BBC Sport, July 27, 2021, https://www.bbc.com/sport/olympics/57982665.

49. Matthew Walker, a professor of psychology and neuroscience at the University of California, Berkeley, has explored this issue in great length in his research and in his best-selling book, Matthew Walker. "Why We Sleep." Simon & Schuster, n.d., https://www.simonandschuster.com/books/Why-We-Sleep/Matthew-Walker/9781501144325.

50. Adam J. Krause et al., "The Sleep-deprived Human Brain," *Nature Reviews. Neuroscience* 18, no. 7 (May 18, 2017): 404–18, https://www.nature.com/articles/nrn.2017.55.

51. Matt Walker, "Sleep Is Your Superpower," n.d., https://www.ted.com/talks/matt_walker_sleep_is_your_superpower?language=en.

52. "Lack of Sleep Disrupts Brain's Emotional Controls," National Institutes of Health (NIH), October 5, 2015, https://www.nih.gov/news-events/nih-research-matters/lack-sleep-disrupts-brains-emotional-controls.

53. Robert Sanders, "Sleepless and Selfish: Lack of Sleep Makes Us Less Generous - Berkeley News," Berkeley News, August 22, 2022, https://news.berkeley.edu/2022/08/23/sleepless-and-selfish-lack-of-sleep-makes-us-less-generous/

54. "Chris Johnstone," Chris Johnstone, n.d., https://chrisjohnstone.info/

55. "Broken Open — Elizabeth Lesser," Elizabeth Lesser, n.d., https://www.elizabethlesser.org/broken-open.

55. Juliet Macur, "A Gymnastics Coach Made the Hall of Fame. Misconduct Complaints Are Trailing Her.," The New York Times, November 6, 2020, https://www.nytimes.com/2020/11/06/sports/gymnastics-coach-misconduct-safesport.html.

56. Dakota London, "USA Gymnastics Suspends Coach Maggie Haney for Eight Years," April 30, 2020, https://www.si.com/more-sports/video/2020/04/30/maggie-haney-suspended-eight-years-emotional-verbal-abuse-athletes.

57. "CONSOLATIONS: The Solace, Nourishment and Underlying Meaning of Everyday Words," David Whyte, n.d., https://davidwhyte.com/pages/consolations.

Chapter 12: Sweet Surrender

1. Cicely Saunders, "The Evolution of Palliative Care," *Journal of the Royal Society of Medicine* 94, no. 9 (September 1, 2001): 430–32, https://www.ncbi.nlm.nih.gov/pmc/articles/PMC1282179/. This led first to the concept of "hospice care," which emphasized end-of-life wishes.

2.	Hallek, M., Cheson, B. D., Catovsky, D., Caligaris-Cappio, F., Dighiero, G., Döhner, H., ... & Kipps, T. J. (2011). Guidelines for the diagnosis and treatment of chronic lymphocytic leukemia: A report from the International Workshop on Chronic Lymphocytic Leukemia updating the National Cancer Institute-Working Group 1996 guidelines. *British Journal of Haematology, 154*(6), 786-804.https://onlinelibrary.wiley.com/doi/full/10.1111/j.1365-2141.2011.08764.

3.	The Origin of Palliative Care" (UPMC, 2014), https://www.upmc.com/-/media/upmc/services/palliative-and-supportive-institute/resources/documents/psi-history-palliative-care.pdf.

4.	ICHA - PEACH – Palliative Education and Care for the Homeless," n.d., https://www.icha-toronto.ca/programs/peach-palliative-education-and-care-for-the-homeless.

5.	Perlita Stroh, "Life on Streets 'a Killer': New Hospice Offers End-of-life Care to the Homeless," *CBC*, July 5, 2018, https://www.cbc.ca/news/health/journey-home-hospice-toronto-homeless-end-of-life-care-1.4715540.

6.	"The process of dying for the homeless is eased with THE GOOD WISHES project," *Newswire.Ca*, December 22, 2018, https://www.newswire.ca/news-releases/the-process-of-dying-for-the-homeless-is-eased-with-the-good-wishes-project-584505261.html.

7.	Perlita Stroh, "Life on Streets 'a Killer': New Hospice Offers End-of-life Care to the Homeless," *CBC*, July 5, 2018, https://www.cbc.ca/news/health/journey-home-hospice-toronto-homeless-end-of-life-care-1.4715540.

8.	Amitha Kalaichandran, "Homelessness Is Not a Choice, so Lose the Apathy," *HuffPost* (blog), March 9, 2015, https://www.huffpost.com/archive/ca/entry/homelessness-is-not-a-choice-so-lose-the-apathy_b_6427646.

9.	"Norman Bethune," The Canadian Encyclopedia, n.d., https://www.thecanadianencyclopedia.ca/en/article/norman-bethune.

10.	"Three Decades of UpToDate," n.d., https://www.wolterskluwer.com/en/solutions/uptodate.

11.	Michael A. Lang et al., "The Haldane Effect," *Diving for Science 2009. Proceedings of the American Academy of Underwater Sciences 28th Symposium*, 2009, https://www.tecvault.t101.ro/Haldane%20effect.pdf.

12.	"Simon's Heart: Preventing Sudden Cardiac Arrest in Children," - Simon's Heart, May 29, 2024, https://simonsheart.org/

13.	Alua Arthur's book, Going with Grace, should be on everyone's list. https://goingwithgrace.com/about-alua/

14.	Death Over Dinner, n.d., https://deathoverdinner.org/

15.	Amitha Kalaichandran, "We're Not Ready for This Kind Of Grief," *The Atlantic*, April 15, 2020, https://www.theatlantic.com/ideas/archive/2020/04/were-not-ready-for-this-kind-of-grief/609856/.

16. The Schwartz Center for Compassionate Healthcare, "Schwartz Rounds - the Schwartz Center," The Schwartz Center, November 16, 2022, https://www.theschwartzcenter.org/programs/schwartz-rounds/

17. Liz Salmi. "The Liz Army: Bringing Punk Rock to Health Care," The Liz Army: Bringing Punk Rock to Health Care, January 27, 2024, https://www.thelizarmy.com/

18. Amitha Kalaichandran, "Glimpsing Our Own Health Secrets: The Coming Revolution in Health-Care Transparency," Quillette, January 26, 2024, https://quillette.com/2019/01/04/glimpsing-our-own-health-secrets-the-coming-revolution-in-health-care-transparency/

19. Another excellent read: Adrian Owen "Into the Gray Zone – a Neuroscientist Explores the Border Between Life and Death," n.d., https://intothegrayzone.com/

20. "Remembering the Life of Klara Boadway.," n.d., https://ottawacitizen.remembering.ca/obituary/klara-boadway-1078937864.

57. American College of Radiology, "ACR Appropriateness Criteria: Headache," n.d., https://acsearch.acr.org/docs/69482/Narrative/.

21. Tate, "'Illustrations to 'The Book of Job'', William Blake, 1825–8 | Tate," n.d., https://www.tate.org.uk/art/artworks/blake-illustrations-to-the-book-of-job-65234.

22. Tate, "William Blake's Songs of Innocence and Experience | Tate," n.d., https://www.tate.org.uk/art/artists/william-blake-39/blakes-songs-innocence-experience.

23. Claire B. Willis, "Opening to Grief | Finding Your Way From Loss to Peace," https://openingtogrief.com/

24. "Willed Body Program," Department of Surgery, n.d., https://surgery.utoronto.ca/willed-body-program

Epilogue: Denouement to Forgiveness & The Future (Tech-enabled Wellness)

1. Corina Knoll, Ali Watkins, and Michael Rothfeld, "'I Couldn't Do Anything': The Virus and an E.R. Doctor's Suicide," The New York Times, July 11, 2020, https://www.nytimes.com/2020/07/11/nyregion/lorna-breen-suicide-coronavirus.html.

2. Amitha Kalaichandran, "During COVID-19, Healers Need Healing, Too," Scientific American, February 20, 2024, https://www.scientificamerican.com/blog/observations/during-covid-19-healers-need-healing-too/

3. Ibram X. Kendi ,"How to Be an Antiracist." https://www.ibramxkendi.com/how-to-be-an-antiracist.

4. Allison P. Davis and Chanda Hall, "The 'Permit Karen' of Montclair, New Jersey," The Cut, December 21, 2020, https://www.thecut.com/article/montclair-new-jersey-permit-karen.html.

5. Ruby Hamad, "How White Women Use Strategic Tears to Silence Women of Colour," The Guardian, May 11, 2018, https://www.theguardian.com/commentisfree/2018/may/08/how-white-women-use-strategic-tears-to-avoid-accountability.

6. Ruby Hamad, "White Tears/Brown Scars," October 6, 2020, https://books.catapult.co/books/white-tears-brown-scars/

7. "I'm Still Here: Black Dignity in a World Made for Whiteness | Podcast - Brené Brown," Brené Brown, January 17, 2024, https://brenebrown.com/podcast/brene-with-austin-channing-brown-on-im-still-here-black-dignity-in-a-world-made-for-whiteness/

8. Years after the death of Chiron, a Centaur in Greek mythology famous for knowledge of medicine, the ancient Greeks came to see suicide as primarily due to malfunctional "humors" – the end result of the build-up of black bile (melancholia) or yellow bile (mania). This is described well in "A Conceptional History of Anxiety and Depression," by Marcel Dekker, ed. J.A. Den Boer and A. Sitsen, *Handbook on Anxiety and Depression* (Marcel Dekker, 2003), https://philpapers.org/archive/GLAACH.pdf.

9. "A Timeline of the Ahmaud Arbery Shooting Case," *The New York Times*, August 8, 2022, https://www.nytimes.com/article/ahmaud-arbery-timeline.html.

10. "Letter From a Birmingham Jail [King, Jr.]," n.d., https://www.africa.upenn.edu/Articles_Gen/Letter_Birmingham.html.

11. Amitha Kalaichandran, "Apple Should Digitize the Medical World With Caution," *HuffPost* (blog), May 11, 2015, https://www.huffpost.com/archive/ca/entry/apple-should-digitize-the-medical-world-with-caution_b_6841298.

12. Apple, "Healthcare," n.d., https://www.apple.com/healthcare/

13. "Amazon Health: Fill a Prescription, Get Medical Care, Shop FSA | HSA," n.d., https://health.amazon.com/

14. "Exceptional Primary Care - Find a Doctor Near You," One Medical, n.d., https://www.onemedical.com/

15. "Oura Ring. Smart Ring for Fitness, Stress, Sleep & Health.," Oura Ring, n.d., https://ouraring.com/

16. "WHOOP | Your Personal Digital Fitness and Health Coach," WHOOP, n.d., https://www.whoop.com/us/en/

17. Google Health, "What Is Google Health? - Google Health," n.d., https://health.google/

18. Internal Family Systems (IFS) therapy is a psychotherapeutic approach that views the mind as composed of multiple sub-personalities or "parts," each with its own perspective and qualities. It aims to harmonize these parts by addressing their concerns and helping the individual achieve a balanced internal system. The therapy also identifies a "Self" that remains calm, compassionate, and confident, which leads the internal family. For more information, visit: https://ifs-institute.com/

19. The poet Yung Pueblo "Letting Go," Goodreads, n.d., https://www.goodreads.com/book/show/59941968-letting-go (from his book Lighter, published in 2022)

Acknowledgements

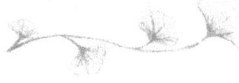

I am deeply grateful to my family, whose unwavering support has been the cornerstone of this journey. To my dearest first readers and cherished friends, Vicki Siu and Robyn Duffus, your insights and encouragement helped shape this book in ways beyond measure. My heartfelt thanks to my publisher, Naomi Rosenblatt, and my agents, Sam and Laura, for guiding me through every step of the publishing process with wisdom and patience. I am especially indebted to Craig Pyette, my first editor and an early believer in this project—your impact on this work is profound, and the publishing world is at a loss without you. A special thank you to my brilliant PR pros, Susan J Marketing and Julia Drake, for helping spread the word with dedication and passion. To the countless other friends, colleagues, mentors, and loved ones who have supported me, both near and far, in person and virtually, you have my endless gratitude. In alphabetical order, they are:

Adam Grant, Adrienne J. Ng, Adrienne Ng, Aliya Dedhar, Andrea Tam, André Picard, Ann Collins, Ann McDougall, Anne Bernard, Atul Gawande, Atritex Technologies, Bernard Simon, Catherine Pound, Cherry May Cabuñag, Chris Richards-Bentley, Chris Johnstone, Christie Smith, Christopher Tidey, Clara Lau, Colin Mackenzie, Craig Pyette, Cyrus Boadway, Dana Corriel, Daniel Lakoff, Danielle Rodin, David Epstein, David Jenkins, Elizabeth White, my editors at the NYT Well/Styles/Opinion sections (Roberta Zeff, Toby Bilanow, Choire Sicha, Jenee Desmond-Harris, Julia Calderone, Peter Catapano), Elena Prozorova, Ellen Bush, Edward Naylor, Eric Topol, Gabrielle Horne, Grace Mammen, Heather Yoshimura, Hilary McClafferty, Jaana Tarma, Jana Glowatz, Jaime Rosenthal, Jennifer Sturm, Jennifer Weinberg, Jenee Desmond-Harris, Jill Czarnik, Joe Reisman, Joe (the cadaver), Joel Cox, Jonathan Kay, Jonathan Swerdlin, Joseph Sullivan, Justin McCarthy, Katie McLaughlin, Kim

Isztwan, KJ Dell'Antonia, Klara Boadway, Kyle McDonald, Lacy Phillips, Ladies of Greenwich, Laura Lee Mattingly, Laura Lynne Jackson, Lindsay McNew, Lisa Simone Richards, Lonny Rosen, Madhuri Sharma, Madhuri Kumar, Malcolm Gladwell, Mamta Gautam, Mark Hyman, Melania Buba, Melanie Roy, Melissa Barall, Michael Kaufman, Michael Osgood, Monica Lamoureux, Nancy Whitmore, Natalie Chan, Natasha Hassan, Nicholas Chadi, Nina Rudnik, Paul Champ, Priya Randev, Rachel Slade, Ramzi Saad, Ric Philipps, Robert Hilliard, Rob Stein, Robert Sargeant, Robin Goldstein, Robyn Duffus, Roger Zemek, Ronya Lola, Rufus Cartwright, Rupa Madhevan, Ruth, Sam Hiyate, Sandeep Jauhar, Sandy Buchman, Sarah Graves, Sarah Kwan, Sara Schwartz, Shuang Shan, Siddhartha Mukherjee, Susan MacRae, Stephanie Pearce, Steve Wozniak, Sunita Vohra, Susan and Bernard Lee, Tara Tucker, Theo Koffler, Uché Blackstock, Vicki Siu, Wanda Jankowski, Wendy Glauser, Yandara Yoga institute, Yavar Hameed, Zak Jason.

Permissions

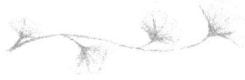

The author and publisher gratefully acknowledge the following sources for permission to use their material:

* Excerpt from "The Body and the Earth" by Wendell Berry, published by Counterpoint Press. Used with permission.
* Excerpt from "Are Doctors People?" (1944 essay) from the New England Journal of Medicine, published by the Massachusetts Medical Society. Used with permission.
* "Mundaka Upanishad" accessed from holybooks.com. Free access provided.
* Diagram from Chapter 9 "Problems Women of Color Face in the Workplace" in COCo-NET, developed by the Safehouse Progressive Alliance for Non-Violence and adapted by the Centre for Community Organizations. Used with permission.
* Excerpt from "The Fearless Organization" by Amy Edmondson, published by John Wiley & Sons, Inc. Used with permission.
* Excerpt from "In the Realm of Hungry Ghosts" by Gabor Maté, published by North Atlantic Books. Used with permission.
* Excerpt from "Consolations" by David Whyte. Used with permission.

Index

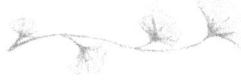

About the Author

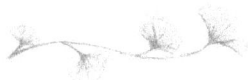

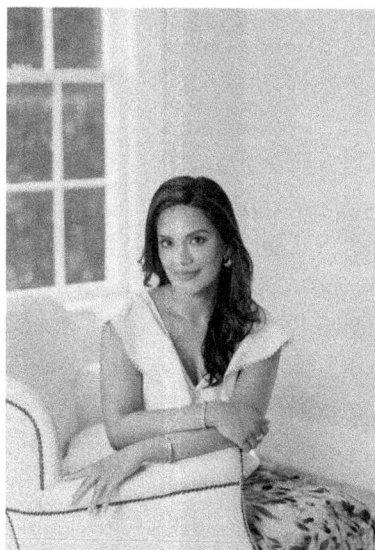

[Amitha Kalaichandran *Photographer: Andre Toro*]

D r. Kalaichandran has given talks at Stanford University, Happify, and South by Southwest, while also regularly contributing to *The New York Times (Well, Opinion,* and *Styles* sections) on topics that deal with medical education, health, and wellness. Her writing also has been featured in a range of national and international publications, including *Wired, Washington Post, New York Magazine, Discover Magazine, Los Angeles Times, The Boston Globe, The Atlantic, The Atavist* (optioned for film), *The Walrus* (Canada), *The Globe and Mail* (Canada), and *New Scientist* (U.K.).

She earned her medical degree (M.D.) from the University of Toronto, and completed a Fellowship in Integrative Medicine through the University of Arizona. In addition, Dr Kalaichandran completed psychotherapy training through the Medical Psychotherapy Association of Canada, Wellness/Lifestyle Coaching through York University, a Journalism Fellowship at the University of Toronto, and a Master's Certificate in Healthcare Management from the Schulich School of Business.

Dr. Kalaichandran has been a mentor for the OpEd Project, which aims to uplift under-represented expert/academic voices — largely women and people of color — in the media via Op-eds. She has served on the advisory boards of Artists Becoming, which strives to improve the well-being of performing artists in New York City, and the Close the Gap Foundation, which pairs first-generation, low-income, immigrant high school students with mentors to guide them through the college application process and job market.

Currently, Dr. Kalaichandran consults in health tech, for companies working on improving healthspan and longevity. She has served as a consultant for the Twitter (now known as X) Health Design Team and served on their health advisory board. She lives in New York City.

-

www.ingramcontent.com/pod-product-compliance
Lightning Source LLC
Chambersburg PA
CBHW020523270326
41927CB00006B/429